AF556875

OXYGEN TRANSPORT TO HUMAN TISSUES

OXYGEN TRANSPORT TO HUMAN TISSUES

A Symposium in honor of Dr. U.C. Luft held 25–27 June 1981 at the Veterans Administration Medical Center, Albuquerque, New Mexico, U.S.A.

Editors:

JACK A. LOEPPKY, Ph.D.
Associate Scientist
Department of Physiology and Biophysics
Research Division, Lovelace Medical Foundation
Albuquerque, New Mexico, U.S.A.

and

MARVIN L. RIEDESEL, Ph.D.
Professor of Biology
Department of Biology
University of New Mexico
Albuquerque, New Mexico, U.S.A.

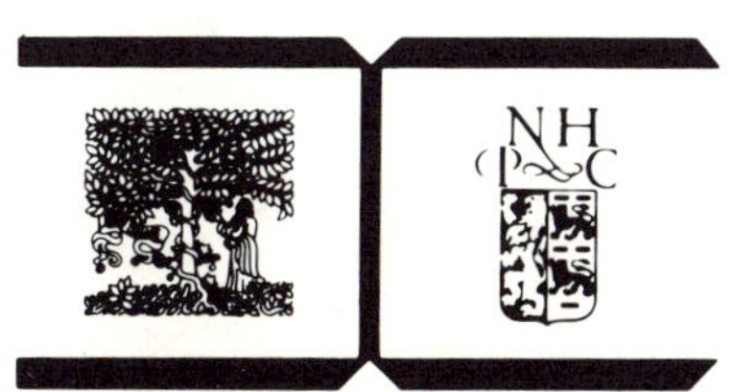

ELSEVIER/NORTH-HOLLAND
NEW YORK • AMSTERDAM • OXFORD

The cover art is a painting entitled "Cumulus Mountain" by Eric Sloane from the permanent collection at the Lovelace Medical Foundation, Albuquerque, New Mexico. The grandeur of this painting reflects the scope of the physiological research presented herewith.

Published by:
Elsevier North Holland, Inc.
52 Vanderbilt Avenue, New York, New York 10017

Sole distributors outside the U.S.A. and Canada:
Elsevier Science Publishers B.V.
P.O. Box 211, 1000 AE, Amsterdam, The Netherlands

Library of Congress Cataloging in Publication Data
Main entry under title:

Oxygen transport to human tissues.

Bibliography: p.
Includes index.
1. Oxygen transport (Physiology)—Congresses.
2. Blood flow—Congresses. 3. Luft, U.C. (Ulrich C.)
I. Luft, U.C. (Ulrich C.) II. Loeppky, Jack A.
III. Riedesel, Marvin LeRoy, 1925- [DNLM:
1. Biological transport—Congresses. 2. Oxygen consumption—Congresses. 3. Oxygen—Blood—Congresses. QV 312
0975 1981]
QP99.3.09093 612′.22 81-19481
ISBN 0-444-00677-X AACR2

Manufactured in the United States of America

Contents

Foreword

When, and if ever, the history of lung biology and pulmonary medicine is written, we will recognize that major advances have often been triggered by unusual events or circumstances. Certainly World War II played a major role in the evolution of new approaches to the study of the respiratory function of the lung. The extensive use of airplanes during the war and the need to reach greater altitudes and higher speeds posed a number of questions for researchers to resolve. Thus, in America and Europe, especially in Germany, new schools of thought were born and the way was paved for intensive investigative work that has led to the explosion of knowledge we are witnessing today.

Lung biology, and more specifically the study of the respiratory function of the lung, attracted a great number of outstanding scientists who have made many remarkable basic contributions. In turn, these contributions have increased our knowledge of the physiopathology of respiratory diseases and, thus, practical medicine has been the ultimate beneficiary.

In many ways, the following proceedings of the symposium on "Oxygen Transport to Human Tissues" are the culmination of nearly 40 years of scientific virtuosity. Many of the participants in the symposium have not only established the landmarks of today's knowledge but they also are the creators of a scenario that is the basis of a new era in lung biology, viz., the study of the nonrespiratory function of the lung.

The dedication of this symposium to Dr. Ulrich C. Luft is a tribute to his foresightedness and to his scientific achievement. His investigative career has been contemporary with the major advances of the 40 years past and he has made many contributions to science which have been an inspiration to others.

Adaptation to hypoxia has been his interest, and a bibliography of over 120 scientific papers is in itself a history of our knowledge of the respiratory functions of the lung. It started in the years just preceding World War II with studies inspired by the problem of acclimatization to mountain climbing. Then Dr. Luft's scientific curiosity turned to the problems encountered by the military fliers. The effect(s) of hypoxia, decompression, increased CO_2, and gravitational forces became familiar topics of investigation. Then came the postwar period! The topics and the questions remained the same, but the studies were broadened to include patients as well as nondiseased subjects.

All who participated in the symposium took great pride in honoring Dr. Luft because we know that directly or indirectly our work has been stimulated by his achievements.

Claude Lenfant, M.D.
Bethesda, Maryland
April 29, 1981

Acknowledgments

We wish to express our deepest appreciation to the contributors to the Luft Symposium and these proceedings and to all those who attended the meeting. The quality and reputation of the participants was assured from the outset because of the many friends and admirers Dr. Luft has accumulated internationally in the course of his career as a dedicated scientist. The gathering of these distinguished individuals and the staging of the Symposium was made possible by financial support from the United States Air Force Office of Scientific Research, the National Aeronautics and Space Administration, the School of Aerospace Medicine, and the W. Randolph Lovelace II Memorial Lectureship Fund. To individuals of these organizations who saw fit to express their indebtedness to Dr. Luft for his many years of service, we are extremely grateful. Additional assistance by Bio-Tech, Inc., the New Mexico Lung Association, and the Maria Teresa Restaurant was also most helpful.

We are also indebted to individuals who volunteered their time and energy in the preliminary arrangements for the meeting. Air travel arrangements were facilitated by the help of David Slaten and Paul Furst. The printing of preliminary programs was made possible by Loralea Anderson and Alice Adams. The preparation and organization of the facilities for the meeting were efficiently carried out by Mary Doris Woltkamp and her Medical Education staff at the Veterans Administration Medical Center. Special assistance in arranging the program and activities during the Symposium was given by Loren Myhre, Karla McKitrick, and Senora Concha Ortiz y Pino de Kleven. The Symposium would not have been what it was without the organizational skills and efforts of Debbie Thomas and other individuals of the Research Division. To Donna Neff and her secretarial staff in the Research Division go

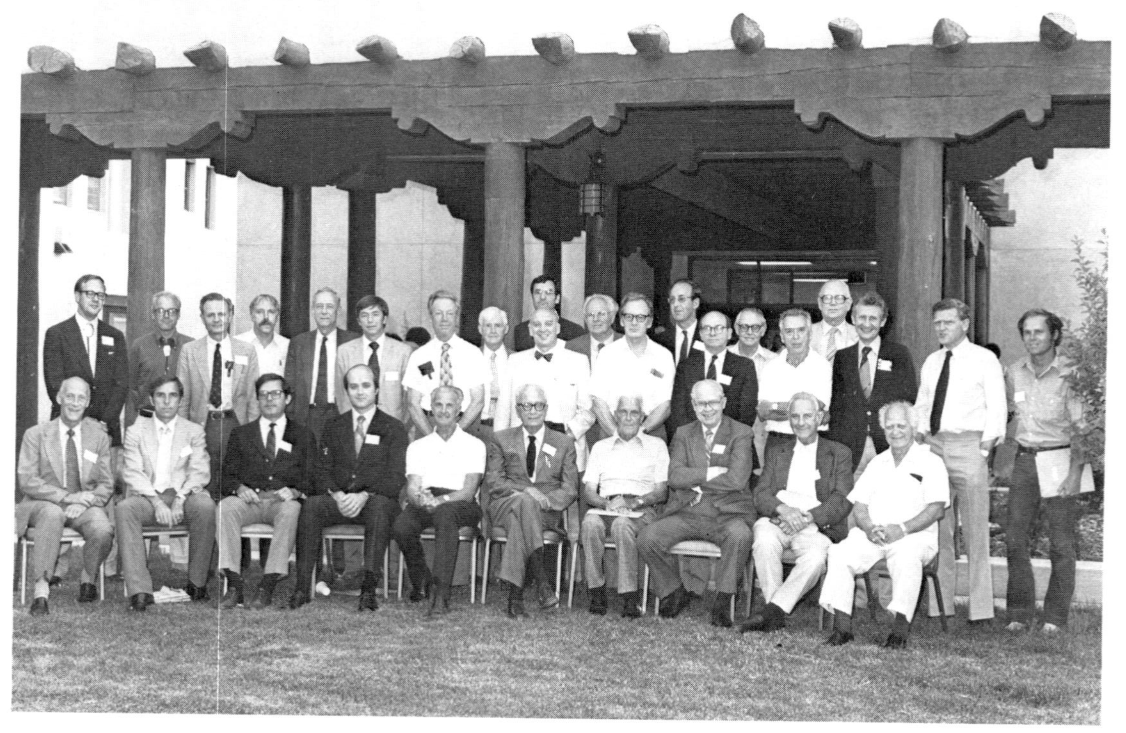

LUFT SYMPOSIUM SPEAKERS: *Seated* (*left to right*): P-O. Åstrand, R. Bone, G. Gurtner, M. Hlastala, B. Balke, U. Luft, D. Dill, C. White, K. Schaefer, S. Horvath. *Standing* (*left to right*): L. Myhre, R. Knudson, G. Filley, J. Loeppky, H. Rahn, I. McMurtry, R. Grover, R. Riley, L. Farhi, J. Green, J. Piiper, J. Severinghaus, J. Grote, J. Mithoefer, H. Hultgren, C. Houston, H. Bjurstedt, K. Kirsch, L. Rowell, E. Greene. *Missing from picture*: E. Robin and J. West.

special thanks for working long hours in preparing the preliminary announcements and for assistance in editing the proceedings. Special mention must be made of Yale Altman and Leesa Stanion of Elsevier North Holland whose efficiency eliminated the usual problems with the editing and publishing process.

The Symposium and these proceedings would not have materialized without the support, administrative skills, and continuing encouragement of Waneta Tuttle, Director of Research of the Lovelace Medical Foundation, in giving this project the priority it deserved. For her and most of us involved in this project, the meeting and these proceedings are an expression of appreciation to Dr. Luft not only for his attributes as a scientist but his human qualities as a kind and compassionate individual. These might well outlive his qualities as a scientific leader for those of us who have had the privilege of knowing him.

Jack A. Loeppky

Marvin L. Riedesel

Luft Symposium Contributors and Participants

Contributors

Per-Olof Åstrand, M.D.
Department of Physiology III, Karolinska Institute, Stockholm, Sweden

Brune Balke, M.D., Ph.D.
Aspen, Colorado

Hilding Bjurstedt, M.D., Ph.D.
Department of Environmental Physiology, Karolinska Institute, Stockholm, Sweden

Roger C. Bone, M.D.
Division of Pulmonary and Critical Care Medicine, University of Arkansas for Medical Sciences, Little Rock, Arkansas

David B. Dill, Ph.D.
Boulder City, Nevada

Leon E. Farhi, M.D.
Department of Physiology, State University of New York at Buffalo, Buffalo, New York

Giles F. Filley, M.D.
Webb-Waring Lung Institute, University of Colorado Health Sciences Center, Denver, Colorado

Jerry F. Green, Ph.D.
Department of Human Physiology, University of California School of Medicine, Davis, California

E. Richard Greene, Ph.D.
Department of Physiology and Biophysics, Lovelace Medical Foundation, Albuquerque, New Mexico

Jürgen Grote, M.D., Ph.D.
Department of Applied Physiology, University of Mainz, Mainz, Germany

Robert F. Grover, M.D., Ph.D.
Cardiovascular Pulmonary Research Laboratory, University of Colorado Health Sciences Center, Denver, Colorado

Gail H. Gurtner, M.D.
Division of Pulmonary Medicine, Johns Hopkins University School of Medicine, Baltimore, Maryland

Michael P. Hlastala, Ph.D.
Department of Medicine, University of Washington School of Medicine, Seattle, Washington

Steven M. Horvath, Ph.D.
Institute of Environmental Stress, University of California, Santa Barbara, California

Charles S. Houston, M.D.
Burlington, Vermont

Herbert N. Hultgren, M.D.
Cardiology Service, Veterans Administration Medical Center, Palo Alto, California

Karl A. Kirsch, M.D.
Department of Physiology, Free University of Berlin, Berlin, Germany

Ronald J. Knudson, M.D.
Division of Respiratory Sciences, University of Arizona Health Sciences Center, Tucson, Arizona

Ulrich C. Luft, M.D., Ph.D.
Albuquerque, New Mexico

Ivan McMurtry, Ph.D.
Cardiovascular Pulmonary Research Laboratory, University of Colorado Health Sciences Center, Denver, Colorado

John C. Mithoefer, M.D.
Pulmonary Division, Medical University of South Carolina, Charleston, South Carolina

Loren G. Myhre, Ph.D.
Crew Protection Branch, USAF School of Aerospace Medicine, Brooks Air Force Base, Texas

Johannes Piiper, M.D.
Department of Physiology, Max-Planck Institute for Experimental Medicine, Göttingen, Germany

Hermann Rahn, Ph.D.
Department of Physiology, State University of New York at Buffalo, Buffalo, New York

Richard L. Riley, M.D.
Petersham, Massachusetts

Eugene D. Robin, M.D.
Department of Physiology, Stanford University Medical Center, Stanford, California

Loring B. Rowell, Ph.D.
Department of Physiology and Biophysics, University of Washington School of Medicine, Seattle, Washington

Karl E. Schaefer, M.D.
Old Lyme, Connecticut

John W. Severinghaus, M.D.
Department of Anesthesia, University of California School of Medicine, San Francisco, California

John B. West, M.D., Ph.D.
Department of Medicine, University of California School of Medicine, La Jolla, California

Clayton S. White, M.D.
Albuquerque, New Mexico

Participants

William I. Christensen, M.D.
Department of Pulmonary Medicine, Lovelace Medical Foundation, Albuquerque, New Mexico (Symposium Chairman)

Albert R. Behnke, Jr., M.D.
San Francisco, California

Donald G. Davies, Ph.D.
Department of Physiology, Texas Tech University Health Sciences Center, Lubbock, Texas

Marlowe W. Eldridge, M.S.M.E.
Department of Physiology and Biophysics, Lovelace Medical Foundation, Albuquerque, New Mexico

Wesley M. Granger, B.A.
Department of Physiology, Medical College of Georgia, Augusta, Georgia

Francois Haas, Ph.D.
Department of Rehabilitation Medicine, New York University Medical Center, New York, New York

Philip P. Hamilton, M.D.
School of Physical and Health Education, Queen's University, Ontario, Canada

Neil B. Kindig, Ph.D.
Webb-Waring Lung Institute, University of Colorado Health Sciences Center, Denver, Colorado

Steven F. Lewis, Ph.D.
Department of Physiology, University of Texas Health Science Center, Dallas, Texas

Lorna G. Moore, Ph.D.
Cardiovascular Pulmonary Research Laboratory, University of Colorado Health Sciences Center, Denver, Colorado

Johannes Piiper, M.D.
Department of Physiology, Max-Planck Institute for Experimental Medicine, Göttingen, Germany

Hilary S. Stanbrook, Ph.D.
Cardiovascular Pulmonary Research Laboratory, University of Colorado Health Sciences Center, Denver, Colorado

Stephen C. Wood, Ph.D.
Department of Physiology, University of New Mexico School of Medicine, Albuquerque, New Mexico

Ulrich Cameron Luft
Curriculum Vitae

1910 Born in Berlin, Germany

1914–1919 With maternal relatives in Edinburgh, Scotland during World War I

1920–1929 Attended Friedenauer Gymnasium in Berlin, Germany

1929–1930 University of Freiburg i. Br.

1930–1931 University of Munich

1931–1935 University of Berlin Medical School

1936 Medical Internship, Krankenhaus am Friedrichshain, Berlin

1936 Licensed as Physician and Surgeon

1937 Doctor of Medicine, University of Berlin. Thesis: "Irreversible structural alterations by hypoxia at low pressures"

Research physiologist, Aeromedical Research Institute of the Air Ministery, Berlin

Physiological studies of acclimation to high altitude during expedition to Nanga Parbat (8126 m) in Western Himalaya

1938 Second expedition to Nanga Parbat

1939 Research at International High Altitude Research Station on Jungfrau-Joch (3300 m) in Swiss Alps

Chief, Physiology Department at Aeromedical Research Institute, Berlin

1942 Physiological Consultant to the Air Force in North Africa on thermal stress

Doctor of physiology, University of Berlin. Inaugural dissertation: "Acclimation to high altitudes"

1943 Appointment as lecturer in Physiology and Aviation Medicine, University of Berlin

Field studies on improvement of tolerance to acute hypoxia by acclimation at medium altitudes in the Alps

1944 Physiological consultant on aerial supply of rations for troops besieged on the Russian front

1945 Staff appointment at Physiology Department, University of Berlin

1946 Acting Director of Physiology Department

1947 Research appointment at U.S. Air Force School of Aviation Medicine, Randolph Field, Texas

1950 Member, American Physiological Society, Society for Experimental Biology and Medicine, Aerospace Medical Society

1953 Associate Professor U.S. Air Force, Air University, School of Aerospace Medicine

1954 Appointed Head of Physiology Department, Lovelace Foundation for Medical Education and Research, Albuquerque, New Mexico

1955 Fellow, American College of Sports Medicine

U.S. Citizenship

1956 Fellow, American College of Chest Physicians

Member, Committee on Space Technology of the National Advisory Committee for Astronautics (later National Aeronautics and Space Administration)

1959 Member of Medical Selection Board of Astronauts for Mercury Program

Adjunct Professor, Biology Department, University of New Mexico

1960 Consulting Physiologist, Veterans Administration Medical Center, Albuquerque, New Mexico

1961 Member International Academy of Astronautics

1962 Member, New York Academy of Sciences

1963 Special Honor Citation of American Medical Association for Medical Support of Manned Space Program

1964 Fellow, Aerospace Medical Association

1965 Member, Medical Advisory Council to the Office of Manned Space Flight, NASA

1968 Adjunct Professor, Physiology Department, University of New Mexico Medical School

1970 Medical Advisor, Department of Health, Education, and Welfare, Bureau of Hearings and Appeals

1974 Citation by American College of Sports Medicine

1976 Eric Liljencrantz Award, Aerospace Medical Association

1980 W.R. Lovelace II Memorial Award, Lovelace Medical Foundation

1981 Honored by symposium on: "Oxygen Transport to Human Tissues" sponsored by W.R. Lovelace Memorial Lectureship Fund, U.S. Air Force, School of Aerospace Medicine and National Aeronautics and Space Administration.

Publications

1936 Buechner, F. and U.C.L. Morphologic changes in the central nervous system induced by experimental hypoxemia. *Beitr. Pathol. Anat.* 96:549–559.

1937 Irreversible structural changes in the organs induced by hypoxemia in decompression. *Beitr. Pathol. Anat.* 98:323–334.

Irreversible structural changes in the organs of adult and immature animals in decompression. *Beitr. Pathol. Anat.* 99:351–368.

Carbon monoxide poisoning. *Verh. Dtsch. Ges. Pathol.* 29. Tagung, p. 101.

1938 The morphologic picture of structural changes in hypoxemia. *Luftfahrtmed.* 2:231–236.

Himalayan Quest. London: Nicholson and Watson (part authorship).

1939 Improvement of altitude-fitness by acclimatization. *Klin. Wochenschr.* 52(37):1–6.

Becker-Freyseng, H., H.H. Loeschcke, U.C.L., and E. Opitz. The arterial oxygen saturation in "time-reserve" experiments. *Luftfahrtmed.* 4:31–41.

Becker-Freyseng, H., H.H. Loeschcke, U.C.L., and E. Opitz. The calibration of the oximeter of Matthes by alveolar air. *Luftfahrtmed.* 4:309–313.

1941 Hartmann, H., G. Hepp, and U.C.L. Physiological observations on Nanga Parbat (Himalayas, 1937–1938). *Luftfahrtmed.* 6:1–44.

On the use of oxygen apparatus on Himalayan expeditions. *Luftfahrtmed.* 6:45–48.

High altitude acclimatization. *Ergeb. Physiol.* 44:256–314.

1942 Hypothermia and protection against cold in high altitude climates. *Zentralbl. Chir.* 69:1775–1779.

Becker-Freyseng, H., H.H. Loeschcke, U.C.L., and E. Opitz. Acclimatization studies on the Jungfrau-Joch: I. Respiration and blood at rest. *Luftfahrtmed.* 7:160–179.

Becker-Freyseng, H., H.H. Loeschcke, U.C.L., and E. Opitz. Acclimatization studies on the Jungfrau-Joch: II. Respiratory volume and carbon dioxide system in acute hypoxemia before and after acclimatization. *Luftfahrtmed.* 7:180–204.

U.C.L. and E. Opitz. Acclimatization studies on the Jungfrau-Joch: III. Increase in high-altitude tolerance during and after acclimatization. *Luftfahrtmed.* 7:205–217.

Loeschcke, H.H., U.C.L., and E. Opitz. Acclimatization studies on the Jungfrau-Joch: IV. Adaptation and acclimatization of breathing during and after acclimatization and the influence of ammonium-chloride. *Luftfahrtmed.* 7:218–227.

1943 Loeschcke, H.H., U.C.L., and E. Opitz. Acclimatization studies on the Jungfrau-Joch: V. Participation of the kidneys in the acid-base balance during sojourn at high altitude and during acute hypoxemia. *Luftfahrtmed.* 8:265–280.

Alveolar Oxygen Pressure in Explosive Decompression to 16,000 Meters. Bericht der Deutschen Akad. Luftfahrtforschung.

Nanga Parbat. Bauer, P., ed. Berlin: Union-Roth (part authorship).

1944 Special problems in the nutrition of flying personnel. In *Wehrhygiene.* Handloser, S. and Hoffmann, W., eds. Berlin: Springer-Verlag. pp. 487–492.

Stimulating drugs in aviation. In *Wehrhygiene.* Handloser, S. and Hoffmann, W., eds. Berlin: Springer-Verlag. pp. 492–493.

Increase in efficiency in mountaineering by drugs. *Klin. Wochenschr.* 23(21/26):237–238.

A Method for Producing Accurate Oxygen-Nitrogen Mixtures. Dtsch. Luftfahrtforsch. No. 1322

Clamann, H.G. and U.C.L. *Experiments with a Pressure-Helmet for Stratosphere Flight.* Forschungsbericht 17/43. Mitteilungen aus dem Gebiet der Luftfahrtmedizin.

Improvements in Altitude Tolerance by Means of Natural Acclimatization for Flights Exceeding 12,000 Meters Altitude. Forschungsbericht 24/44. Mitteilungen aus dem Gebiet der Luftfahrtmedizin.

1949 U.C.L., H.G. Clamann, and H.F. Adler. Alveolar gases in rapid decompression to high altitudes. *J. Appl. Physiol.* 2:37–48.

1950 Kramer, K., U.C.L., and O. Krayer. Action of epinephrine and veratramine upon heart and oxygen consumption in heart-lung preparation of the dog. *Fed. Proc.* 9:292.

Altitude tolerance. In *German Aviation Medicine, World War II, Vol. I.* Washington, D.C.: Government Printing Office. pp. 304–320.

Acute hypoxia and natural acclimatization. In *German Aviation Medicine, World War II. Vol. I.* Washington, D.C.: Government Printing Office. pp. 409–413.

1951 Kramer, K. and U.C.L. The mobilization of red cells and oxygen from the spleen in severe hypoxia. *Am. J. Physiol.* 165:215–228.

U.C.L., H.G. Clamann, and E. Opitz. The latency of hypoxia on exposure to altitude above 50,000 feet. *J. Aviat. Med.* 22:117–122A.

Pichotka, J., R.B. Lewis, and U.C.L. Influence of general hypoxia on local cold injury. *Tex. Rep. Biol. Med.* 9:601–612.

Hetherington, A.L., U.C.L., L.E. Moses, S.S. Wilkes, H.B. Hale, H.G. Clamann, D.W. Aiken, and R.W. Briggs. *The Cardiovascular and Respiratory Responses of Personnel Suddenly Exposed to Very Low Temperature Windblast.* Project No. 21-23-028 (July). USAF School of Aviation Medicine, Randolph Field, Texas.

Tuttle, A.D., J.P. Marbarger, and U.C.L. The K-S disposable oxygen mask. *J. Aviat. Med.* 22:265–277, 1951.

1952 Physiological limitations in cabin environment and human adaptations. In *Physics and Medicine of the Upper Atmosphere.* White, C.S. and Benson, O.O., eds. Albuquerque: University of New Mexico Press. pp. 567–574.

U.C.L. and W.K. Noell. Anoxic survival of cerebral activity in sudden exposure to high altitudes. *Am. J. Physiol.* 171:745.

Boothby, W.M., U.C.L., and O.O. Benson. Gaseous nitrogen elimination. *J. Aviat. Med.* 23:141–158.

1953 Physiological aspects of prolonged flight at high altitudes and survival in emergencies. *Aeronaut. Eng. Rev.* 12:1–6.

Bancroft, R.W. and U.C.L. *Effective Tracheal and Intrathoracic Pressures Obtained with the D-1 Pressure-Demand Regulator.* Report No. 1, Project No. 21-1201-008. USAF School of Aviation Medicine, Randolph Field, Texas.

U.C.L., R.W. Bancroft, and E.T. Carter. *Rapid Decompression with Pressure Demand Oxygen Equipment.* Report No. 2, Project No. 21-1201-008. USAF School of Aviation Medicine, Randolph Field, Texas.

1954 Balke, B., G.P. Grillo, E.B. Konecci, and U.C.L. Work capacity after blood donation. *J. Appl. Physiol.* 7:231–238.

Physiological aspects of pressure cabins and rapid decompression. In *Handbook of Respiratory Physiology in Aviation.* Boothby, W.M., ed. Randolph Field, Texas: USAF School of Aviation Medicine. pp. 129–142.

1955 Bancroft, R.W., E.T. Carter, and U.C.L. *Evaluation of a Hypoxia Warning Device.* Report No. 55-60. USAF School of Aviation Medicine, Randolph Field, Texas.

Expiratory resistance as determined from transthoracic pressure during rapid decompression. *Fed. Proc.* 14:96.

U.C.L., E.H. Roorbach, and R.E. MacQuigg. Pulmonary nitrogen clearance as a criterion of ventilatory efficiency. *Am. Rev. Tuberc.* 72:465–478.

1956 U.C.L. and W.K. Noell. Manifestations of brief instantaneous hypoxia in man. *J. Appl. Physiol.* 8:444–454.

Goddard, R.F. and U.C.L. Intermittent positive pressure-aerosol therapy in pediatrics. *Dis. Chest.* 29:616–632.

U.C.L. and R.W. Bancroft. Transthoracic pressure in man during rapid decompression. *J. Aviat. Med.* 27:208–220.

Goddard, R.F. and U.C.L. Therapy for respiratory dysfunction. *Modern Medicine* 24:133–134.

The effectiveness of ventilation in healthy adults. *Abstracts of Communications, XXth International Physiological Congress.* Brussels, Belgium. p. 596.

The efficiency of ventilation in pulmonary disease. *Abstracts of Fourth International Congress on Diseases of the Chest.* Cologne, Germany, p. 560.

1957 U.C.L. and E.H. Roorbach. Physical competence of men from 20–45 years of age. *J. Aviat. Med.* 28:209.

Roorbach, E.H., T.P.K. Lim, and U.C.L. Cardiac and metabolic response of nonathletes to graded exercise. *Physiologist* 1(1):72–73.

1958 Lim, T.P.K., U.C.L., and F.S. Grodins. Effects of cervical vagotomy on pulmonary ventilation and mechanics. *J. Appl. Physiol.* 13:317–324.

Spirometric methods. In *Aviation Medicine—Selected Reviews.* (AGARDograph 25). London: Pergamon Press. pp. 8–22.

Lim, T.P.K. and U.C.L. Functional residual capacity and elastic properties of lungs after vagotomy. *Fed. Proc.* 17:97.

Lim, T.P.K. and U.C.L. Changes in lung compliance and functional residual capacity with posture. *Physiologist* 1(4):48–49.

1959 Lim, T.P.K. and U.C.L. Alterations in lung compliance and functional residual capacity with posture. *J. Appl. Physiol.* 14:164–166.

1960 Cardus, D.P., T.P.K. Lim, E.C. Anderson, J.L. Howarth, and U.C.L. Aerobic capacity in relation to body size and composition. *Fed. Proc.* 19:238.

Cartwright, R.S., T.P.K. Lim, U.C.L., and W.E. Palich. A study of the physiological changes in the lungs during cardiopulmonary bypass. *Surg. Forum* XI:226–228.

Schwichtenberg, A.H., U.C.L., and K.L. Stratton. Altitude physiology: air travel in the jet age. In *Clinical Cardiopulmonary Physiology*. Gordon, B.L. and Kory, R.C., eds. New York: Grune and Stratton. pp. 936–957.

Lim, T.P.K. and U.C.L. Body temperature regulation in hypoxia. *Physiologist* 3(3):105.

U.C.L., J.W. Grossman, and E.H. Roorbach. Functional and radiological changes in the lung following Cobalt-60 radiation therapy. *Proceedings of the Sixth International Congress on Diseases of the Chest.* Vienna, Austria.

1961 U.C.L., R.F. Goddard, and E.H. Roorbach. Characteristics of respiratory flow and pressure in newborn infants. *Fed. Proc.* 20:429.

Altitude sickness. In *Aerospace Medicine.* Armstrong, H.G., ed. Baltimore: Williams and Wilkins. pp. 120–142.

Lim, T.P.K. and U.C.L. Body density, fat and fat-free weight (Editorial). *Am. J. Med.* 30:825–832.

Pulmonary ventilation and alveolar gas exchange. In *Handbuch der Allgemeinen Pathologie. Vol. V, Part I.* Buechner, F., Letterer, E., and Roulet, F., eds. Berlin: Springer-Verlag. pp. 276–294.

U.C.L. and T.P.K. Lim. Modified procedure for the determination of body volume by hydrostatic weighing. In *Techniques for Measuring Body Composition*. Brožek, J. and Henschel, A., eds. Washington, D.C.: National Academy of Sciences, National Research Council. p. 107.

Blood and Other Body Fluids. Altman, P.L. and Dittmer, D.S., eds. Washington, D.C.: Federation of Societies for Experimental Biology and Medicine, Committee on Biological Handbooks (contributor and reviewer).

1962 Lovelace, W.R., II, A.H. Schwichtenberg, U.C.L., and R.R. Secrest. Selection and maintenance program for astronauts for the National Aeronautics and Space Administration. *Aerosp. Med.* 33:667–684.

Cardus, D.P., U.C.L., W.A. Spencer, and H.E. Hoff. Considerations on appraisal of physical fitness. *Arch. Phys. Med. Rehabil.* 43:222–227.

Cartwright, R.S., T.P.K. Lim, U.C.L., and W.E. Palich. Pathophysiological changes in the lungs during extracorporeal circulation. *Circ. Res.* 10:131–141.

Lim, T.P.K. and U.C.L. *Influence of Hypoxia on Thermal Homeostasis in Man*. Tech. Doc. Rep. AAL-TDR-61-55. Arctic Aeromedical Laboratory, Fort Wainwright, Alaska.

U.C.L., T.P.K. Lim, D.P. Cardus, J.L. Howarth, and E.C. Anderson. Physical competence in relation to body size and composition. *Proceedings of the International Union of Physiological Sciences*. XXII International Congress, Leiden, The Netherlands. II.

1963 Cardus, D., U.C.L., and B. Beck. Measurements of total circulating hemoglobin with the carbon monoxide rebreathing method. *J. Lab. Clin. Med.* 61:944–952.

U.C.L., D.P. Cardus, T.P.K. Lim, E.C. Anderson, and J.L. Howarth. Physical performance in relation to body size and composition. *Ann. N.Y. Acad. Sci.* 110:795–808.

Lim, T.P.K. and U.C.L. *The Effect of Induced Hypoxia on Thermoregulation and Cardiopulmonary Function*. Tech. Doc. Rep. AAL-TDR-62-19. Arctic Aeromedical Laboratory, Fort Wainwright, Alaska.

1964 Allison, R.D. and U.C.L. Cardiopulmonary dynamics and electrical resistance changes in the thorax. *Fed. Proc.* 23:116.

Laboratory facilities for adaptation research: low pressures. In *Handbook of Physiology. Section 4, Adaptation to the Environment.* Dill, D.B., ed. Washington, D.C.: American Physiological Society. pp. 329–341.

1965 Aviation physiology—the effects of altitude. In *Handbook of Physiology. Section 3. Respiration, Vol. II.* Fenn, W.O. and Rahn, H., eds. Washington, D.C.: American Physiological Society. pp. 1099–1145.

Lovelace, W.R., II, U.C.L., A.H. Schwichtenberg, T.O. Nevison, R. Proper, E.M. Roth, and G.S. Woodson. The selection of astronauts including dynamic testing. In *First International Symposium on Basic Environmental Problems of Man in Space*. Bjurstedt H., ed. Vienna: Springer-Verlag. pp. 35–64.

Lim, T.P.K. and U.C.L. Thermal homeostasis under hypoxia in man. In *First International Symposium on Basic Environmental Problems of Man in Space*. Bjurstedt, H., ed. Vienna: Springer-Verlag. pp. 132–145.

1967 Early detection of deteriorative trends in pulmonary function. In *The Art of Predictive Medicine*. Marxer, W.L., ed. Springfield, Illinois: Charles C. Thomas. pp. 163–174.

1968 U.C.L. and S. Finkelstein. Hypoxia: a clinical-physiological approach. *Aerosp. Med.* 39:105–110.

Mostyn, E.M., S. Finkelstein, and U.C.L. Emphysema at medium altitude. *Proceedings of the International Union of Physiological Sciences*. XXIV International Congress, Washington, D.C. VII, p. 306.

Mostyn, E.M. and U.C.L. Alveolar-arterial gradients for oxygen and carbon dioxide in pulmonary embolization. In *Current Research in Chronic Obstructive Lung Disease*. Public Health Service Publication 1787. Washington, D.C.: U.S. Government Printing Office. pp. 135–144.

McGill, F. and U.C.L. Physical performance in relation to fat-free weight in women compared to men. In *Physiological Aspects of Sports and Physical Fitness*. Balke, B., ed. Chicago: Athletic Institute. p. 82.

1969 Physiologic alterations of altitude in aviation. In *Clinical Cardiopulmonary Physiology*. Third Edition. Gordon, B.L., ed. New York: Grune and Stratton. pp. 631–649.

Rapid decompression. In *Orbital International Laboratory and Space Sciences Conference Proceedings*. (Cloudcroft, New Mexico). Stapp, J.P., von Beckh, H.J., Howard, J., and Steinhoff, E.A., eds. Alamogordo, New Mexico: Publications Branch, Holloman A.F.B. pp. 30–42.

Effects of altitude climates on human performance: a review. In *Physiological Systems in Semiarid Environments*. Riedesel, M.L., ed. Albuquerque, New Mexico: The University of New Mexico Press. pp. 187–190.

Elliott, J.C., S. Finkelstein, and U.C.L. Modified rebreathing procedure for mixed venous gas tensions. *Physiologist* 12(3):214.

1970 Damon, E.G., J.T. Yelverton, U.C.L., and R.K. Jones. *Recovery of the Respiratory System Following Blast Injury*. Tech. Prog. Rep. Contract No. DA-49-146-XZ-372, DASA 2580. Albuquerque, New Mexico.

1971 Damon, E.G., J.T. Yelverton, U.C.L., K. Mitchell, Jr., and R.K. Jones. Acute effects of air blast on pulmonary function in dogs and sheep. *Aerosp. Med.* 42:1–9.

Respiratory system. In *Health Related Problems in Arid Lands*. Symposium number 14. Riedesel, M.L., ed. Tempe, Arizona: Arizona State University Press. pp. 9–17.

1972 Nunneley, S.A., S. Finkelstein, and U.C.L. Longitudinal study on physical performance of ten pilots over a ten-year period. *Aerosp. Med.* 43:541–544.

Muggenburg, B.A., J.L. Mauderly, J.A. Pickrell, T.L. Chiffelle, R.K. Jones, U.C.L., R.O. McClellan, and R.C. Pfleger. Pathophysiologic sequelae of bronchopulmonary lavage in the dog. *Am. Rev. Respir. Dis.* 106:219–232.

Principles of adaptations to altitude. In *Physiological Adaptations—Desert and Mountain*. Yousef, M.K., Horvath, S.M., and Bullard, R.W., eds. New York: Academic Press. pp. 143–156.

1973 Pickrell, J.A., M.E. Light, J.L. Mauderly, P.B. Beckley, B.A. Muggenburg, and U.C.L. Certain effects of sampling and storage on canine blood of different oxygen tensions. *Am. J. Vet. Res.* 34:241–244.

Coester, N., J.C. Elliott, and U.C.L. Plasma electrolytes, pH, and ECG during and after exhaustive exercise. *J. Appl. Physiol.* 34:677–682.

U.C.L., L.G. Myhre, and J.A. Loeppky. Validity of Haldane calculation for estimating respiratory gas exchange. *J. Appl. Physiol.* 34:864–865.

Pulmonary function, body composition and physical fitness of 415 airline pilots in relation to age. In *Physical Fitness*. Seliger, V., ed. Prague: University Karlova. pp. 237–243.

1974 U.C.L., S. Finkelstein, and J.C. Elliott. Respiratory gas exchange, acid-base balance, and electrolytes during and after maximal work breathing 15 mm Hg $PICO_2$. In *Carbon Dioxide and Metabolic Regulations*. Nahas, G. and Schaefer, K.E., eds. New York: Springer-Verlag, pp. 282–293.

U.C.L. Aerospace environments. In *Environmental Physiology*. Slonim, N.B., ed. St. Louis: C.V. Mosby. pp. 376–398.

Loeppky, J.A. and U.C.L. Shifts in O_2 stores with posture affecting apparent O_2 intake. *Proceedings of the International Union of Physiological Sciences*. XXVI International Congress, New Delhi. XI:77.

1975 Loeppky, J.A. and U.C.L. Fluctuations in O_2 stores and gas exchange with passive changes in posture. *J. Appl. Physiol.* 39:47–53.

1976 U.C.L., L.G. Myhre, and M.D. Venters. Tolerance to lower body negative pressure before and after acute dehydration in the heat. *Fed. Proc.* 35:725.

Myhre, L.G., U.C.L., and M.D. Venters. Heat acclimation and responses to acute dehydration and lower body negative pressure. *Fed. Proc.* 35:725.

Loeppky, J.A. and U.C.L. O_2 stores and ventilation in response to lower body negative pressure. *Physiologist* 19(3):275.

Myhre, L.G., U.C.L., and M.D. Venters. Responses of athletes and nonathletes to lower body negative pressure and acute dehydration. *Med. Sci. Sports Exer.* 8:53–54.

How good is exercise for astronauts? In *The Eagle has Returned*. Steinhoff, E.A., ed. Science and Technology, Vol. 43. Proceedings of the Dedication Conference of the International Space Hall of Fame, Alamogordo, New Mexico. American Astronautical Society. pp. 176–180.

1977 Loeppky, J.A., L.G. Myhre, M.D. Venters, and U.C.L. Total body water and lean body mass estimated by ethanol dilution. *J. Appl. Physiol.* 42:803–808.

Scientific facts in support of euthanasia by the high altitude-low pressure method: human experiences in rapid decompression. *Proceedings of the Euthanasia Symposium*. Denver, Colorado (October): The American Humane Association.

Tuttle, W.C., J.A. Loeppky, and U.C.L. Effect of gas density on total respiratory conductance measured by forced oscillation. *Fed. Proc.* 36:614.

1978 Loeppky, J.A., M.D. Venters, and U.C.L. Gravitational effects on blood distribution, ventilation, and gas exchange at the onset and termination of exercise. In *Environmental Stress: Individual Human Adaptations*. Folinsbee, L.J., Wagner, J.A., Borgia, J.F., Drinkwater, B.L., Gliner, J.A., and Bedi, J.F., eds. New York: Academic Press. pp. 225–245.

Tuttle, W.C., S.A. Murphy, and U.C.L. Simple measurement of density dependence of total respiratory conductance in young asthmatic children. *Am. Rev. Respir. Dis.* 117:303.

Loeppky, J.A., M.D. Venters, and U.C.L. Blood volume and cardiorespiratory responses to lower body negative pressure. *Aviat. Space Environ. Med.* 49:1297–1307.

1979 U.C.L., J.A. Loeppky, and E.M. Mostyn. Mean alveolar gases and alveolar-arterial gradients in pulmonary patients. *J. Appl. Physiol.* 46:534–540.

Loeppky, J.A., Y. Kobayashi, M.D. Venters, and U.C.L. Effects of regional hemoconcentration during LBNP on plasma volume determination. *Aviat. Space Environ. Med.* 50:763–767.

Loeppky, J.A., K.L. Richards, E.R. Greene, M.W. Eldridge, D.E. Hoekenga, M.D. Venters, and U.C.L. Instantaneous stroke volume in man during lower body negative pressure (LBNP). *Physiologist.* 22(6):S81–S82.

1980 Kobayashi, Y., J.A. Loeppky, M.D. Venters, and U.C.L. Circulation and respiration response to arm exercise and lower body negative pressure. *Med. Sci. Sports Exer.* 12:244–249.

Loeppky, J.A. and U.C.L. Effect of lower body negative pressure release on hyperpnea induced by inhaled gas. *Respir. Physiol.* 41:349–365.

Famous fallacies in altitude physiology. In *Environmental Physiology: Aging, Heat, and Altitude.* Horvath, S.E. and Yousef, M.K., eds. New York: Elsevier North Holland. pp. 229–232.

Hoekenga, D.E., E.R. Greene, J.A. Loeppky, E.C. Mathews, K.L. Richards, and U.C.L. A comparison of noninvasive Dopplercardiographic and simultaneous Fick measurements of left ventricular stroke volume in man. *Circulation* 62(Part II):III–199.

1981 U.C.L., E.M. Mostyn, J.A. Loeppky, and M.D. Venters. Contribution of the Haldane effect to the rise of arterial PCO_2 in hypoxic patients breathing oxygen. *Crit. Care Med.* 9:32–37.

Loeppky, J.A., E.R. Greene, D.E. Hoekenga, A. Caprihan, and U.C.L. Beat-by-beat stroke volume assessment by pulsed Doppler in upright and supine exercise. *J. Appl. Physiol.* 50:1173–1182.

Appendix

Specialized Physiological Studies in Support of Manned Space Flight. A research program performed under contract with the NASA L.B. Johnson Space Center, Houston, Texas from 1967 to 1980.

Report No. NASA9-7009, February 1970

Part I-A: The effects of breathing low concentrations of CO_2 on exercise tolerance.

Part I-B: The effects of breathing low concentrations of CO_2 on respiratory gas exchange, acid-base balance, and electrolytes during and after exhaustive exercise.

Part II: Evaluation of respiratory measurements for application in space operations
A: The forced oscillation method for measuring total respiratory resistance
B: Estimation of mixed venous gas tensions by a short rebreathing method.

Part III: Validation tests on automatic devices for metabolic rate measurements
A: The Oxygen Consumption Computer (OCC-Technology, Inc.)
B: The Metabolic Rate Monitor (MRM-Webb Assoc.).

Report No. NASA9-7009, December 1971

Section A: The effects of low concentrations of CO_2 on metabolic, respiratory, and circulatory measurements during work and at rest.

Section B: The relationship between heart rate and metabolic rate.

Section C: Alterations in acid-base and electrolytes during exhaustive exercise and recovery.

Report No. NAS9-12572, February 1973

Part A: Evaluation of the single-breath method (Kim et al.) for determining cardiac output using direct Fick procedure as standard.

Part B: Optimum protocol for the assessment of cardiopulmonary competence.

Part C: Body fluids and electrolytes under conditions of single and combined stress.

Part D: Reevaluation of the open-circuit (Haldane) method for measuring metabolic rate with regard to the alleged metabolic production of gaseous nitrogen.

Part E: The use of the forced oscillation method to determine total respiratory conductance in healthy adults, children, and pulmonary patients.

Report No. NAS9-12572, February 1974

Part I: Circulatory and respiratory transients during and after orthostasis and the effects of beta-adrenergic blockade.

Part II: The determination of total body water by a noninvasive ethanol dilution method.

Part III: Increased total respiratory conductance breathing 100% O_2 (Forced oscillation method).

Report No. NAS9-12572, February 1975

Part I: Fluctuations in O_2 stores and gas exchange with passive changes in posture.

Part II: A comparison of the closing volume test with other pulmonary function measurements.

Part III: Total body volume estimated by stereophotogrammetry and by hydrostatic weighing.

Report No. NAS9-14472, February 1976

Part I: A study of factors affecting tolerance of gravitational stress simulated by lower body negative pressure (dehydration by heat and exercise).

Part II: Total respiratory conductance by the forced oscillation method using air and Heliox (20% He + O_2) as a screening test.

Part III: Validation of the alcohol dilution method for total body water and fat-free mass compared with tritium dilution and hyodrstatic weighing.

Report No. NAS9-14920, December 1977

Part I: Blood volume shifts and cardiorespiratory fluctuations in response to lower body negative pressure (LBNP).

Part II: Gravitational effects on blood distribution, ventilation, and gas exchange at the onset and termination of exercise.

Part III: Forced oscillations with air and Heliox to determine the site of airway obstruction.

Part IV: A new method for determining closing volume using forced oscillations.

Report No. NAS9-15483, December 1978

Part I: Effects of acute diuresis with Lasix on the volume and composition of body fluids and the responses to LBNP.

Part II: Effects of peripheral blood sequestration during LBNP on plasma volume determinations.

Part III: Effect of LBNP release on transient hyperpnea induced by inhaled gas mixture.

Part IV: Cardiorespiratory responses to arm exercise with and without LBNP.

Report No. NAS9-15483, July 1980

Part A: Tolerance to LBNP in endurance runners, weightlifters, swimmers, and nonathletes.

Part B: Noninvasive aortic blood flow by pulsed Doppler echocardiography (PDE) compared to cardiac output by direct Fick measurements.

Part C: Beat-by-beat stroke volume assessment by PDE in upright and supine exercise.

Part D: Instantaneous changes in stroke volume by PDE during and after constant LBNP (−50 Torr).

Part E: Changes in cardiac output and tibial artery flow during and after progressive LBNP.

OXYGEN TRANSPORT TO HUMAN TISSUES

SECTION I:

Historical Perspectives

J.A. Loeppky and M.L. Riedesel, editors
OXYGEN TRANSPORT TO HUMAN TISSUES

The Lovelace Years

Clayton S. White

It is a pleasure to participate in this symposium honoring a colleague over many years, Dr. Ulrich C. Luft, one of the world's outstanding and remarkably productive scientists. Beyond introducing him, I would like to sketch some of the historical highlights of the Lovelace Clinic and the Lovelace Foundation for Medical Education and Research. As Dr. William R. Lovelace (1883–1968) died on December 4, 1968 and his nephew, Dr. W. Randolph Lovelace II (1907–1965) was lost with his wife, Mary, and their pilot, Milton Brown, in an airplane accident near Aspen, Colorado, on December 12, 1965, my remarks will be mostly limited to deal selectively with events prior to these dates in highlighting progress subsequent to the founding of the Lovelace organization.

Organization

The Lovelace Clinic, appearing in Albuquerque as a partnership involving Dr. William R. Lovelace and his brother-in-law, Dr. Edward T. Lassetter in 1922, initiated the group practice of medicine into New Mexico. The clinic grew steadily and currently continues to flourish. It has grown from three M.D.s in 1923 to 86 M.D.s, four Ph.D.s and one Nurse Practitioner in 1980, staffing the Lovelace Medical Center on Gibson Boulevard and three additional Satellite locations in the Albuquerque Metropolitan Area. In addition, three Associated Group practices operate in New Mexico at Roswell (1978), Gallup (1979), and Grants (1979).

W. Randolph Lovelace II became a third partner to the Lovelace Clinic following his decision to leave the surgical staff of the Mayo Clinic in 1946. A year later, as a consequence of prior understandings between Dr. Lovelace II and his uncles, the partnership was dissolved and the clinic reorganized as an association of physicians. There were 15 physicians on the clinic staff in 1947 including Clayton S. White, who reported in August of that year to establish a section of Internal and Aviation Medicine and to accept an appointment as Director of Research of the still unformalized Foundation. Concurrently, the Lovelace Foundation for Medical Education and Research was founded for educational, scientific, benevolent, and charitable purposes. The certificate of incorporation was filed September 24, 1947 naming 14 individuals including the three Lovelace Clinic incorporators and Trustees. Trustees were distinguished members of the professional, business, and ranching communities. All except four resided in New Mexico. Five were physicians (four Lovelace Clinic doctors, and the Dean of the University of Colorado School of Medicine). Among the nine lay individuals were a Federal Judge, two bankers, two ranchers, and four businessmen. The nonprofit New Mexico Corporation, later to become tax-exempt, received the assets of the Lovelace Clinic as a gift. At the first meeting of the Board of Trustees, Mr. Floyd B. Odlum was elected President, Dr. W. Randolph Lovelace II, Vice President, Dr. W.R. Lovelace, Treasurer, and Mr. Jack A. Korber, Secretary. In 1949, Mr. Odlum was elected Chairman of the Board of Trustees and Dr. W. Randolph Lovelace II was named President and Director of the Foundation, a post he held until his death in 1965. Mr. Odlum served continuously as Chairman of the Board until he requested retirement in February of 1967. At that time, Mr. Robert O. Anderson of Roswell, New Mexico accepted the Chairmanship, a position he currently holds.

Early Concepts

Dr. Lovelace II, in initial discussions with the Board of Trustees, emphasized that, among other things, the founding Charter of the Foundation specified activities in medical education and research at both clinical and basic levels. Undeterred by the statewide absence of important essentials to carry out such objectives, he proposed a plan to assemble systematically in Albuquerque the elements necessary for education and research in medical schools and medical centers. The Board members proved their optimism by reacting favorably to the plan. From the beginning, at least six functional entities were recognized as essential; a clinic for outpatients, a hospital for inpatients, facilities for research and instruction in the basic and paramedical sciences including appropriate laboratories, suitable equipment, qualified personnel, and operating funds.

The Lovelace plan to push research ahead of education (the reverse of the convention in medical schools and academic medical centers prior to 1950) marked the Albuquerque operation as different. This approach proved timely and advantageous. For example, the view prioritizing research in a medically-oriented environment, advertised a certain dissatisfaction with the status quo, placed the current inventory of biomedical information under critical scrutiny and emphasized a resolve to upgrade and enhance the quality of patient care available to citizens of Albuquerque, New Mexico and neighboring states. In addition, the comprehensive approach to short- and long-term objectives placed efficacious constraints upon the choice of personnel because only those experienced in a clinical mileau and talented enough to pursue independent investigations and later to teach would do for the key laboratory disciplines. Also those to be recruited in the paramedical and more physically-oriented disciplines would have to be unusually gifted, flexible, and either proven achievers or judged high on the work-potential scale. Indeed, better all hands be adventuresome, for unless that were the case, who would join those audaciously envisioning the emergence of a major medical center in a town of 40,000 (Albuquerque population in 1947) centrally located in the sparsely settled state of New Mexico?

Significant also was the post-World War II feeling and mood and the accompanying realization by many that the conceptual and technical advances associated with military operations in the United States and abroad provided a potent stimulus for making constructive use of all that was new and yet unapplied. The Lovelace Trustees understood this and their "lay-it-on-the-line" actions engendered a reciprocal response from the staff. Communications were good enough to stimulate an observer on one occasion to say "it seems both Trustees and staff are trying to teach each other the art of leading by example."

Facilities

One outcome of this spirit on the part of the Trustees was immediate approval and implementation of a long-term construction program following the donation of a tract of land on Gibson Boulevard by Dr. W.R. Lovelace. The site chosen for Foundation headquarters was near the Veterans Hospital which had just opened a new 300-bed addition to the facility. Seven construction projects placed six new buildings on the site between 1950 and 1968. The Trustees tended to favor an overbuilding policy which proved immeasurably useful when extramural funds became available to support research of interest to the staff. For example, Albert K. Mitchell told the Trustees in 1954 he was arranging a series of contributions to equip a machine shop because he was tired of hearing the Director of Research complain that none was at hand. This and similar events involving Dr. Lovelace, Mr. Odlum, and other Trustee members prompted Dr. Lovelace II to note, "he was beginning to understand better what friends and Trustees were for."

Also, the Lovelace family, Trustees, and friends were active in obtaining funds and pledges to aid the Methodist Church to build Bataan Memorial Methodist Hospital adjacent to the Foundation property. The hospital opened in 1952 and in 1969 it was acquired by the Lovelace Foundation.

Always cautious and considerate, the Board's reactions were at the same time remarkably farsighted and visionary. Typical, for example, was their discussion to move ahead with the W.R. Lovelace building project which was begun on April 24, 1961. The structure, more than doubling space at headquarters and integrating the hospital with the Lassetter, OB-Gyn and Radiation Therapy buildings, was planned with fourth and fifth floor options. Overbuilding as a policy was maintained much through the generosity of Mr. Robert O. Anderson whose substantial contributions made possible building the fifth floor as a "shell" which was finally utilized in 1978, some 17 years after it was constructed at substantially reduced cost.

Early Personal Recollections

That there was a clinic to operate and patients to see was always very much on Dr. W.R. Lovelace's mind. His concerns were such that for years he routinely directed the clinic operator to direct all night calls to his home. I recall receiving a ring one morning near two A.M. "Hello Sambo," he said. "There is a lady out in the North valley who thinks she is having a heart attack." "How old is she," I asked. He replied, "Twenty-two." I said, "She is probably fighting with her husband." His authoritative interruption was, "Don't you think you better go out there and see?" I did and she was.

Not long after arriving in Albuquerque, my wife and I attended a Saturday afternoon staff picnic held on the far east mesa up against the mountains. A vehicle appeared and parked about 200 yards away. It was noticed and there was much asking and wondering among the new hands until an old-timer remarked: "Uncle Doc always hires a radio-equipped taxi to stand by on occasions like this. There are, after all, clinic physicians and surgeons up here and there's Lovelace patients and competitors down there."

Dr. Jack Grossman, the very competent clinic radiologist, and I were called into Randy Lovelace's office in 1948 and told the Lovelace Foundation had a contract to explore the need for an Aviation Biophysics Facility possibly to be constructed at the Arnold Engineering Development Center (AEDC). The work was to encompass conceptual facilities design and a local architect was to help. Jack went to Berkeley and I went to Los Alamos and Rochester, New York. The architect went where architects go and, I believe Randy went to Washington, D.C. and Oak Ridge. On returning to Albuquerque, we compared notes and discussed and outlined a report. It became clear to me then that Randy Lovelace knew information and data might be contained in books and libraries, but wisdom was found elsewhere. The biophysics facility was not built at AEDC, but Lovelace, Grossman, and White learned a lot.

The Symposium on the Physics and Medicine of the Upper Atmosphere

Dr. Lovelace II, as a consequence of his Mayo clinic contacts and his directing the Aeromedical Laboratory at Wright Field during the war, knew an amazing number of influential people. He was active on the Air Force Scientific Advisory Board and in organizing the Air Research and Development Command projects led by Professor Theodor Von Karman of Cal Tech. Also, Randy Lovelace possessed an extraordinary sense of opportunity and timing, not unrelated to his telling me early in 1950 about discussions he had with General Otis Benson, the Commanding officer of the USAF School of Aviation Medicine at San Antonio, Texas. It developed that the Lovelace Foundation was to plan, organize, and document a symposium on the Physics and Medicine of the Upper Atmosphere. The objective was to collect available data and information essential to planning future research necessary for manned flight towards the top of the earth's atmosphere. The contract was signed in June of 1960. Thirty-four scientists who were knowledgeable in the fields of astrophysics, aeronautical engineering, biology, radiobiology, toxicology, and aviation medicine were invited. In retrospect, I probably enjoyed this assignment and the associations developed with the several participants more than any other assignment during my association with the Lovelace Foundation. The highly successful symposium, was held November 6 to 9, 1951 in San Antonio. Most major participants had turned in their manuscripts prior to the meeting, but without exception all picked them up afterwards saying they had learned so much from others present that only significant revisions would do. The cooperation was amazing, and a report of the symposium in the form of a textbook published by the University of New Mexico Press, was available the following June. The book was just in time for delivery to NATO country representatives, who were to assemble in the fall of 1952 to organize the Aeromedical Panel of the Advisory Group for Aeronautical Research and Development (AGARD). You might surmise that Dr. Lovelace II thought C.S. White, as a reward for working so hard on the symposium, should go to Paris and work for another pleasant and stimulating slave driver, Professor Von Karman, who was then Chairman of AGARD. I did, but what was unusual, unexpected, and very welcome was that my boss had, through contributions to a travel fund, made it possible for my wife, Peggy, also to accompany me on the trip. Randy Lovelace said, "That was what understanding friends were for."

Major Programs

Seizing the opportunities opened by Lovelace leadership the staff subsequently developed a number of major research programs.

The Blast and Biology Program initiated in 1951 under contract with the Atomic Energy Commission, was concerned with the biological effects of rapid variations of environmental pressure induced by explosive events, the damage produced by energized debris, and the consequences of accelerative and decelerative whole-body displacement. Relevant research on the pathophysiology, prevention, and therapy required following blast-induced injuries is still being carried out.

Also currently active are activities stemming from the Fission Product Inhalation Program, implemented in 1960 under contract with the Division of Biology and Medicine of the Atomic Energy Commission. Concerned with the hazards of inhaling radioactive liquid and particulate aerosols, the effort has been expanded to include the inhalation toxicology of effluents from fuel cycles of interest to the Department of Energy.

The Aging Program, beginning in 1960 under contract with the FAA and subsequently grant-supported by the NIH over a period of almost 10 years, involved serial studies of pilots using a battery of physiological, psychological, and clinical tests. The aim was to evaluate the levels of normal function in American males as they might vary as a function of time and age. Dr. Luft was intimately involved in the physiological aspects of this program and he utilized the data to develop invaluable standards for physical and physiological variables (e.g., Luft, U.C. 1973. Pulmonary function, body composition and physical fitness of 415 airline pilots in relation to age. In *Physical Fitness*. V. Seliger, ed. Praha: Universita Karlova. pp. 237–243.).

Started in 1962, under the auspices of the National Aeronautical and Space Administration, the Aerospace Support Program undertook as an early objective the collection and analysis of information from all disciplines, biological as well as physical, which might relate to the biomedical aspects of operating manned space craft. A thesaurus embodying over 12,000 descriptions were prepared, computerized, and automated to allow retrieval of over 30,000 coded documents. Also a three-volume compendium for development of Human Standards in Space System Design was completed. The outstanding work represented an unsurpassed contribution to the Nation's space effort. Follow-up work under NASA support continued until 1980, mainly under the direction of Dr. Luft, in specialized physiological studies in support of manned space flight.

Though there were many other research activities, particularly of a clinical nature, that were of interest up to 1968 with some continuing to the present day, those will not be noted here. Figure 1 shows research costs on a cumulative basis, and how these were interrelated with personnel, publications, salary, and equipment metrics. More impressive than the consistent uptrend in the variables chosen to assess progress over the years, is the evidence that the interplay between the Board of Trustees and staff was so effective and so viably sound as to survive the loss of the Foundation's two key leaders between 1965 and 1968. Had this not been true, I am certain I would have had a "Hello Sambo" message from Uncle Doc and word from Randy saying "You've forgotten what I said interested Trustees and colleagues were for."

Dr. Ulrich Cameron Luft

After coming to Albuquerque in 1954, Dr. Luft played a vital role in the Lovelace saga. In the course of doing the 1951 symposium and book, I became acquainted with him and his wife, Alice. I recall enjoying dinner and an

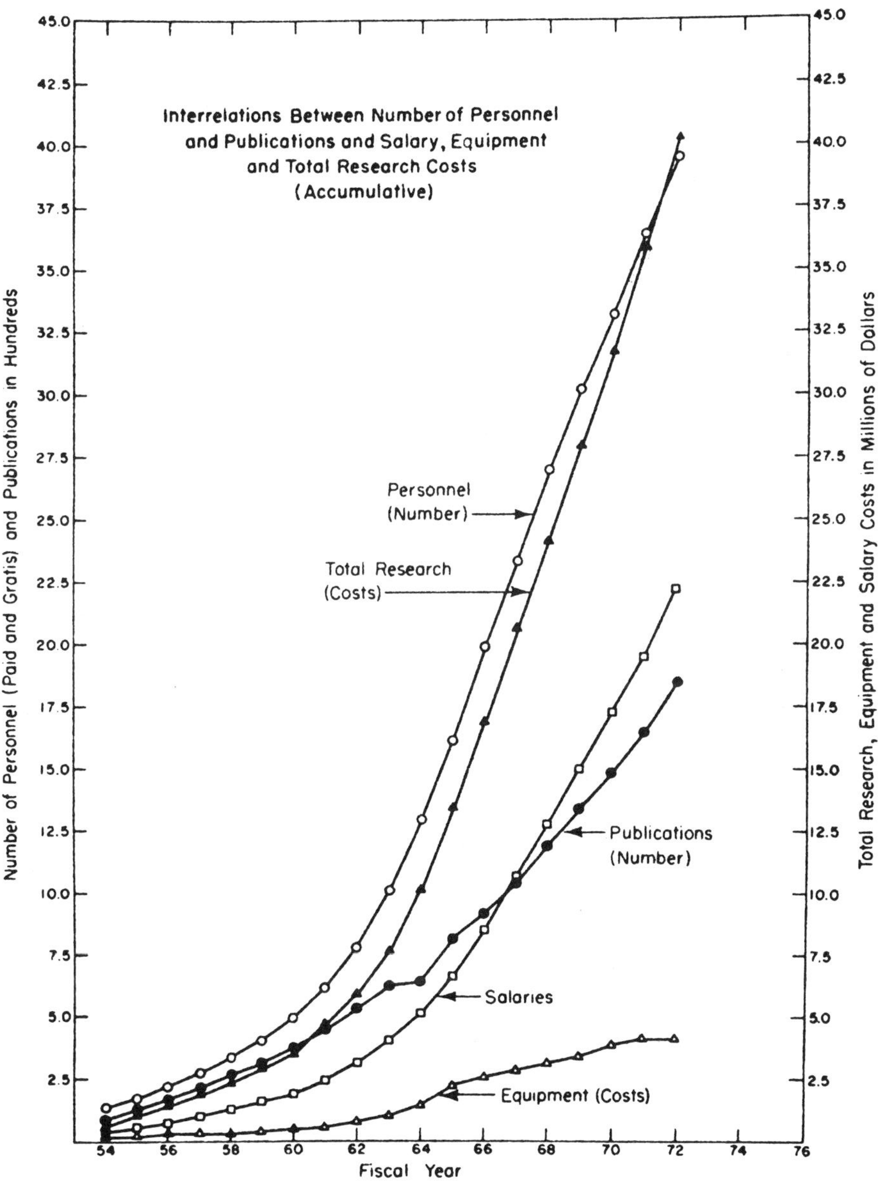

Figure 1. Research progress indices for the Lovelace Foundation, 1954 to 1972.

evening in their home in San Antonio, along with John Dornacker, the Foundation Administrator. I'm sure they thought we both were working too hard and being hospitable and friendly they prescribed relaxation in their homelike atmosphere and manner. Subsequent contacts ensued because a collaborator of Dr. Luft's at the School of Aviation Medicine, Dr. Walter M. Boothby, had moved to Albuquerque in 1950 to head the Department of Physiology at the Lovelace Foundation. At that time, Dr. Nils Lundgren from Sweden was in the midst of a postdoctoral fellowship and the first three graduate students were completing work on their M.S. degrees. Dr. Boothby launched a project to produce a 10-chapter Handbook on Aviation Physiology under contract with the School of Aviation Medicine. Dr. Luft contributed a chapter and thus kept informed about the Lovelace adventure in Albuquerque. In passing, I am pleased to note that counting Ulrich Luft and myself, five of those who contributed to the Boothby Handbook are participating in this symposium: Dr. Charles Houston, Dr. Hermann Rahn, and Dr. Richard Riley.

Dr. Walter Boothby died in July of 1953. Dr. Lundgren was leaving to go to the World Health Laboratory in Calcutta. Lovelace people had just completed participating in the 1953 Nuclear Test Series at the Nevada Test Site and were planning to continue there in 1955. We were desperately short of personnel and I and other hands were delighted when Dr. Luft agreed to leave San Antonio and head the Foundation's Department of Physiology. Other team players were Dr. Bernard B. Longwell in Biochemistry, Dr. W. Everett Clapper in Microbiology, and Dr. Thomas L. Chiffelle in Pathology. All these compatible men were experienced in clinical laboratory work in medical schools and hospitals and they brought distinction, class, and accuracy into clinical and hospital operations. What came out of their "shops" was always of research caliber and such precision was enthusiastically welcomed by those responsible for clinical care.

Dr. Luft, Alice, and their son Friedrich (now a practicing physician and researcher in nephrology at the University of Indiana) arrived in Albuquerque the day the Hopkins Radiation Laboratory and Therapy Center was dedicated on January 16, 1954. There must have been some Providence at work for housed therein was the second rotational cobalt therapy unit to operate in the U.S., having been commissioned the previous fall. Dr. Jack W. Grossman in Radiology and Dr. John Howarth, a radiation physicist recruited from Sheffield, England, were already present and now, with Dr. Luft aboard, the stage was set for what was to be a scientific first; namely, the demonstration in humans that high energy gamma radiation produced a radiation pneumonitis and a partially reversible fall in pulmonary function, the severity of which was associated with the radiation dose. The study, supported by NIH was reported by Dr. Luft in Vienna in 1960 at the International Congress on Chest Diseases. The findings were not unexpected as similar data were obtained at Rochester University in dogs, but the work in Albuquerque helped define and punctuate a caution for Radiation therapists to heed. Whom do you think it was that donated the funds for Dr. Luft's trip to Vienna? None other than Mr. John J.

Hopkins, who also generously supported the construction of the Radiation Therapy Laboratory housing the Cobalt unit, which in turn was a gift from another Trustee, Mr. Ellis A. Hall. "That," Randy Lovelace said, "was what perceptive Trustees were for."

Dr. Luft first became interested in medicine as a consequence of making rounds as a youngster with an uncle who practiced surgery near London. His mother was born Mary Wilson in Edinburgh, Scotland. His father, Friedrich J. Luft, was a teacher of modern languages in Berlin, Germany, but they frequently spent the summer vacations in Edinburgh with their family. One such trip—it happened to be the summer of 1914—was destined to be an unexpectedly long one for Ulrich. His family returned to Berlin in July for the beginning of the school term while he, not being of school age, was to return later in the year accompanied by his aunt. World War I broke out in August and Ulrich was separated from his parents until 1920. On returning to Berlin at the age of 10, Ulrich had to relearn German, a task enhanced by learning and playing violin with his father who was an accomplished violinist. Ulrich's mother was a pianist and singer and his sister later played concert class cello. Dr. Luft's interest in music had endured and remains an attractive facet of his personality.

Dr. Luft started medical school at Freiburg in the fall of 1929. He was persuaded by a boyhood friend interested in mountaineering to transfer to the University of Munich Medical School. There he joined the Alpine Club. Upon the death of his father in 1931, he returned to Berlin and entered the University of Berlin Medical School taking his M.D. in 1935. After a year of internship in a large city hospital in Berlin (1935–36), he was licensed to practice medicine in Germany. He then took a residency in Pathology at the Medical School in Freiberg (1936–37), an aspect of his training which was intimately associated with his first research publication. In 1937 and 1938, he spent three months each year on expeditions to the Himalayas, working for and with Dr. Hans Hartmann. Both expeditions were sponsored by the Aeromedical Research Institute of the Air Ministry. During 1938–42, Dr. Luft worked as a Research Physiologist at the Aeromedical Research Institute in Berlin and in 1942 took his Ph.D. in Physiology at the University of Berlin. His thesis was titled "High Altitude Acclimitization." From 1942 to 1945, he served as Chief of Aviation Physiology at the Aeromedical Research Institute and held the rank of Associate Professor of Physiology at the University of Berlin Medical School. In 1945, he was appointed Associate Professor and Acting Director of the Department of Physiology at the reactivated University of Berlin Medical School, a post he held until 1947 when he elected to leave Germany. He arrived in San Antonio to join the staff of the USAF School of Aviation Medicine in June 1947 as a Research Physiologist and Associate Professor. His wife and son joined him there later that year.

There is so much more that could be said about Dr. Luft; his publications totalling some 120 papers or book chapters over 55 years (27 at the Lovelace Foundation in Albuquerque) attest to his unflagging energy and productivity.

He is a superb methodologist as those who work in his department soon learn. His contribution to the fine judgment required to define the line between normality and disease has been outstanding. Beyond this and the high regard with which his career is viewed by those who know and read his work, I suspect his greatest contribution and satisfaction will stem from what he has imparted to the pre- and postdoctoral fellows he has trained. The Albuquerque list indicates 16 postdoctorates from 11 different countries: Canada, Czechoslovakia, Denmark, England, Germany, India, Japan, Spain, Sweden, Thailand, and the U.S.A. Four have taken their Ph.D. and three their M.S. degrees under his watchful eye. Odds are high you will hear from all these individuals over the years ahead, but maybe not with the force with which Dr. Ulrich Luft has impacted science. Men of his caliber are rare indeed. I am honored to introduce a scientist and a friend whose quiet competence is as impressive as his works are great.

J.A. Loeppky and M.L. Riedesel, editors
OXYGEN TRANSPORT TO HUMAN TISSUES

Adventures in Hypoxia

Ulrich C. Luft

An important aspect of this symposium on "O_2 Transport to Human Tissues" will be the disturbance or limitation of O_2 supply to the cells, be this due to exogenous or endogenous causes, which lead to hypoxia. By way of introduction to this theme, I intend to recall several episodes in my career that may appear to be entirely unrelated except for the fact that they all involve hypoxia.

I encountered the first adventure, when I was working on my doctoral thesis in 1935. After graduating from medical school in Berlin, I took my mandatory medical/surgical internship and then decided to take a residency in pathology at the largest municipal hospital in Berlin. There were two other residents in the department and we had to perform all the autopsies of which there were 8 to 10 every day. This was an excellent experience and we were kept very busy because we also had to do all the histological studies ourselves. In my "spare time," I began a series of animal experiments for my doctoral thesis which I had been contemplating for some time. While I was studying in Munich, I had spent my weekends climbing and skiing in the Alps with a friend, Hans Hartmann. He was a brilliant young physiologist who had taken part in a Himalayan expedition to Kangchenchunga in 1931 and had done studies on himself and the other climbers at altitudes up to 7700 m. At that time, I wondered whether any morphological changes might occur to various organ tissues at these altitudes, so I set up a simple arrangement to expose guinea pigs to low pressure. I got a piece of sewer pipe 60 cm in diameter and 60 cm long and had an iron plate welded onto the bottom end. The rim at the top was milled off smoothly and I placed a large piece of plate glass 3 cm thick on it with a strong rubber gasket as a seal. Not having any experience with low or high pressure, I believed that the glass would withstand at least one atmosphere of negative pressure. The pressure was reduced by an ordinary suction pump on the water line and any desired pressure could be set by a vent-valve triggered by a variable mercury column. This arrangement also supplied continuous ventilation. In the first test, fortunately without any animals, everything went beautifully until the pressure in the chamber had dropped to about 200 Torr. Then there was a tremendous bang and large and small splinters of glass were flying all over the room. I escaped with only one gash across my wrist, which fortunately did not sever the artery. After this adventure, I consulted with a glass blower and found out that only tension-free glass is suitable for working with high or low pressures and that solved the problem. After 3 days staged ascent at lower "altitudes," several animals were exposed together to pressures of 250 to 300 Torr for an average of 5 days. The animals were recompressed to ambient pressure for one hour every day for feeding and cleaning. The most widespread and uniformly distributed changes after exposure were found in the liver (Figure 1) where there was necrosis surrounding the vein in the center of each lobulus with fatty degeneration (Sudan stain) in the cells in the periphery. Of the various parts of the central nervous system

Figure 1. Necrosis around the center of a liver lobulus surrounded by cells with fatty degeneration.
SOURCE: *Luft, 1938.*

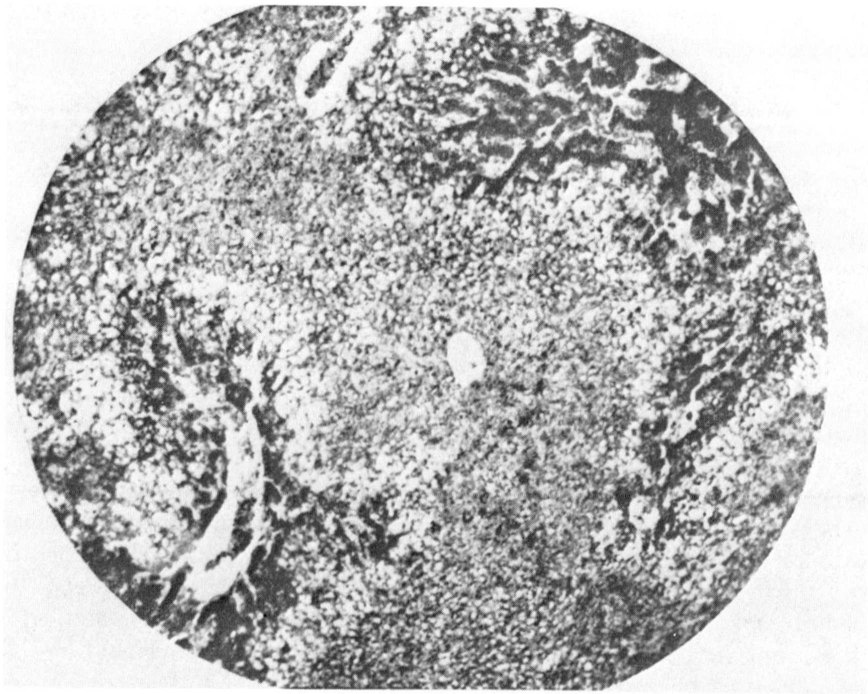

that were examined (Nissl method), no lesions were found in the cerebral cortex. However, manifest degenerative lesions were seen below the fourth ventricle such as shown in Figure 2. Another organ that was consistently affected by the simulated altitude exposure was the heart muscle. Disseminated necroses were found in the walls of the left and right ventricle, in the papillary muscles, and the apex (Figure 3). In the affected areas, the muscle cells were dissolved into homogenous hyaline globs without any visible nuclei. In the specimen shown, there is also some infiltration by leukocytes. Incidentally, this was the first time it had ever beeen demonstrated that myocardial necrosis can be caused by hypoxia alone without any pathology in the coronary vasculature (Luft, 1937, 1938).

Certainly my most memorable adventures with hypoxia I experienced on two expeditions to the Himalayas in 1937 and 1938. The objective of these expeditions was the summit of Nanga Parbat (8125 m, 26,659 ft) located at the western end of the main Himalaya in the state of Kashmir (Figure 4). It is one of the 16 peaks higher than 8000 m, none of which had ever been climbed at that time. My friend, Hans Hartmann, who was at that time chief physiologist at the Aeromedical Research Institute in Berlin, asked me to join the expedition in 1937 and help him with his physiological studies on the mountain. Early in May, the German and Austrian climbers started on the trek from

Figure 2. Right: Motor ganglion cell from the floor of the fossa rhomboidea with severe degeneration of the nucleus and alterations of the "Nissl" bodies after 5 days exposure to 230 Torr. Left: Ganglion cell from the same region in control animal.
SOURCE: *Luft, 1938.*

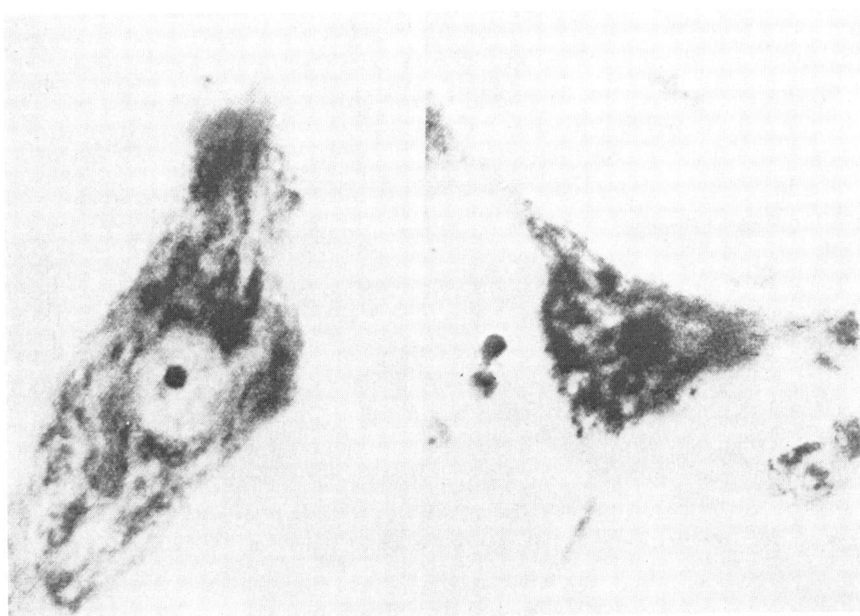

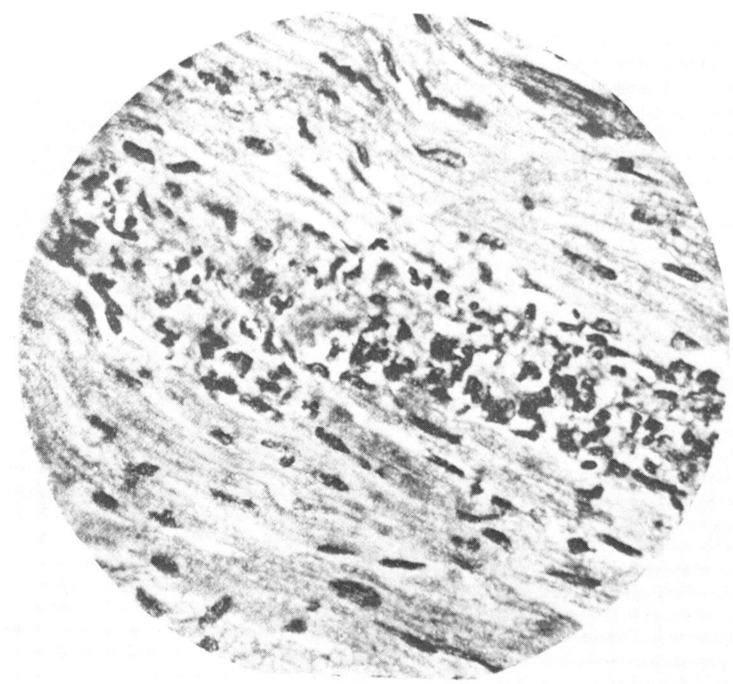

Figure 3. Dissolution of fibers of papillary heart muscle into homogenous debris. Reactive infiltration with leukocytes and isolated fibroblasts.

SOURCE: *Luft, 1938.*

Srinagar through the foothills to the Indus river on the north side of Nanga Parbat and reached the base camp (3700 m) two weeks later with 150 porters carrying the provisions and equipment. At first, the ascent was hampered by repeated heavy snow falls, forcing the assault group to retreat to base camp. Early in June, however, conditions improved and by the 6th camp IV (6270 m) was established and in the next few days all the necessary resources for the final assault were assembled there. I remained at base camp with instructions to await the arrival of mail from Gilgit, the nearest post office, before proceeding to camp IV with more provisions. The camp was not visible from the base, but on the morning of June 14th I could see a party of climbers slowly moving up toward a shelf where camp V was to be built. The same afternoon our British liaison officer arrived at base camp with two sick porters. He reported that heavy snowfall had again delayed their progress and that 7 climbers and 9 porters were still waiting impatiently for it to clear up. Two days later, the mail runner arrived and I started early next morning, followed by 7 porters carrying supplies. After spending the night at Camp II (5380 m), we proceeded up the mountain at daybreak eagerly looking forward to joining

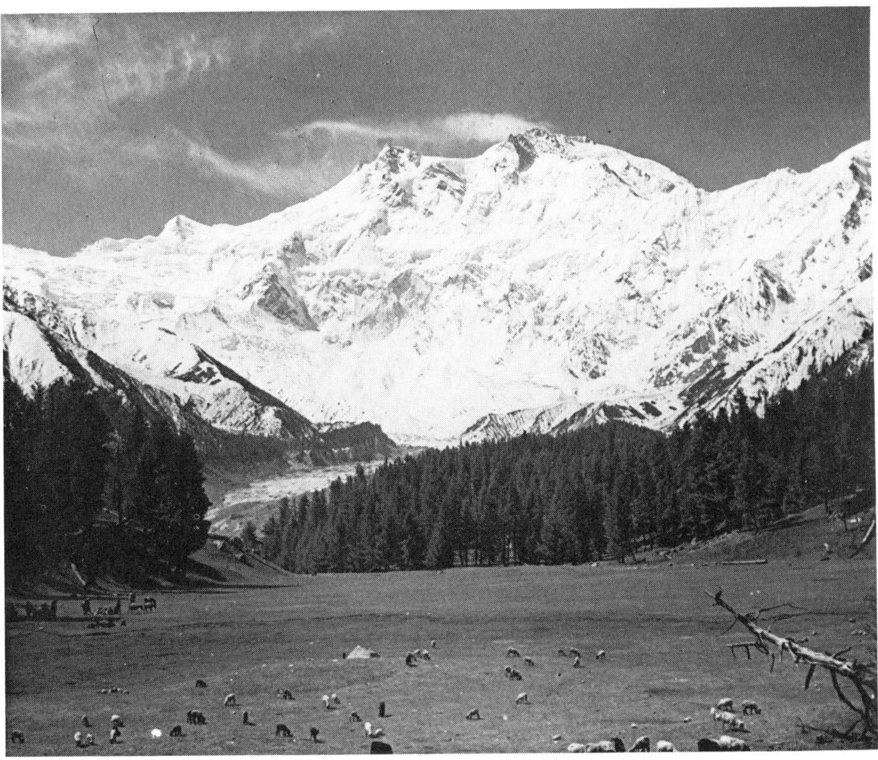

Figure 4. Nanga Parbat (8,125 m) in Kashmir from the "Fairy Meadow" below base camp.
SOURCE: *German Himalaya Foundation.*

our friends by noon. The porters were lagging behind under their heavy loads and with increasing altitude, so I hurried ahead alone. Soon I reached a vantage point with a view over the slopes where I knew Camp IV had been located. But there were no signs of life. Getting close, I realized that an avalanche of ice blocks and compressed snow had completely covered an area of about 15 acres. In the meantime, the porters who had been here before confirmed my worst fears. Far above I could see old tracks leading toward the summit ridge, presumably from the party I had seen from base camp by telescope on June 14th. But, obviously there could be no survivors, or they would have signalled for help immediately after the catastrophe. Any attempt to reach the victims that day was out of the question without the proper equipment. Furthermore it was getting late and we were without shelter for the night. So I ordered the porters to cache their loads and we hurried downhill reaching base camp well after dark. An urgent telegram to our headquarters in Munich alerted a rescue party of three experienced mountaineers who left by air a few days later and were flown to Gilgit from Delhi by the Royal Air Force. I was greatly relieved to have them join us on July 8th at the base camp. In the meantime, the tracks up the glacier had been obliterated by snow fall and more avalanches and it was with great difficulty that we managed to reach the site of the tragedy, particularly since the newcomers had not had time to acclimatize. On July 15th, a month after the accident, we began the laborious task of excavation in the ice at 6270 m with picks, shovels, and avalanche probes. After searching for 5 days in vain, we finally located the camp and were able to uncover 5 of the 7 climbers and locate the 9 porters. All of them were in their sleeping bags and had apparently been smothered instantaneously under 10 to 12 ft of ice and snow. We recovered their scientific records and diaries. Hans Hartmann had written his last diary on the evening of June 14th. The watch he wore on his wrist had stopped at 12:20, but started to run again in the warmth of my pocket. After 7 days of exhausting labor, we were at the end of our endurance and were running out of supplies and fuel. We buried our friends under a mound of snow, marked it with an ice-axe and climbing rope. Before taking our leave with sad hearts, we had already resolved to return to Nanga Parbat the following year.

On June 1, 1938, a team of 10 climbers from Germany and Austria arrived at our old base camp ready to renew the assault. Bruno Balke, a friend of mine from medical school, was team physician and joined me in the physiological studies planned for the previous year by Hans Hartmann, which had been so tragically interrupted. A radically new departure was the participation of a transport aircraft assigned to us by the Air Ministry to supply the base and higher camps from Srinagar so as to reduce the number of porters required, of whom 9 had lost their lives the year before. Weather conditions were even worse than the year before and, after reaching Camp IV, a group of climbers and porters were marooned for 6 days without any communication with base camp after a heavy snowstorm. Here the airlift proved invaluable by dropping supplies at 6270 m on the first clear morning on alert by radio. The assault continued despite several more setbacks and Camp VI was established at 7000 m on the summit ridge. In view of the weather reports from Srinagar that the monsoon season was already in progress and more storms were to be expected around Nanga Parbat, further attempts on the summit had to be abandoned. All climbers and porters returned safely.

The physiological observations of 1937 and 1938 reported in detail elsewhere (Hartmann et al., 1942) can be summarized as follows. It was already well known at that time that animals and man become polycythemic at altitude. We wanted to find out how rapid the erythropoietic response was at various altitudes and also how soon it abated after return to lower altitudes. The results are shown in Figure 5. During the 65-day sojourn at altitude between 4000 and 7000 m, there was a continuous rise in the red cell count and in hemoglobin, but the former increased more rapidly than the latter, resulting in a reduçed Hb/Hct ratio and the disparity persisted even 30 days after descent.

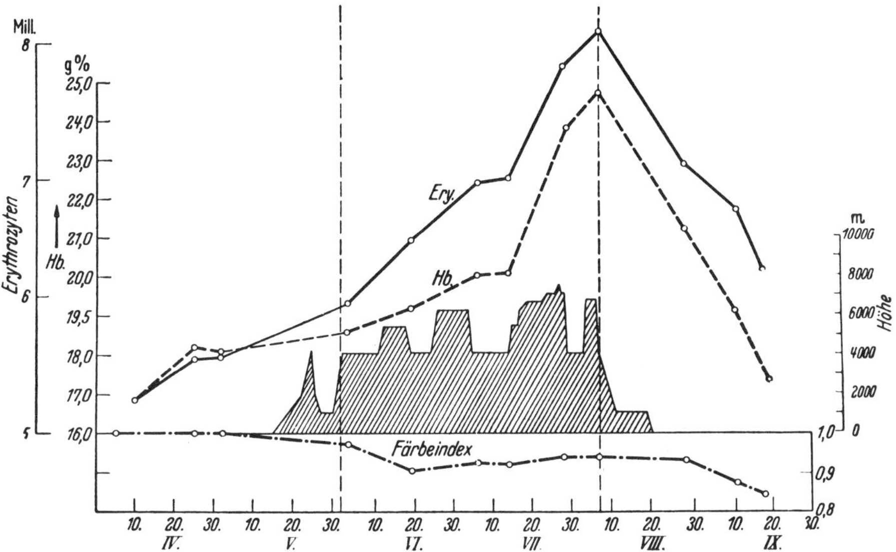

Figure 5. Erythrocyte counts, hemoglobin concentration and Hb/Hct ratio (Färbeindex) in the course of the Nanga Parbat expedition, 1938. Mean values on 5 subjects.
SOURCE: *Hartmann et al., 1942.*

Earlier studies by Hartmann on Kangchenchunga had shown that the resting heart rate was a very sensitive indicator of an individual's state of acclimation at a given altitude. This was borne out in 1937 where heart rates were taken daily in the morning before rising by all members of the expedition (Figure 6). The lower curve in this figure shows average heart rates at rest for 7 climbers of the main expedition from sea level to 6200 ft where the accident happened and the upper curve shows mean values on 3 members of the rescue group who reached the site of the accident within 10 days from sea level, while the others had taken 40 days (Luft, 1941; Hartmann et al., 1942).

Another entirely different aspect of hypoxia that we got involved with in Berlin in the late 30s and during the war was the effect of rapid or explosive decompression during flight at high altitude on gas exchange in the lungs and on subsequent mental performance and consciousness. In a specially designed small compression chamber attached to a larger chamber which acted as a vacuum reservoir, the small chamber could be decompressed to 50,000 ft in 1 to 2 sec by an electrically operated valve. End-tidal samples were collected by the subject into evacuated burettes for analysis on the Haldane Apparatus. Table 1 (Luft et al., 1949) shows gas concentrations in alveolar gas after rapid decompression (RD) from sea level to equivalent altitudes ranging from 16,000 to 50,000 ft. The O_2 values increase from approximately 14% at sea level with altitude and reached that of the inspired air at about 35,000 ft. At higher

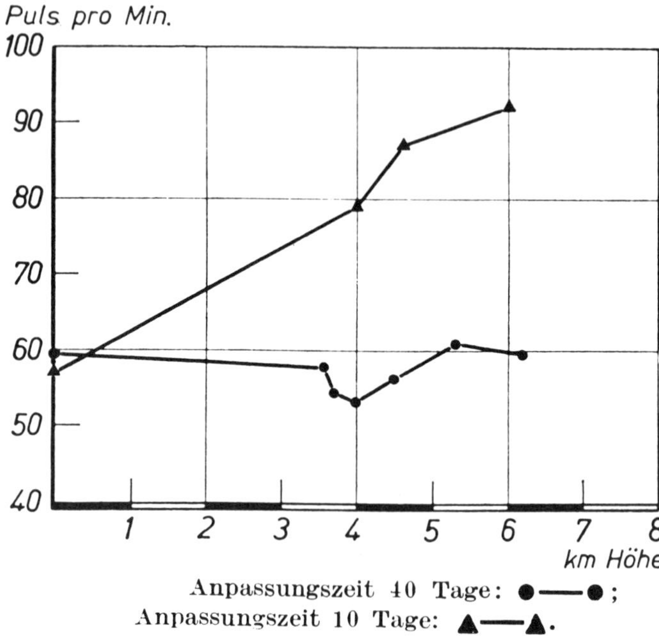

Figure 6. Heart rate at absolute rest, average of 7 climbers who had acclimatized for 40 days on reaching Camp IV (6270 m) (●-●). Upper curve (▲-▲) gives mean values on 3 climbers of the rescue team who reached the same altitude in only 10 days.
SOURCE: *Luft, 1941.*

Table 1. Composition of Alveolar Gas 2 to 5 Sec After Rapid Decompression from Sea Level Breathing Air.

Altitude ft	O_2 %	CO_2 %	N_2 %	P_B Torr
0	14.3	5.6	80.1	760
16,400	13.7	8.9	77.3	405
19,700	14.4	11.1	74.5	354
21,700	14.8	11.8	73.5	325
23,300	15.0	10.8	74.2	309
26,300	15.3	14.8	69.9	267
29,500	15.4	16.4	68.2	231
31,200	16.3	17.7	66.0	214
32,800	19.3	22.3	58.4	199
33,000	19.8	22.0	58.0	197
34,500	20.5	24.2	55.8	184
39,500	23.7	30.7	45.6	144
40,000	23.4	29.1	47.5	141
45,900	24.7	41.6	34.4	106
46,000	26.0	42.0	32.0	106
50,000	27.0	40.3	32.7	87

altitudes, the O_2 concentration was consistently above 21% and reached 27% at 50,000 ft. This strongly suggests that O_2 uptake is nonexistent after RD to 35,000 ft and that at higher altitudes there is a significant influx of O_2 from the mixed venous blood into the alveoli due to the reversal of the PO_2 gradient. It should be remembered that these experiments were performed just a few years after J.S. Haldane, in the last edition (1935) of his classic text "Respiration," still advocated his theory of active secretion of O_2 in the lungs. Rapid decompression offers unique opportunities for studying the effects of a transient anoxic state on body functions by reducing the partial pressure of O_2 instantaneously at the blood-gas interface in the alveoli to levels where O_2 uptake ceases or is even reversed. Furthermore, the duration of the exposure can be controlled precisely by rapid recompression to specific O_2 pressures. Previous observations (Luft et al., 1951) had shown that although loss of consciousness occurs faster with increasing altitude, a minimum time of consciousness of 15 ± 1 (S.D.) sec is reached at 50,000 ft (87 Torr) which remains constant at higher altitudes. The experiments described below involved RD breathing 100% O_2 from a total pressure of 200 Torr, where O_2Hb saturation is still normal, to 68 to 70 Torr in 0.2 sec (Luft and Noell, 1956). A typical recording is shown in Figure 7 where the barograph indicates an exposure to 68 Torr with recompression to 200 Torr in 2 sec. Throughout the

Figure 7. Oscillograph recording during decompression from 200 to 68 Torr in 0.2 sec breathing O_2. Recompression after 12 sec exposure. From top: Barograph, response to audio signal on Morse key, ear opacity, O_2 saturation (Oximeter), and respiration. Subject was unconscious from 14th to 24th sec.

SOURCE: *Luft and Noell, 1956.*

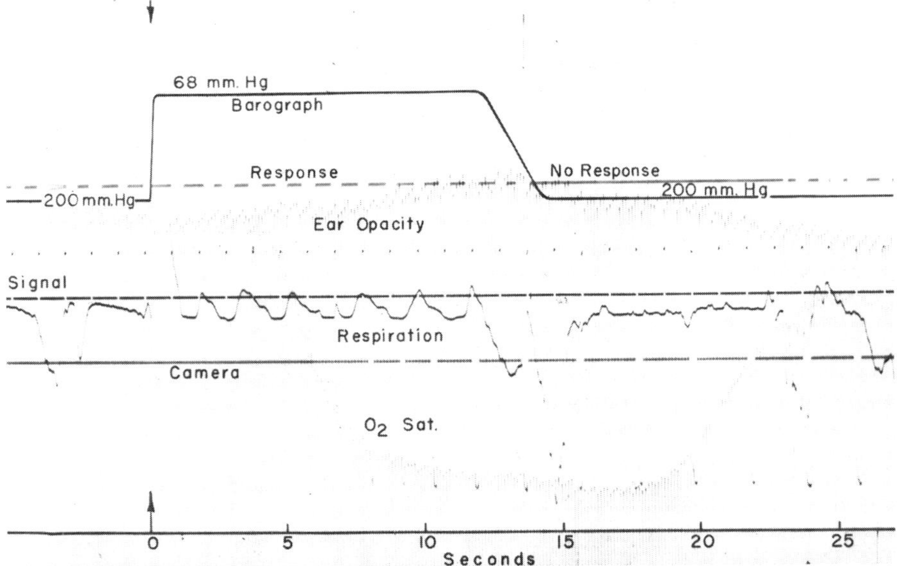

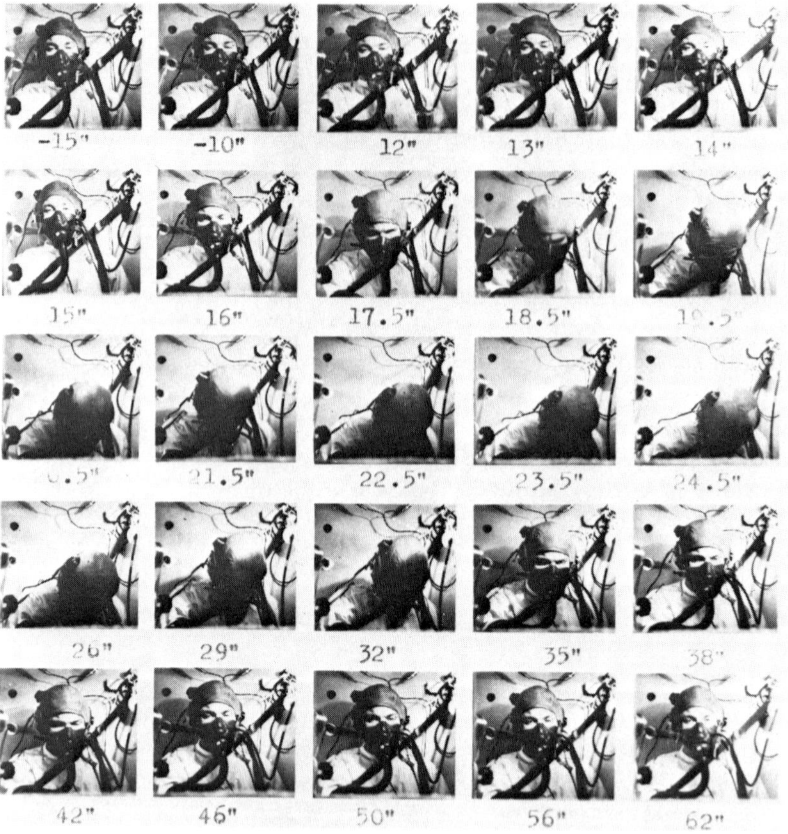

Figure 8. Pictures taken before (−15 sec) and during 18-sec exposure to 68 Torr. Postural failure beginning at 17.5 sec with intermittent upward movements. Gradual recovery from 26 sec to 35 sec. Response to audio signal was absent between 14 sec and 24 sec.

SOURCE: *Luft and Noell, 1956.*

experiment, the subject was required to reply to an audio signal from his earphones by pressing a Morse key. Failure to respond signified onset of unconsciousness. The tracing from the ear-oximeter shows no change for the first 5 sec after RD followed by a precipitous drop during the following 5 sec. Conversely, resaturation did not begin until 5 sec after recompression. This delay is compatible with the lung-to-ear circulation time. Respiration was increased immediately after decompression but was absent during the phase of unconsciousness (9 sec) after recompression. Similar experiments, where the duration of exposure to anoxia was varied between 6 and 18 sec, demonstrated that loss of consciousness occurred in all exposures of more than 6 sec, but not before 14 to 16 sec had elapsed, regardless of the duration of exposure. In the example in Figure 7, unconsciousness occurred at 14 sec, at a time when recompression was nearly complete. Individual frames taken from a continuous movie during an 18-sec exposure are shown in Figure 8. Postural failure is apparent 17 to 18 sec after RD and lasted for 18 sec after recompression, while unconsciousness (no signal) lasted only 10 sec (14 to 24 sec). The time which elapsed between recompression and recovery of cerebral activity increased with the duration of the anoxic exposure. Not clearly visible from the photographs is a staring or a glazed appearance of the eyes which signifies cerebral arrest as in a petit mal seizure. This phase coincided closely with postural failure.

I could give more examples of my adventures in hypoxia, but these may suffice to illustrate the infinite variety of its manifestations and the physiological responses to it. And that is why hypoxia has been the "leitmotiv" in my scientific endeavors over the years.

References

Haldane, J.S. and Priestley, J.G., 1935. *Respiration*. Oxford: Clarendon Press. p. 293.

Hartmann, H., Hepp, G., and Luft, U.C., 1942. Physiologische Beobachtungen am Nanga Parbat 1937/1938. *Luftfahrtmed.* 6:10–44.

Luft, U.C. 1937. Irreversible Organveränderungen durch Hypoxämie im Unterdruck. *Beitr. Pathol. Anat.* 98:323–334.

Luft, U.C. 1938. Das morphologische Bild hypoxämischer Organveränderungen. *Luftfahrtmed.* 2:231–238.

Luft, U.C. 1941. Die Höhenanpassung. *Ergeb. Physiol.* 44:256–314.

Luft, U.C., Clamann, H.G., and Adler, H., 1949. Alveolar gases in rapid decompression to high altitudes. *J. Appl. Physiol.* 2:37–48.

Luft, U.C., Clamann, H.G., and Optiz, E. 1951. The latency of hypoxia on exposure to altitude above 50,000 feet. *J. Aviat. Med.* 22:117–122A.

Luft, U.C. and Noell, W.K., 1956. Manifestations of brief instantaneous anoxia in man. *J. Appl. Physiol.* 8:444–454.

J.A. Loeppky and M.L. Riedesel, editors
OXYGEN TRANSPORT TO HUMAN TISSUES

Oxygen Transport In Aging

D.B. Dill, M.K. Yousef, Aaron Goldman, Terry S. Vitez, Noble S.R. Maluf, Robert Patzer, Lawrence A. Golding, and Al F. McDaniels.

Introduction

I plan to trace the development of methods for measuring aerobic capacity (max $\dot{V}O_2$). Sid Robinson was a pioneer, first in perfecting the method and next in measuring change in max $\dot{V}O_2$ with age. A study of black and white sharecroppers in Mississippi in 1941 revealed equality of these samples of the two races with respect to max $\dot{V}O_2$. This proved crucial to interpretation of later findings on Blacks. Bruno Balke became a celebrity in post-WWII days: During his stay at Brooks AFB, he developed a stepwise method for measuring max $\dot{V}O_2$. On retirement in 1961, Dill joined Robinson for 5 years of research including a comparison of response of max $\dot{V}O_2$ in acute and chronic exposure to equally reduced barometric pressures, "acute" in Robinson's altitude chamber and "chronic" on White Mountain in California. Fifteen years at Boulder City followed. Studies of O_2 transport in a group of Caucasians of both sexes, old and young, in 1979 and a similar study of Blacks in 1980, will be presented.

Measuring Oxygen Consumption in 1925

Measuring the rate of oxygen consumption ($\dot{V}O_2$) was carried out routinely by 1925 in Arlie Bock's laboratory in the Bulfinch Building, Massachusetts General Hospital (MGH). Equipment included a bicycle ergometer, gasometers, Douglas bags, and a portable gas analysis apparatus of the Haldane design. Subjects in exercise experiments were the investigators and Clarence DeMar, the great marathon runner of that day. He won the Boston Marathon 7 times. DeMar enjoyed taking part in Brock's program. He did many steady state rides on the bicycle ergometer during which we estimated cardiac output and made related metabolic measurements. Then he ran around a path in the little park in front of the Bulfinch Building breathing into a Douglas bag that one of the staff carried. The pace was too slow for an aerobic capacity: he used 4.13 liter/min but his run was aerobic since his RQ was 0.89 and his blood lactate elevation only about one mEq/liter. His aerobic $\dot{V}O_2$ was 57.2 ml/min/kg; this was at age 39. Results were reported by Bock et al. in 1928.

Opening the Fatigue Laboratory

Thanks to the concept of L.J. Henderson (LJ) and the backing of Dean David Edsall of the Harvard Medical School and Dean Wallace Donham of the Harvard Business School, funds were obtained in 1926 from the Rockefeller Foundation to equip and underwrite for 10 years a laboratory in the Harvard Business School for expanding research that had been initiated by Bock. Dill was given charge of the research program responsible to LJ and his committee, which included Bock.

The laboratory was opened in the fall of 1927. Based on experience acquired at the MGH, the "Fatigue Laboratory" soon became a stimulating environment for research in exercise physiology for studies on what LJ called "physicochemical properties of blood" and in comparative physiology. Besides bicycle ergometers such as that at the MGH, we borrowed the motor-driven treadmill that had been used years before at the Carnegie Nutrition Laboratory of Boston for physiological studies of level and grade walking. Based on our experiences with it, arrangements were made with a belt-conveyor company in Cambridge to make a rugged treadmill on which men could run at intermediate or high speeds horizontally or on an incline.

Marathoner Clarence DeMar

In his fastest marathon at age 36, DeMar averaged 282 m/min. At age 40 and weight 61.5 kg, he ran on the treadmill for 20 min aerobically; his $\dot{V}O_2$ was 63.7 ml/min/kg. On another occasion at age 49, he ran at 233 m/min on a grade of 8.6% with an apparent RQ of 1.17. His $\dot{V}O_2$ was 58.6 ml/min/kg, clearly his aerobic capacity at 49 yr. In his last marathon at age 66, he averaged 176 m/min, about 6.5 mph. Those findings and an account of his post-mortem have been summarized (Dill, 1965).

Robinson at the Fatigue Laboratory

Robinson was a pioneer at persuading champion runners to run all-out on the treadmill. In 1937 as a fellow in the Fatigue Laboratory, he had an opportunity to work for a Ph.D. He had come from Indiana University where he had held a dual appointment as Assistant Professor of Physiology and assistant track coach. By that time our laboratory had a treadmill with a Reeves drive which permitted a continuous range of speeds and grades. Robinson persuaded several great distance runners competing in the Boston Garden Saturday to come to the laboratory Sunday to run on our treadmill. Don Lash, who had set a record in the indoor two-mile race, agreed. At 360 m/min, his pace in setting his world's record, his max $\dot{V}O_2$ was 81.3 ml/min/kg, at that time a record aerobic capacity (Robinson et al., 1937).

During that year, Robinson completed a study of physiological changes with age, including aerobic capacity, in 93 males ranging in age from 6 to 91 yr. This was accepted as part of the requirement for his Ph.D. and was published in the leading journal of exercise physiology of that day (Robinson, 1938).

Before Robinson returned to Indiana, others in the laboratory joined him in planning a field study of sharecroppers in his home state of Mississippi for the summer of 1939. In June 1939, his treadmill was taken by truck from Bloomington, Indiana to Benoit, Mississippi. Several of us from the Fatigue Laboratory arrived with other laboratory supplies; a laboratory was set up in the high school gymnasium. Robinson was responsible for observations on max $\dot{V}O_2$ on 23 black and 8 white sharecroppers (Robinson et al., 1941). The 23 black sharecroppers had virtually the same max $\dot{V}O_2$ (49.9), as that of the 8 white sharecroppers (49.6 ml/min/kg). Since occupation and environment were the same, it is evident that these samples of the two races were about equal in respect to capacity for supplying oxygen to tissues.

Robinson at Indiana

Robinson's early studies of champion runners became the basis for longitudinal studies of aerobic capacity. These runners were studied again about 25 yr later and again, recently, 43 yr after their competitive careers (Robinson et al., 1976). Decline in max $\dot{V}O_2$ in the former runners was compared with its decline in nonathletes. When young, the runners' mean max $\dot{V}O_2$ was 71.4 compared with 50.6 ml/min/kg in nonathletes. In the recent study, and at comparable ages the value for max $\dot{V}O_2$ had dropped to 46.6 in runners and to 35.5 ml/min/kg in the others. In two of the runners who had been cigarette smokers and who had led sedentary lives, max $\dot{V}O_2$ had dropped below the average for nonathletes of their age.

The Balke Test

Bruno Balke's system was designed to measure $\dot{V}O_2$ as the subject walked at a fixed rate on the treadmill; but with the grade raised a fixed amount each minute. His procedure was well standardized so that he could make a good estimate of max $\dot{V}O_2$ from the duration of the test. The procedure has been in general use since then, sometimes with modifications, but it remains the "Balke Test."

Danish Longitudinal Study

In the period 1925–1930, Asmussen measured max $\dot{V}O_2$ in a large number of Danish physical education students. He did follow-up measurements in 1959 and 1971 of those subjects who were still available. The last paper (Asmussen et al., 1975) summarizes earlier findings. His max $\dot{V}O_2$ expressed as liter/min was estimated from heart rates measured at several submaximal work rates, a common practice in Scandinavia. His mean values for max $\dot{V}O_2$ in 19 males in chronological order for ages 24, 49, and 61 yr and weight 70, 76, and 78 kg, respectively, were 3.5, 2.9, and 2.7 liter/min. Corresponding values for 6 females for ages 24, 51, and 63 yr and weight 60, 62, and 58 kg, respectively, were 3.0, 1.9, and 1.8 liter/min. These men and women learned their lessons well in their days as students of physical education. Their stable body weight and their maintainance of a nearly stable max $\dot{V}O_2$ for 12 years after age 50 is remarkable.

Five Years at Indiana University

Dill had the good fortune to spend the period 1961–66 as a research scholar at Indiana University with Robinson. During that period, four of us made use of the altitude chamber in the newly-completed environmental room. Aerobic capacity was measured at ambient barometric pressure and barometric pressures equal to those of three laboratories of the White Mountain Research Station at 535, 484, and 455 Torr. Each of us did three Balke tests at each pressure in random order. This study of acute exposure to altitude formed the basis for a study of chronic exposure to altitude carried out on White Mountain in 1966. The decrease in max $\dot{V}O_2$ was significantly greater in the chronic exposure which is still unexplained (Dill et al., 1967).

Boulder City—1966 to Present

Fifteen happy and productive years of research in environmental, exercise, and comparative physiology in Boulder City, Nevada followed. Aerobic capacity measurements were done on the Monark bicycle ergometer until 1972 when a Quinton treadmill was acquired. Research on physiological changes with aging man resumed during this period.

In 1977, Dill with Yousef as co-investigator submitted the proposal to the National Institute on Aging (NIOA) for a comparative study of three racial groups, Caucasions, Blacks, and Chicanos. In that summer, observations were made of thermoregulation, sweat rate, and composition of sweat in aerobic walks in desert heat. Correlated measurements were made of body fat and aerobic capacity. The subjects were 7 male and 4 female laboratory assistants all of whom were superior in scholarship and in athletics. That study served as a pattern for the NIOA study. In final form, the proposal called for a physician supervising measurement of aerobic capacity with the volunteer riding a bicycle ergometer.

Whites and Blacks: Max $\dot{V}O_2$

During the summer of 1979, the study began. Fifty-eight men and women volunteered, many of whom had been members of jogging classes in previous years sponsored by the University's Continuing Education Department. The first measurement was aerobic capacity. Those who were judged fit by the physician did three 1-hr desert walks with ambient temperature up to or above 40° C. Based on previous findings on youths, the rate of walking was adjusted to require about 40% of aerobic capacity. Body fat was determined by the K-40 method. Some of the findings will be presented here together with findings on Blacks in 1980.

There was an important difference in backgrounds of the two groups. Many of the Whites had maintained exercise programs after their participation in jogging classes. Only a minority of the Blacks were committed to any exercise. Many did participate in a jogging program in the spring of 1980 prior to our study. During the summer, 48 completed the three walks, 19 men ages 17 to 61 years and 29 women ages 16 to 56 yr.

Results

Values for percentage of body fat for male and female Blacks and Whites are given in Table 1. There were no significant differences between these samples of the two races.

Measurements of max $\dot{V}O_2$ for Blacks are presented (Figure 1). These indicate the decline in max $\dot{V}O_2$ with age. The dimensions of each rectangle correspond to S.D. for age on the horizontal axis and S.D. for max $\dot{V}O_2$ on the vertical axis. In Figure 2, mean values for Whites are shown in the center of the rectangles by hollow squares. Solid triangles in Figure 2 correspond to mean values for max $\dot{V}O_2$ of Blacks (Figure 1).

Discussion

The basis for measuring aerobic capacity was laid in Bock's laboratory in Boston. All necessary equipment was on hand and techniques had been perfected when Dill arrived in 1925. Observations were made on DeMar the marathoner in aerobic rides on the bicycle ergometer and in a run. The Fatigue Laboratory was opened in 1927. It was ten years before Robinson arrived and directed our attention to all-out exercise. He was the senior author of the first paper from the Fatigue Laboratory dealing primarily with aerobic capacity (Robinson et al., 1937). He used a combination of speed and grade that brought the subject to his endpoint in 5 to 10 min. The criterion for the subject having attained his limiting $\dot{V}O_2$ was apparent with RQ values well above unity and an elevation of blood lactate 5 to 10 times above resting. These criteria proved less reliable in old age where the capacity for such increases in RQ and in lactate are lost.

Table 1. Body Fat, Age and Max $\dot{V}O_2$ in Whites and Blacks.

Group		Whites	Blacks	Difference in max $\dot{V}O_2$
	n	32	6	
< 30 yr	Age	18.1 ± 1.4	20.5 ± 3.9	Whites > Blacks
Male	Fat	12.6 ± 6.1	17.6 ± 9.1	$p < 0.005$
	n	26	11	
< 30 yr	Age	17.4 ± 1.2	20.7 ± 4.6	Whites > Blacks
Female	Fat	25.1 ± 6.3	21.3 ± 11.9	$p < 0.001$
	n	9	14	
30–39 yr	Age	36.1 ± 2.1	33.4 ± 2.9	Whites > Blacks
Male	Fat	28.6 ± 9.0	26.7 ± 9.6	$p < 0.2$ (NS)
	n	12	9	
30–39	Age	34.1 ± 3.7	33.8 ± 3.0	Whites > Blacks
Female	Fat	37.5 ± 9.2	37.5 ± 6.9	$p < 0.2$ (NS)
	n	4	10	
40–49 yr	Age	42.8 ± 1.0	44.5 ± 2.9	Whites > Blacks
Female	Fat	38.0 ± 6.7	42.1 ± 14.1	$p < 0.001$

NOTE: Mean values ± S.D. are shown for age (yr) and Fat (percent of body weight). Differences for max $\dot{V}O_2$ can be seen in Figure 2.

One is required by the Institutional Committee on Human Safety to explain all details of the plan and emphasize to the subject that he can stop at any time. This is an onerous task if the investigator has been a track coach accustomed to urging the runner to "Keep going, don't quit!"

That constraint and authorities' concern about possible accidents led to the decision to utilize in recent studies the bicycle ergometer for aerobic capacity following the Balke practice of stepwise increase in load. Studies by Taguchi et al. (1974) indicate aerobic capacity of men is significantly less (over 8%) on the ergometer than on the treadmill. There was a mean difference of 3% in the same direction in women, but it was not significant. The differences in the case of the men, however, should be taken into account when comparing values for max $\dot{V}O_2$ with findings on the treadmill.

Table 1 shows that there was little if any difference in percentage of body fat between groups of Blacks and Whites that were studied.

In the case of max $\dot{V}O_2$, there were highly significant differences among some groups of Blacks and Whites of the same sex and age range based on the t-test, those of the Whites always exceeding Blacks' (Table 1).

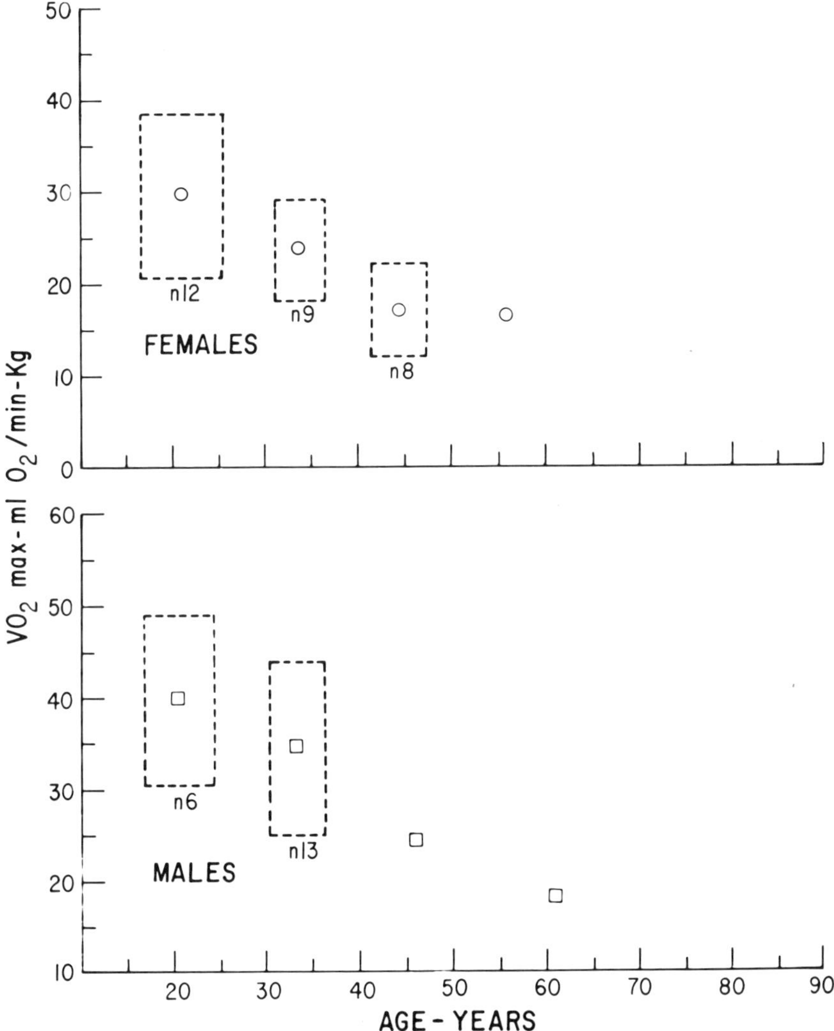

Figure 1. Aerobic capacity vs age in Blacks. Aerobic capacity (max $\dot{V}O_2$) was determined on the bicycle ergometer. Means are indicated by open symbols in the center of the rectangle. S.D.s are indicated by length and width of rectangles. Open symbols outside the rectangles are individual values.

The early study of max $\dot{V}O_2$ of black and white sharecroppers had shown equality of max $\dot{V}O_2$. Those two groups were comparable in economic status, in environment, and in occupation. Hence, it is reasonable to conclude that the difference in max $\dot{V}O_2$ observed between the Whites of 1979 and the Blacks of 1980 depends on differences in living habits. It may be that the participation

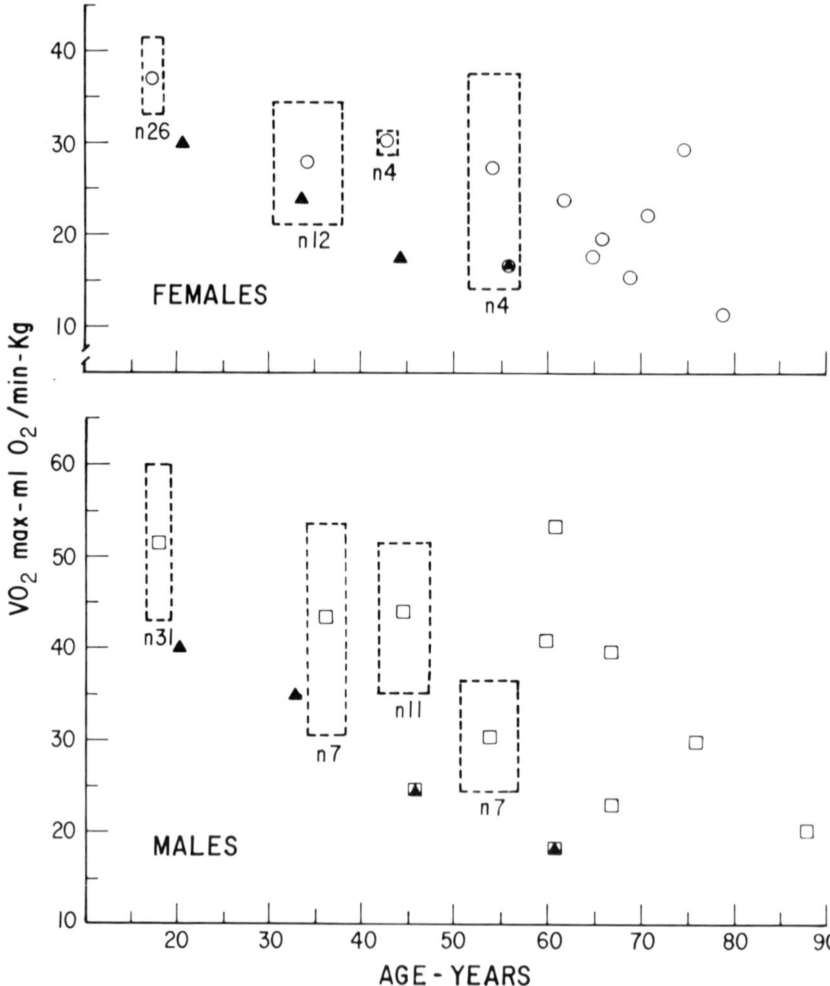

Figure 2. Aerobic capacity vs age, Blacks, and Whites. Aerobic capacity (max $\dot{V}O_2$) was determined on the bicycle ergometer. The rectangles show means and S.D.s for groups of Whites; open symbols in the older age range are individual values for Whites. Solid triangles are mean values for groups of Blacks; they correspond to the open symbols in the rectangles of Figure 1. Solid triangles in closed squares are individual values for Blacks.

by many of the Whites in organized jogging classes and their continued regular exercise slowed down the decline in max $\dot{V}O_2$ with age. This certainly was true of several of the white males and one female who competed in long distance races.

ACKNOWLEDGMENTS
We acknowledge the support of the National Institute on Aging, Grant AG00037-08. We are indebted to Scott Martin for valuable statistical assistance and to the following skilled laboratory assistants who played essential roles: Robert Tucker and Chris Barton, Darnell Frazier, Valerie Gaines, Nancy Gronfeldt, and Kim Fiero.

References

Asmussen, E., Fruensgaard, K., and Norgaard, S. 1975. A follow-up longitudinal study of selected physiological functions in former physical education students—after forty years. *J. Am. Geriatr. Soc.* 23:442–480.

Bock, A.V., van Caulaert, C., Dill, D.B., Folling, A., and Hurxthal, L.M., 1928. Studies in muscular activity. Dynamical changes occurring in man at work. *J. Physiol.* (*London*). 66:136–161.

Dill, D.B. 1965. Marathoner DeMar: physiological studies. *J. Natl. Cancer Inst.* 35:185–191.

Dill, D.B., Myhre, L.G., Brown, D.K., Burrus, K., and Gehlsen, G., 1967. Work capacity in chronic exposures to altitude. *J. Appl. Physiol.* 23:555–560.

Robinson, S. 1938. Experimental studies of physical fitness in relation to age. *Arbeitsphysiol.* 10:251–323.

Robinson, S., Dill, D.B., Harmon, P.M., Hall, F.G., and Wilson, J.W., 1941. Adaptations to exercise of negro and white sharecroppers in comparison with northern Whites. *Hum. Biol.* 13:139–158.

Robinson, S., Dill, D.B., Robinson, R.D., Tzankoff, S.P., and Wagner, J.A., 1976. Physiological aging of champion runners. *J. Appl. Physiol.* 41:46–51.

Robinson, S., Edwards, H.T., and Dill, D.B., 1937. New records in human power. *Science* 85:409–410.

Taguchi, S., Raven, P.B., Drinkwater, B.L., Kaneko, M., and Katusi, H., 1974. Comparative physiological response to a bicycle ergometer and a treadmill walking maximum capacity test. *J. Hum. Ergol.* (*Tokyo*) 3:67–74.

SECTION II:

Alveolar-Capillary Gas Equilibration

J.A. Loeppky and M.L. Riedesel, editors
OXYGEN TRANSPORT TO HUMAN TISSUES

Dilution Methods for Measurement of Cardiac Output: A Review

Leon E. Farhi

Because the function of the circulatory system is to supply adequate tissue blood flow, the cardiac output is obviously one of the major indices of that system's performance. It is not surprising, therefore, that a great number of investigators should have devoted considerable effort to devise and perfect methods for determining this variable; the purpose of this article is to review recent progress in this field. In order to allow the reader to evaluate these developments in their proper context, they will be presented in the framework of a general description of dilution methods. It is fortunate that three scholarly reviews (Hamilton, 1962; Guyton, 1963; Butler, 1965) which are as important today as when they were published provide both a thorough description of essential classical methods and a complete survey of the literature unnecessary.

Cardiac output can be directly measured only by temporarily diverting the blood flow into a container where the amount of blood accumulated per unit time can be determined. Consequently, all methods of measurement used routinely for clinical or research purposes are necessarily indirect. Some of these rely on the positioning of flowmeter probes around vessels and are therefore applicable to human study only under extremely rare surgical conditions. Other methods of measurement like those based on pulse pressure studies, yield results of questionable accuracy and still others like those derived from measurements of the heart chambers using angiocinefluorography are too complex for routine use. Because all these methods are well-discussed in both Hamilton's comprehensive review (1962) and Guyton's book (1963) they will not be considered any further. An interesting technique with great potential has recently been described by Loeppky et al. (1981). Some of its features are discussed in this book by E.R. Greene. In this presentation, we will concentrate on the dilution techniques with which the vast majority of data in the literature have been obtained.

The basic principle on which these methods are based was clearly and succinctly presented by Adolph Fick nearly a century ago (1870). If a substance X is injected at a rate $\dot{V}$ into the blood flowing at a rate $\dot{Q}$, the concentration of X beyond the point of injection, C, must be equal to $\dot{V}/\dot{Q}$. When considering addition of a substance already present in the blood stream, the *difference* between C_1, the concentration of X upstream of the injection point and C_2, the downstream concentration, is equal to $\dot{V}/\dot{Q}$. Obviously, this relationship also pertains if X is withdrawn rather than added, a condition in which C_1 is larger than C_2 and $\dot{V}$ is negative. In either case, the blood flow can be calculated from:

$$\dot{Q}=\frac{\dot{V}}{C_2-C_1} \tag{5.1}$$

This basic relationship (which can be applied to any individual vascular bed) may be used to measure total cardiac output provided that X is distributed uniformly into the total blood flow. It is notable that when dealing with any unsteady state, as is the case in single injection techniques, the equation is still valid at any one instant and the time integral may be used to calculate flow. All the dilution methods used in the clinic rely on Fick's basic approach and differ only in the nature of X (which can be a gas, a dye, a radioactive tracer, or even a physical characteristic such as temperature or electrical conductivity) and consequently in the methods for determining C_2 and C_1. Table 1 lists various dilution methods and supplies information on the nature of the tracer and site of sampling.

Methods Requiring Cardiac Catheterization and/or Arterial Puncture

"Direct Fick"

The dilution equation set by Fick lay untested for nearly 20 years, until first used by Grehant and Quinquaud (1886). At the turn of the century, Zuntz and Hagemann (1898) used this approach on resting and exercising horses, another 30 years elapsing before the first self-catheterization by Forssmann (1929) was introduced to the modern era. In the "direct Fick" technique, oxygen is usually the tracer gas, with the O_2 uptake from the alveolar gas representing $\dot{V}$, and the O_2 concentration in pulmonary arterial and pulmonary venous blood giving C_1 and C_2, respectively. It is noteworthy that Zuntz and Hagemann had already recognized the pitfall created by the difference in O_2 content of blood returning from the various organs, and indicated that a mixing chamber, the right heart, was required. Similarly, the value corresponding to C_2 can be determined only after the contents of the four main pulmonary veins have been mixed in the left heart, which acts as a second mixing chamber. Because these safeguards are incorporated in the direct Fick technique, it is still widely used as the standard against which new approaches are tested.

Dye-Dilution Techniques

In this method, a dye is infused into a peripheral vein at a known rate and allowed to mix into the cardiac output in the right ventricle. The changing arterial concentration yields C_2 and $\dot{V}$ is the rate of dye infusion. Before recirculation occurs, C_1 should remain zero. Unfortunately, it is seldom if ever possible to obtain a dye plateau before recirculation takes place (Hamilton, 1962).

One can also inject a single slug of dye in a peripheral vein, and follow changes in dye concentration by continuous sampling, giving C_2. The value of $\dot{V}$ is related to the amount of dye injected and C_1 is measured by withdrawing an aliquot of blood (into which dye from previous injections is now uniformly diluted) from either the arterial cannula or the vein used for injection. In the single injection technique, as with continuous infusion, recirculation occurs before the measurements are completed and appropriate corrections must be introduced.

Injection of Poorly Soluble Inert Gases

This approach has been described by Rochester and coworkers (1961), Cornell, Braunwald, and Brochenbrough (1961) and by Klocke and associates (1968), who injected krypton and hydrogen, respectively, in a systemic vein. As in the case of dye, $\dot{V}$ is obtained from the volume of solution injected. Here the right heart serves as a mixing chamber, and C_2 is obtained by sampling blood from the pulmonary artery. The advantage of this approach resides in the fact that gases of low solubility are practically eliminated completely in the lung. The small amount retained and recirculated (which gives C_1) can be measured in systemic arterial blood, or a small correction factor may be substituted. It is possible to infuse the solution continuously, or to simulate the single injection of the dye-dilution technique.

Thermodilution Methods

The dilution principle has been applied to conditions where heat is the tracer ($\dot{V}$) and downstream blood temperature (C_2) is monitored. Both a steady state technique with introduction of heat in the pulmonary artery and measurement of blood temperature downstream (Fronek and Ganz, 1960) and single injection in the pulmonary artery, with measurement of temperature in the aorta (Fegler, 1954), have been described. Although blood temperature is measured in situ and no samples are required, right heart catheterization is necessary.

Table 1. Dilution Methods for Determining Blood Flow.

	Nature and site of measurement of variables		
Method	$\dot{V}$	C_2	C_1
Steady state direct Fick			
O_2	O_2 uptake, measured at mouth	O_2 content, systemic arterial blood	O_2 content pulmonary arterial blood
CO_2	CO_2 output, measured at mouth	CO_2 content, systemic arterial blood	CO_2 content, pulmonary arterial blood
Non-volatile tracers (dye, PAH, etc.)	Rate of infusion of tracer in systemic vein	Concentration of tracer past the right ventricle, which acts as a mixing chamber	Assumed equal to zero *or* concentration of tracer in systemic artery after abrupt cessation of infusion *or* calculated from arterial concentration vs time curve
Gases of low solubility	Rate of infusion, systemic vein	Concentration, pulmonary artery	Concentration, systemic artery *or* calculated
Thermodilution	Heat supplied to blood by catheter in pulmonary artery	Blood temp. in pulmonary artery beyond point of heating, measured by thermistor on catheter	Blood temp. before heat is supplied
Non-steady state methods requiring blood analysis			
Dyes and non-volatile tracers	From amount injected in systemic vein	From changing concentration in systemic artery	Level in blood before injection
Gases of low solubility	From amount injected in systemic vein	From changing concentration in pulmonary artery	Essentially zero

Thermodilution	From volume and temp. of liquid injected in pulmonary artery	Changing temp. in aorta	Aortic temp. after equilibration
"Indirect Fick", O_2 or CO_2			
One-step methods	O_2 uptake or CO_2 output, lungs	Arterial O_2 or CO_2 content, calculated from blood dissociation curve and alveolar gas tensions	Mixed venous O_2 or CO_2 content from blood dissociation curves and gas tensions in occluded alveoli
Two-step methods: Equilibrium techniques	O_2 uptake or CO_2 output, lungs (step 1)	Arterial O_2 or CO_2 content, calculated from blood dissociation curve and alveolar gas tensions (step 1)	Mixed venous O_2 or CO_2 content from blood dissociation curves and alveolar gas tensions after breath-holding or rebreathing (step 2)
Rate of change techniques	O_2 uptake or CO_2 output, lungs (step 1)	Arterial O_2 or CO_2 content, calculated from blood dissociation curve and alveolar gas tensions (step 1)	Mixed venous O_2 or CO_2 content from blood dissociation curve and alveolar gas tension calculated by interpolation or extrapolation (step 2)
Inert gas methods			
Uptake: Unsteady state	Inert gas uptake, at mouth	Arterial inert gas content calculated from solubility and alveolar tension	Assumed to be zero
Steady state	Inert gas uptake, at mouth	Arterial inert gas content calculated from solubility and alveolar tension	Mixed venous content, calculated from solubility and mixed venous tension, estimated in a second step
Infusion of very soluble gases	Rate of infusion, systemic vein	Mixed venous inert gas content, calculated from solubility and alveolar tensions during rebreathing	Estimated from rate of rise of alveolar tension during rebreathing

"Noninvasive Techniques"

A didactic presentation must start with the description of the basic direct Fick methods, in which all necessary variables are measured, and lead to the noninvasive methods, where some of the variables are assessed indirectly or assumed. In fact, because adequate methods for catheterization and blood analysis were not available initially, some indirect methods were developed and used long before the direct techniques.

Methods Based on O_2 and CO_2 Exchange

The fact that Fick's original concept was enunciated in terms of the lung oxygen uptake and carbon dioxide output probably explains the numerous attempts to indirectly assess the arterial and venous O_2 and CO_2 values required for the calculations. In nearly all cases, this is done by measuring alveolar gas tensions under conditions where this gas reflects the composition of the blood either entering or leaving the lung.

Use of the same organ to sample both C_1 and C_2 is made possible by either of two procedures. In the first, the lung is physically divided, so that some respiratory elements reflect arterial blood while others mirror mixed venous blood. In the second, the two measurements are taken in succession, resulting in a 2-step technique.

The divided lung was first described in 1871 by Wolfberg who isolated part of a dog's lung and allowed it to reach equilibrium with the mixed venous blood perfusing it. Gas tensions in the remainder of the lung allowed the investigator to determine arterial gas values. Forty years later, Loewy and Von Schrotter (1903) were able to apply this method to humans. Although the "aeronometer" has the advantage of allowing simultaneous measurement of arterial and venous blood, catheterization of a lobe or segment of the lung is by no means an easy procedure, especially in man, and most methods separate measurement of C_1 and C_2 in time rather than spatially.

In these 2-step methods, gas exchange and arterial gas composition are usually measured first. In a second step, gas exchange is interrupted, the total lung volume is allowed to equilibrate with mixed venous blood and C_1 is determined. Normally, $P\bar{v}CO_2$ is about 10 Torr higher than $PaCO_2$. This means that in order to bring alveolar PCO_2 to the level of mixed venous blood, approximately 10 ml of CO_2 will have to be added (from the circulation or from a rebreathing bag) to each liter of alveolar gas. Since the corresponding oxygen tension difference is six times higher (which means that re-equilibration can be expected to occur sooner for CO_2 than for O_2), most indirect methods have dealt with carbon dioxide.

However, even with this gas, equilibration is not rapid enough to obtain mixed venous-alveolar equilibrium by simple breath-holding before the mixed venous blood composition starts to change. In fact, it has been stated (Richards and Strauss, 1930) that equilibrium may occur prior to recirculation only if the initial composition of the alveolar gas is artifically readjusted so that PCO_2 is less than 2mm Hg removed from $P\bar{v}CO_2$.

Haldane's group (Christiansen et al., 1914) must be credited with being the first to use CO_2 equilibration on a large scale. Their subjects performed several breath-holding maneuvers, the initial CO_2 content of the lung being varied between experiments. The equilibrium $P\bar{v}CO_2$ value must lie between that of the highest alveolar gas composition at which PCO_2 increases during breath-holding and that of the lowest alveolar PCO_2 which decreases during breath-holding. Collier (1956) adapted this method to modern day technology by monitoring continuously, with an infrared CO_2 analyzer, the carbon dioxide fraction at the mouth of rebreathing subjects.

An ingenious method for starting with an initial alveolar CO_2 in near equilibrium with mixed venous PCO_2 uses the subject to "prepare" his own breathing mixture by prebreathing in a bag. A rest period allows the mixed venous blood composition to return to its previous value, after which there is a second rebreathing period. This is essentially what Richards and Strauss (1930) did, and later the widely used technique of Campbell and Howell (1960) emphasized the same approach.

In all these methods, hypoxia is avoided by keeping adequately high O_2 tension in the lung (in case of breath-holding) or in the rebreathing bag. Therefore, the equilibrium value obtained is not "true" venous PCO_2 but rather "oxygenated" venous PCO_2.

O_2 Equilibration Methods

As indicated above, the considerable difference between alveolar and mixed venous O_2 has not encouraged the development of methods for obtaining $P\bar{v}O_2$ from alveolar gas composition. Nevertheless, this approach has been tried, notably by Plesch (1909) and later by Burwell and Robinson (1924). In both cases, subjects rebreathed a low O_2 mixture until equilibrium was achieved. Because the O_2 dissociation curve has a lower slope than the CO_2 dissociation curve, it is more easily affected by recirculation, and the O_2 plateau is of rather short duration. Thus, former investigators, lacking the current methods for rapid O_2 analysis, could easily miss the fleeting O_2 equilibrium.

The advent of the respiratory mass spectrometer which allows continuous monitoring of respiratory gases allowed Cerretelli and coworkers (1966a) to develop a rapid maneuver. A bag containing approximately 7 or 8% CO_2 in N_2 is prepared and the subject, having expired to residual volume, rebreathes from the bag while the gas tensions at the mouth are monitored continuously. If the bag volume is properly selected, after 2 or 3 breaths a plateau is found for both O_2 and CO_2. Note that in this case, the CO_2 value obtained corresponds to true venous CO_2 because blood passing though the lungs is no longer gaining oxygen. Mass spectrometers are expensive, cumbersome, and not entirely trouble free. It is fortunate therefore that the method or Cerretelli et al. (1966a) could be adapted to other instrumentation. Introduction of minor modifications into standard laboratory O_2 electrodes has been shown to increase the response speed to the point where they can be used to measure the level of the O_2 plateau (Farhi et al., 1966). Although doubts have been expressed about the validity of the CO_2 level during rebreathing (Gurtner et al., 1967), mixed venous O_2 and the O_2 obtained by application of the Cerretelli method seem to be in agreement.

Methods Based on Rate of Change of Alveolar Gas Composition

It has been suggested that even with an initial bag PCO_2 approximating $P\bar{v}CO_2$, the time required for adequate mixing of alveolar and bag contents approaches or exceeds the time available before recirculation occurs, and consequently the CO_2 tension at which the alveolar gas stabilizes may not indicate the $P\bar{v}CO_2$ that prevailed before the rebreathing maneuver. It is also extremely difficult to distinguish between a true plateau and a gentle ascending slope due to recirculation. This lends interest to methods where the mixed venous CO_2 is calculated from *the rate* of change of PCO_2 during expiration, breathholding, or rebreathing. All these techniques are based on the linear relationship between the CO_2 movement across the alveolar wall and the driving pressure responsible for this transfer.

At constant lung volume, the rate of change of $PaCO_2$ will be proportional to the CO_2 movement and therefore to ($P\bar{v}CO_2 - PaCO_2$). The exponential equation describing this relationship was first published by DuBois, Fenn, and Britt (1952) and Defares (1958) later used the rate of change to calculate $P\bar{v}CO_2$.

Knowles, Newman, and Fenn (1960) had their subjects perform standardized breath-holding maneuvers. The initial PCO_2 was varied by changing the composition of the gas inspired before breath-holding. At the end of the breathhold, PCO_2 was determined again. The CO_2 output was estimated by the change in PCO_2 and was plotted against the initial PCO_2. The interpolated value, at which there would be no change in PCO_2 must represent $P\bar{v}CO_2$.

Although the technique described by Fenn and Dejours (1954) is also based on the relationship between $PaCO_2$ and $\dot{V}CO_2$, these variables are assessed in an entirely different fashion. The $PaCO_2$ is varied by altering breath-holding time rather than inspired gas composition. As long as the oxygen tension in the alveoli remains adequate, the oxygen uptake is constant, and changes in $\dot{V}CO_2$ are reflected by proportional changes in R, the gas exchange ratio, the variable actually measured in this experiment. By plotting $PaCO_2$ versus R, one obtains a straight line, and extrapolation to $R=0$ determines the alveolar tension at which $P\bar{v}CO_2 - PaCO_2$ would be zero.

The method of Kim, Rahn, and Farhi (1963) is essentially a contraction of the technique of Fenn and Dejours to a single breath. During a very slow expiration, several aliquots are collected and analyzed, and each is then treated as if it represented one of the values obtained with the multiple breath technique. Implicit in this technique is the assumption (validated by Sikand,

Cerretelli, and Farhi in 1966 for normal upright man) that the changes during expiration are due to a difference in the time spent by the gas in the lungs and not to sequential emptying of elements having different patterns of gas exchange.

In addition to the substantial advantage resulting from continuous sampling during *one* expiration, an additional bonus is the determination of true venous $P\bar{v}CO_2$. This is based on an old observation by Haldane that the O_2-CO_2 interaction on the hemoglobin molecule is such that deoxygenation of hemoglobin allows it to load an additional amount of carbon dioxide without changing PCO_2, the ratio between the CO_2 added and the oxygen removed being 0.32. Kim et al. (1963) reasoned therefore that when the instantaneous alveolar gas exchange ratio is 0.32, the alveolar PCO_2 must be equal to the true venous value.

Cerretelli, Sikand, and Farhi (1966b) were able to perfect the Kim technique by using a mass spectrometer, sampling continuously from the mouth during expiration. They found that during exercise the changes in alveolar PCO_2 were rapid enough to allow them to use the method without resorting to an artificial prolongation of expiration. Although this appears at first glance to be only a technical improvement, it does represent a major advance in the sense that all three values required for determining cardiac output could now be obtained from a single breath.

A single step technique has been reported from the same laboratory (Farhi et al., 1976). At the end of a normal expiration, the subject is asked to rebreathe in and out of a bag, containing initially a CO-free mixture for 15 to 25 sec. Tidal volume and frequency during the rebreathing maneuver are selected so as to provide a slight hyperventilation; as a consequence, alveolar PCO_2 drops initially and then rises asymptotically toward its equilibrium value. All the values necessary for calculating the pulmonary blood flow are obtained from bag volume and from the CO_2 fraction at the mouth at different times. The method is of interest not only because it is simple and convenient, but also because it overcomes certain nagging problems, such as those caused by the ability of lung tissue to store CO_2 as PCO_2 increases. The technique has been validated and applied to problems such as the readjustment in cardiovascular variables during water immersion (Farhi and Linnarsson, 1977) or following changes in posture (Matalon and Farhi, 1979).

Methods Based on Uptake of Soluble Inert Gases

The first method based on this principle was suggested by Markoff, Muller, and Zuntz (1911). The principle is that large quantities of soluble gas can be taken up via the lungs before the body stores become equilibrated. Thus, it would be easy to measure $\dot{V}$ during the initial stages of breathing a mixture containing such a gas; acetylene and nitrous oxide have received the attention of most investigators. The assumption that end-capillary blood and alveolar gas are in equilibrium makes it possible to determine C_2 indirectly by sampling alveolar gas. In most methods (a notable exception being the steady state technique of Becklake et al., 1962), C_1 has been assumed to remain zero because the measurements are made before recirculation takes place. The problems of this assumption have been underlined by both Hamilton (1962) and Butler (1965).

It is not the object of this paper to discuss in detail established methods but it may be useful to point out that they fall into two categories. In the first, gas uptake is measured during steady state conditions with the subject breathing through an open circuit. In this case, the alveolar-capillary equilibrium level will depend on the ratio of ventilation to perfusion ($\dot{V}A/\dot{Q}$) of the elements in which the exchange takes place. The better ventilated elements (where the partial pressure of the inspired inert gas remains high) contribute proportionally more to ventilation than to perfusion, while the opposite is true for the better perfused alveoli. Consequently, the mixed alveolar gas tension will be higher than the arterial value it is supposed to mirror. In the normal erect resting man, a 10% difference can be calculated, resulting in a similar error in measured cardiac output, and this difference may be so much greater in patients and in certain experimental conditions as to limit the usefulness of the technique.

This pitfall is avoided in the second category of methods where uptake is measured during rebreathing from a bag containing initially a measurable fraction of the inert gas. Since rebreathing tends to create a homogeneous alveolar gas composition, the effects of uneven $\dot{V}A/\dot{Q}$ distribution are eliminated. However, a new problem is generated by this technique, namely that as the inert gas tension in the system decreases during uptake, a similar change takes place in the lung parenchyma, which now releases some of the gas that had been dissolved. Thus, the total volume of exchange is not limited to the gas phase, but includes an unknown tissue component. Thus, judicious analysis of the data supplies information on additional aspects of cardiopulmonary function. The technique has been refined to the point where it can be used to measure pulmonary blood flow, FRC, lung tissue volume, and diffusing capacity (Sackner et al., 1975).

Enormous strides in knowledge have been made on the basis of inert gas uptake studies, and it is noteworthy that the very elegant demonstration by Lee and DuBois (1955) of the pulsatile nature of pulmonary capillary blood flow was obtained by studying the N_2O uptake.

Possible Sources of Error in Noninvasive Methods

Since the pitfalls of these methods have been reviewed some time ago (Farhi and Haab 1967), they will be presented here only very briefly. Measurement of $\dot{V}$ is usually no different in direct or indirect methods and necessitates either a comparison of inspired and expired gas or, as is the case in the infusion or injection techniques, knowledge of the amount of tracer that is added to the system.

All the indirect methods require caution because the blood gas content is obtained by measuring an alveolar tension. To obtain the blood content, one must first assume partial pressure equilibrium between gas and blood, and then convert partial pressure into blood gas content. We have already alluded to the danger of assuming alveolar-arterial pressure equilibrium in the methods based on steady state uptake of soluble inert gases. This is, of course, not unique to these methods but pertains to any technique in which differences in ventilation-perfusion ratios cause an inhomogeneous alveolar gas composition. In order to go from pressure to content, it is necessary to know the solubility exactly (if one deals with an inert gas) or the shape of the dissociation curve, if either O_2 or CO_2 is considered. It is because of the variability and alinearity in the dissociation curves that the indirect methods are always regarded with suspicion. Farhi and Haab (1967) have, however, pointed out that although the calculated cardiac output may be in error, the indirect O_2 and CO_2 methods give a good estimate of mixed venous tensions, which is precisely the factor that circulation regulates.

References

Becklake, M.R., Vavis, C.J., Pengelly, L.D., Kenning, S., McGregor, M., and Bates, D.V. 1962. Measurement of pulmonary blood flow during exercise using nitrous oxide. *J. Appl. Physiol.* 17:579–586.

Burwell, C.S. and Robinson, G.C. 1924. A method for the determination of the amount of oxygen and carbon dioxide in the mixed venous blood of man. *J. Clin. Invest.* 1:47–63.

Butler, J. 1965. Measurement of cardiac output using soluble gases. In *Handbook of Physiology, Sec. 3: Respiration, Vol. II.* Fenn, W.O. and Rahn, H., eds., Washington, D.C.: Am. Physiol. Soc. pp. 1489–1503.

Campbell, E.J. and Howell, J.B. 1960. Simple rapid methods of estimating arterial and mixed venous PCO_2. *Brit. Med. J.* 1:458–462.

Cerretelli, P., Cruz, J.C., Farhi, L.E., and Rahn, H. 1966a. Determination of mixed venous O_2 and CO_2 tensions and cardiac output by a rebreathing method. *Respir. Physiol.* 1:258–264.

Cerretelli, P., Sikand, R., and Farhi, L.E. 1966b. Readjustments in cardiac output and gas exchange during onset of exercise and recovery. *J. Appl. Physiol.* 21:1345–1350.

Christiansen, J., Douglas, C.G., and Haldane, J.S. 1914. The absorption and dissociation of carbon dioxide by human blood. *J. Physiol. (London).* 48:244–271.

Collier, C.R. 1956. Determination of mixed venous CO_2 tensions by rebreathing. *J. Appl. Physiol.* 9:25–29.

Cornell, W.P., Braunwald, E., and Brockenbrough, E.C. 1961. Use of $krypton^{85}$ for the measurement of cardiac output by the single-injection indicator-dilution technique. *Circ. Res.* 9:984–988.

Defares, J.G. 1958. Determination of $P\bar{v}CO_2$ from the exponential CO_2 rise during rebreathing. *J. Appl. Physiol.* 13:159–164.

DuBois, A.B., Fenn, W.O., and Britt, A.G. 1952. CO_2 dissociation curve of lung tissue. *J. Appl. Physiol.* 5:13–16.

Farhi, L.E., Chinet, A., and Haab, P. 1966. Pression partielle d'oxygene du sang veineux mele chez l'homme, en plaine et haute altitude. *J. Physiol. (Paris)* 58:516.

Farhi, L.E. and Haab, P. 1967. Mixed venous blood gas tensions and cardiac output by "bloodless" methods; recent developments and appraisal. *Respir. Physiol.* 2:225–233.

Farhi, L.E. and Linnarsson, D. 1977. Cardiopulmonary readjustments during graded immersion in water at 35°C. *Respir. Physiol.* 30:35–50.

Farhi, L.E., Nesarajah, M.S., Olszowka, A.J. Metildi, L.A. and Ellis, A.K. 1976. Cardiac output determination by simple one-step rebreathing technique. *Respir. Physiol.* 28:141–159.

Fegler, G. 1954. Measurement of cardiac output in anesthetized animals by a thermodilution method. *Quart. J. Exper. Physiol.* 39:153.

Fenn, W.O. and Dejours, P. 1954. Composition of alveolar air during breath-holding with and without prior inhalation of oxygen and carbon dioxide. *J. Appl. Physiol.* 7:313–319.

Fick, A. 1870. Über die Messung des Blutquantums in den Herzenventrikeln. *Sitzungsber. Phys.-Med. Ges. Würzburg.* July 9, p. 36.

Forssmann, W. 1929. Die Sondierung des rechten Herzens. *Klin. Wchschr.* 8:2085–2087.

Fronek, A. and Ganz, V. 1960. Measurement of flow in single blood vessels including cardiac output by local thermodilution. *Circ. Res.* 8:175–182.

Grehant, H. and Quinquaud, C.E. 1886. Recherches experimentales sur la mesure du volume de sang qui traverse les poumons en un temps donne. *Compt. Rend. Soc. Biol.* 30:159.

Gurtner, G.H., Song, S.H., and Farhi, L.E. 1967. Alveolar-to-mixed venous PCO_2 difference during rebreathing. *Physiologist* 10(3):190.

Guyton, A.C. 1963. *Circulatory Physiology: Cardiac Output and Its Regulation*. Philadelphia: W.B. Saunders.

Hamilton, W.F. 1962. Measurement of the cardiac output. In *Handbook of Physiology, Sec. 2: Circulation, Vol. I.* Hamilton, W.F., ed. Washington, D.C.: Am. Physiol. Soc. pp. 551–584.

Kim, T.S., Rahn, H., and Farhi, L.E. 1963. *Estimation of true venous and arterial PCO_2 and cardiac output by gas analysis of a single breath*. Report AMRL-TDR-63-1031, Wright-Patterson AFB, Ohio. pp. 58–73.

Klocke, F.J., Greene, D.G., and Koberstein, R.C. 1968. Indicator-dilution measurement of cardiac output with dissolved hydrogen. *Cir. Res.* 22:841–853.

Knowles, J.H., Newman, W., and Fenn, W.O. 1960. Determination of oxygenated mixed venous blood CO_2 tension by a breath-holding method. *J. Appl. Physiol.* 15:225–228.

Lee, G.deJ., and DuBois, A.B. 1955. Pulmonary capillary blood flow in man. *J. Clin. Invest.* 34:1380–1390.

Loeppky, J.A., Greene, E.R., Hoekenga, D.E., Caprihan, A., and Luft, U.C. 1981. Beat-by-beat stroke volume assessment by pulsed Doppler in upright and supine exercise. *J. Appl. Physiol.* 50:1173–1182.

Loewy, A. and Von Schrötter, H. 1903. Ein Verfahren zur Bestimmung der Blutgasspannungen, der Kreislaufgeschwindigkeit und des Herzschlagvolumens am Menschen. *Arch. Anat. Physiol. Abth.*, p. 394.

Matalon, S.V. and Farhi, L.E. 1979. Cardiopulmonary readjustments in passive tilt. *J. Appl. Physiol.* 47:503–507.

Markoff, I., Müller, F., and Zuntz, N. 1911. Neue Methoden zur Bestimmung der im menschlichen Körper umlaufenden Blutmenge. *Z. Balneol.* 4:14–16.

Plesch, J. 1909. Hamodynamische Studien. *Z. Exptl. Pathol. Therap.* 6:380–618.

Richards, D.W. and Strauss, M.L. 1930. Carbon dioxide and oxygen tensions of the mixed venous blood of man at rest. *J. Clin. Invest.* 9:475–532.

Rochester, D.F., Durand, J., Parker, J.O., Fritts, H.W., Jr. and Harvey, R.M. 1961. Estimation of right ventricular output in man using radioactive krypton (Kr^{85}). *J. Clin. Invest.* 40:643–648.

Sackner, M.A., Greenletch, D., Heiman, M.S., Epstein, S., and Atkins, N. 1975. Diffusing capacity, membrane diffusing capacity, capillary blood volume, pulmonary tissue volume, and cardiac output measured by rebreathing technique. *Am. Rev. Respir. Dis.* 111:157–165.

Sikand, R., Cerretelli, P., and Farhi, L.E. 1966. Effects of $\dot{V}A$ and $\dot{V}A/\dot{Q}$ distribution and of time on the alveolar plateau. *J. Appl. Physiol.* 21:1331–1337.

Wolffberg, S. 1871. Uber die Spannung des Blutgasse in den Lungencapillarien. *Arch. Ges. Physiol.* 4:465–469.

Zuntz, N. and Hagemann, O. 1898. Untersuchungen über den Stoffwechsel des Pferdes bei Ruhe und Arbeit. *Land: Jb. 27* (Ergänz. Bd 3): p. 1.

J.A. Loeppky and M.L. Riedesel, editors
OXYGEN TRANSPORT TO HUMAN TISSUES

Alveolar-Capillary Equilibration of O_2 and CO_2 in Lungs Studied by Rebreathing

J. Piiper, M. Meyer, and P. Scheid

The conductance of alveolar-capillary transfer of gases is characterized by pulmonary diffusing capacity (transfer factor). A reliable determination of the pulmonary diffusing capacity (D) is rendered difficult by the disturbing effects of functional inhomogeneities in the lungs (Piiper and Scheid, 1980). Therefore, we attempted to measure D during a rebreathing procedure which is expected to homogenize lung gas and thus to reduce (or eliminate) the inhomogeneity artefacts (Piiper et al., 1979).

The aim of this paper is to briefly describe the procedure, the results, and the consequences resulting from comparison of D values for O_2, CO, and CO_2. In the second part, the completeness of blood-gas equilibration, which depends on D as well as on pulmonary capillary blood flow, and the slope of the blood dissociation curves, will be analyzed.

Determination of Pulmonary Diffusing Capacity by Rebreathing Techniques

Principle

The kinetics of the approach of alveolar gas partial pressures to the mixed venous ($P_{\bar{v}}$) values is recorded during rebreathing of suitable gas mixtures, before the onset of recirculation (Figure 1). From the rate constant, k, the diffusing capacity can be calculated provided a number of further parameters are known or can be determined simultaneously: rebreathing bag volume, V_R (known); lung or distribution volume, V_L (from He dilution for D_{O_2} and D_{CO} and from CO_2 dilution for D_{CO_2}); effective ventilation, V_{eff} (from He dilution

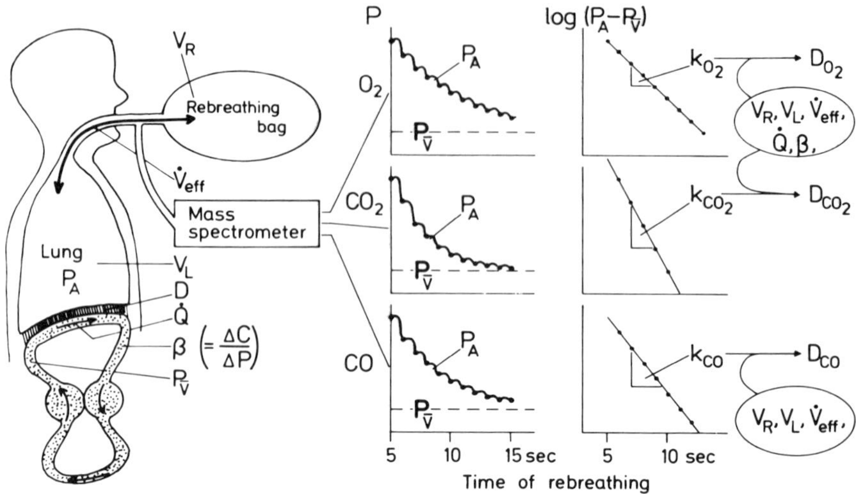

Figure 1. Principle and experimental design for determination of pulmonary diffusing capacity (D) for O_2, CO_2, and CO. See text for symbols.

and equilibration kinetics); pulmonary capillary blood flow, $\dot{Q}$ (from acetylene dilution and equilibration kinetics); effective solubility or slope of blood dissociation curve, β; capacitance coefficient in the gas phase, β_g (Piiper and Scheid, 1980).

The value for D is calculated using the following formulae, which are easily derived considering that the lung and the rebreathing bag constitute a two-compartment system open at the lung to mixed venous blood (Adaro et al., 1973; Piiper et al., 1980; Piiper and Scheid, 1981):

$$D_{O_2} = -\beta_{O_2} \cdot \dot{Q} \cdot \ln\left[1 - \frac{k_{O_2} \cdot \beta_g \cdot V_L}{\beta_{O_2} \cdot \dot{Q}}\left(1 + \frac{V_R/V_L}{1 - k_{O_2} \cdot V_R/\dot{V}_{eff}}\right)\right] \tag{6.1}$$

$$D_{CO} = \beta_g \cdot V_L \cdot k_{CO} \cdot \left(1 + \frac{V_R/V_L}{1 - k_{CO} \cdot V_R/\dot{V}_{eff}}\right) \tag{6.2}$$

$$D_{CO_2} = -\beta_{CO_2} \cdot \dot{Q} \cdot \ln\left[1 - \frac{k_{CO_2} \cdot \beta_g \cdot V_L}{\beta_{CO_2} \cdot \dot{Q}}\left(1 + \frac{V_R/V_L}{1 - k_{CO_2} \cdot V_R/\dot{V}_{eff}}\right)\right] \tag{6.3}$$

Advantages of Using Stable Isotopes of O_2 CO, and CO_2

In principle, D for O_2, CO_2, and CO can be determined from rebreathing equilibration kinetics of the naturally abundant isotopes $^{16}O_2$, $^{12}C^{16}O_2$, and $^{12}C^{16}O$. Stable, naturally occurring but rare isotopes of these gases ($^{18}O_2$, $^{13}C^{16}O_2$, $^{12}C^{18}O$) reveal important advantages over their abundant components for the following reasons.

1. Mixed venous partial pressure, which constitutes the asymptote for equilibration of alveolar (P_A) and bag partial pressures, is practically zero. Conversely, $P_{\bar{v}}$ for the naturally abundant component of O_2 and CO_2 varies with metabolic conditions and is generally not known or cannot be determined with high enough accuracy by noninvasive techniques. Also $P_{\bar{v}}$ for CO ("back pressure") may be elevated in smokers.
2. The use of isotopic CO, e.g., $^{12}C^{18}O$ (mass 30) or $^{13}C^{18}O$ (mass 31) is indispensable when a conventional respiratory mass spectrometer is used as a gas analyzer because the abundant isotope of CO, $^{12}C^{16}O$, cannot be separated from the abundant N_2 isotope which has about the same molecular mass.
3. For determination of D_{O_2} and D_{CO_2}, the slope of the blood dissociation curve, β (dC/dP), can be regarded as constant when there is partial replacement of the naturally abundant component, e.g., $^{16}O_2$, by the rare component $^{18}O_2$ at constant (combined) O_2 content (C_{O_2}). In this condition the slope of the effective dissociation curve (β_{eff}) is constant for all values of $p^{16}O_2$ and $P^{18}O_2$ and equal to the ratio $(C_{\bar{v}}/P_{\bar{v}})_{O_2}$. Experimentally, this condition is met if the major abundant component is in rebreathing equilibrium and P_A for the rare isotopic component is small compared with the naturally abundant isotope. The condition of constant effective solubility, validating the use of an effective straight line dissociation curve, applies also to CO_2, e.g., for replacement of $^{12}C^{16}O_2$ by $^{13}C^{16}O_2$.

Experimental Procedure

After breathing a mixture of 21% O_2 in N_2 (used instead of room air to wash out disturbing ^{36}Ar from lung gas), the subject takes two rapid priming breaths of an oxygen-free hypercapnic mixture and thereafter rebreathes for 15 sec a gas mixture containing 0.07% $^{18}O_2$, 0.07% $^{12}C^{18}O$, 1.0% He (for determination of lung volume and effective ventilation), 1% C_2H_2 (for determination of pulmonary blood flow) and 8% CO_2 and 1 to 3% $^{16}O_2$ to establish gas/blood equilibrium for these gases during rebreathing.

While $^{16}O_2$ and CO_2 are in equilibrium, C_2H_2, $^{18}O_2$, and $^{12}C^{18}O$ steadily decline as they are taken up by pulmonary capillary blood. From the slopes of the apparently exponential part of these curves, after initial mixing and before onset of recirculation, the equilibration rate constants (k) are obtained and used to calculate blood flow and D according to the equations listed.

For determination of D_{CO_2} the same set-up and techniques were used replacing $^{18}O_2$ and $^{12}C^{18}O$ by the stable isotope $^{13}C^{16}O_2$.

Results

The mean values of D_{O_2}, D_{CO}, and D_{CO_2} obtained in healthy young male subjects are shown in Table 1.

Relationship between D_{O_2} and D_{CO}. The ratio of D_{O_2}/D_{CO}, about 1.2, is in agreement with the prediction based on Fick's diffusion equation, since the

Table 1. Measurements of Pulmonary Diffusion Capacity (D) on Healthy Young Male Subjects.

	n	Rest	Exercise
D_{O2}	6	54 ± 10	63 ± 13
D_{CO}	6	47 ± 11	52 ± 10
D_{CO2}	3	178 ± 20	305 ± 9
D_{O2}/D_{CO}		1.2	1.2
D_{CO2}/D_{O2}		3.3	4.8

NOTE: Mean values ± S.D. are shown at rest and during bicycle ergometer exercise at 50 to 125 W. n: number of subjects; D: expressed ml/min/Torr (STPD).

ratio of Krogh's diffusion constants, K (diffusion coefficient×solubility) for O_2/CO is also about 1.2.

If the processes in the red cell (diffusion and chemical reaction with hemoglobin, θ) prevailed as limiting factors, the D_{O_2}/D_{CO} ratio should approach the θ_{O_2}/θ_{CO} ratio which according to generally accepted values equals about 3.0 (Piiper and Scheid, 1980). Thus one may conclude that simple diffusion appears to be the limiting process. However, when extreme literature values for θ_{O_2} are considered, a θ_{O_2}/θ_{CO} ratio as low as 1.1 may be obtained. If this is true, analysis of D_{O_2}/D_{CO} ratio allows no differentiation as to the site of gas transfer resistance.

It should be pointed out that in most previous investigations, the ratio D_{O_2}/D_{CO} has been found to be less than unity. This finding cannot be easily explained by a diffusion-reaction model and is probably due to the fact that functional inhomogeneities lead to a more pronounced underestimation of D_{O_2} as compared to that of D_{CO} (Chinet et al., 1971; Piiper and Scheid, 1980; Savoy et al., 1980).

Relationship between D_{CO_2} and D_{O_2}. The D_{CO_2} values, 180–300 ml/min/Torr, (Table 1) appear to be high. Indeed, Hyde et al. (1968), attempting to determine D_{CO_2} using the stable isotope $^{13}CO_2$ with a breath-holding technique, could not show D_{CO_2} to be statistically different from infinity. But Krogh's diffusion constant ratio, K_{CO_2}/K_{O_2}, for tissue is about 20. Thus alveolar-capillary CO_2 equilibration is slower than expected if O_2 equilibration is assumed to be purely diffusion-limited and much slower if O_2 equilibration is in part reaction-limited. Recent experimental results have shown the reequilibration of the $H^+/HCO_3^-/CO_2$ in blood, in particular the HCO_3^-/Cl^- exchange between red cells and plasma, to limit the capillary-alveolar CO_2 transfer in lungs (Klocke, 1980).

Thus, although a complete equilibration of pulmonary capillary blood with alveolar gas may be attained with respect to molecular CO_2, i.e., equalization of PCO_2, the CO_2 content of blood is expected to stay at a higher level than the equilibrium value (Figure 2). The internal reequilibration of the $CO_2/H^+/HCO_3^-$ system in blood after the blood has left the pulmonary capillaries would raise blood PCO_2, thus producing secondarily, a PCO_2 equilibration deficit measurable as an arterial-alveolar PCO_2 difference.

Diffusing Capacity vs Equilibration Conductance

Since the major limiting process in alveolar-capillary equilibration of CO_2 is not diffusion of molecular CO_2, the term "CO_2 diffusing capacity" is inappropriate if not misleading. More appropriate terms would be "equilibration capacity" or "equilibration conductance," where the term "equilibration" encompasses both diffusive processes and chemical reactions involved in the approach to an equilibrium state. These terms should also be preferred for D_{O_2} and D_{CO}. The well-known dependence of D_{CO} upon P_{O_2} clearly shows that CO equilibration is reaction-limited, at least in the hyperoxic range.

Alveolar-Capillary Equilibration Deficit

The degree of completeness of equilibration and its counterpart, the equilibration deficit, depends not only on the diffusive (or equilibration) conductance of the alveolar-capillary barrier, but also on pulmonary blood flow and blood dissociation curves.

Figure 2. Schematic representation of blood-gas CO_2 equilibration in lungs. C_{CO_2}: total blood CO_2 content; eq A: in equilibrium with alveolar gas (A).

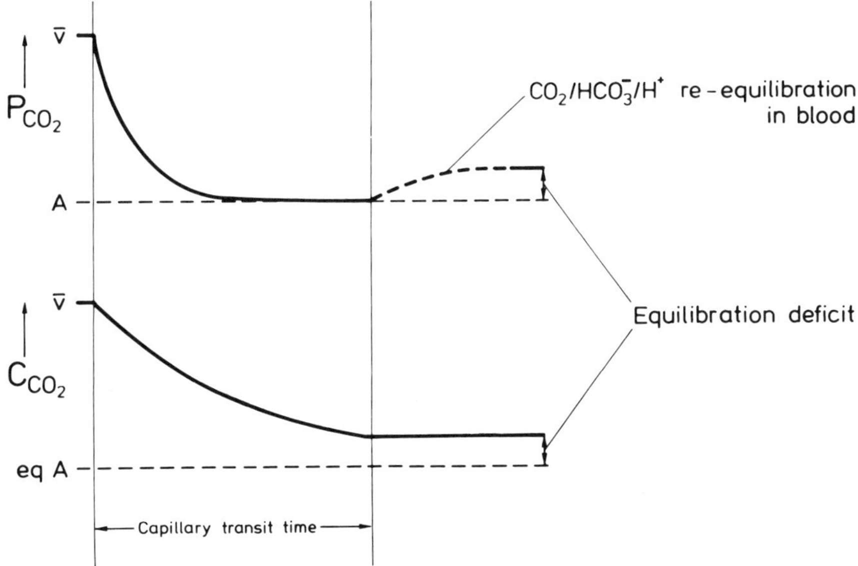

The simplest possible model for study of alveolar-blood equilibration is shown in Figure 3. The relative equilibration deficit, the ratio $(P_A - P_a)/(P_A - P_{\bar{v}})$, is determined by the ratio $D/(\dot{Q}\beta)$, where $\dot{Q}$ is the blood flow and β is the slope of the dissociation curve (Piiper and Scheid, 1981):

$$\frac{P_A - P_a}{P_A - P_{\bar{v}}} = e^{-D/(\dot{Q}\beta)} \tag{6.4}$$

Since the product $\dot{Q}\beta$ may be considered as the perfusive conductance (transfer rate/arteriovenous partial pressure difference), the decisive parameter is the ratio of diffusive to perfusive conductance.

Three ranges may be distinguished with regard to the limiting process: (1) $D/(Q\beta) > 3$, the equilibration deficit is less than 5% and gas transfer is limited by perfusion, (2) $3 > D/(Q\beta) > 0.1$, gas transfer limited by both diffusion and perfusion, (3) $D/(Q\beta) < 0.1$, gas transfer is limited by diffusion only and the increase of $Q\beta$ leads to an increase of transfer rate of less than 5%.

When the behavior of different gases is to be compared, it is useful to consider that according to Fick's law of diffusion, D for a flat and homogeneous sheet is given by the relationship,

$$D = d \cdot \alpha \cdot F/g \tag{6.5}$$

where d is the diffusion coefficient; α, the solubility; F, the surface area; and g, the thickness of the barrier to diffusion.

Figure 3. Model for analysis of diffusion-perfusion limitation in alveolar-capillary gas transfer. See text for symbols.

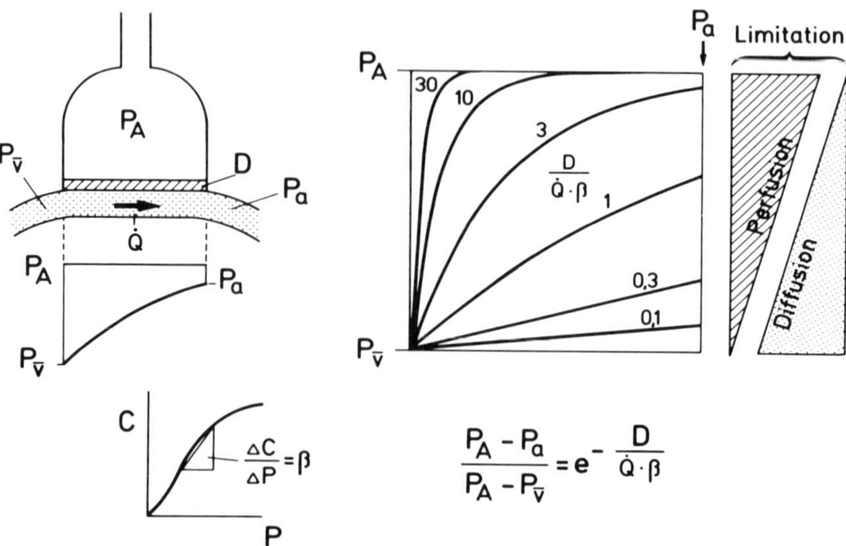

Evidently for two gases, I and II, one obtains:

$$\frac{\left[D/(\dot{Q}\beta)\right]_{II}}{\left[D/(\dot{Q}\beta)\right]_{I}} = \frac{[d\cdot\alpha/\beta]_{II}}{[d\cdot\alpha/\beta]_{I}} \tag{6.6}$$

The most important variable is the α/β ratio. For O_2, the slope of the dissociation curve increases markedly upon transition from the normoxic range into the hypoxic range. The ensuing decrease of the α/β ratio, with the concomitant decrease of the $D/(\dot{Q}\beta)$ ratio, is the reason why the diffusion limitation for O_2 becomes apparent in hypoxia as shown in Figure 4. It is seen that at this level of hypoxia a very low $D/(\dot{Q}\beta)$ value of 0.4 is calculated, meaning that pulmonary gas transfer is much more limited by diffusion that by perfusion. The question of diffusion limitation in alveolar-capillary transfer of O_2 in normoxia is difficult due to changing β and the unknown extent of possible reaction limitations in the P_{O_2} range.

For CO, the $D/(\dot{Q}\beta)$ ratio may be estimated to be about 10^{-2}. Therefore, CO uptake in lungs is diffusion and reaction limited and practically independent of pulmonary blood flow.

For CO_2, the effect d is reduced by slowness of the reequilibration of the $H^+/HCO_3^-/CO_2$ system in blood and the α/β ratio is small due to steepness of the blood CO_2 dissociation curve. Thus, an equilibration deficit on the basis of D_{CO_2} estimates can be calculated to reach about 20% in heavy exercise.

An important fact, not considered in the above analysis, is the interdependence of O_2 and CO_2 reactions in blood. These are usually analyzed, for equilibrium conditions, as Bohr and Haldane effects. When O_2 equilibration in hypoxia is slow, the CO_2 equilibration, specifically the portion corresponding to the Haldane effect, should also be slowed down relative to normoxia. For all inert gases the α/β ratio is close to unity, meaning that in lungs (where the

Figure 4. Application of the model of Figure 3 to man in high altitude hypoxia.

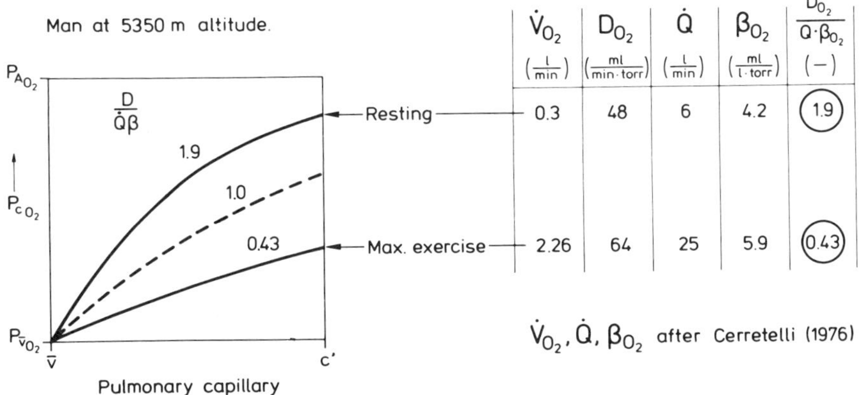

F/g ratio is sufficiently high to enable O_2 transfer in hypoxia) equilibration deficits for inert gases are not expected to occur.

Summary

The pulmonary diffusing capacity (D) is reinvestigated by rebreathing techniques using stable isotopes of O_2, CO, and CO_2 as test gases. Whereas the ratio D_{O_2}/D_{CO} in hypoxia averaged 1.2, which is close to the prediction from Krogh's diffusion constants or tissue, the ratio D_{CO_2}/D_{CO} was about 4.0, probably due to alveolar-capillary CO_2 equilibration being in part limited by incomplete equilibration of the $H^+/HCO_3^-/CO_2$ system in blood. On the basis of the $D/(\dot{Q}\beta)$ ratio ($\dot{Q}$, pulmonary capillary blood flow; β, effective solubility in blood), it is shown that alveolar-capillary equilibration of O_2 is strongly diffusion-limited in hypoxia, but not in normoxia. Alveolar-capillary equilibration of CO_2 is expected to slightly limit CO_2 exchange at rest, but in heavy exercise considerable limitation may arise.

References

Adaro, F., Scheid, P., Teichmann, J., and Piiper, J. 1973. A rebreathing method for estimating pulmonary D_{O_2}: theory and measurements in dog lungs. *Respir. Physiol.* 18:43–63.

Cerretelli, P. 1976. Limiting factors to oxygen transport on Mount Everest. *J. Appl. Physiol.* 40:658–667.

Chinet, A., Micheli, J.L., and Haab, P. 1971. Inhomogeneity effects on O_2 and CO pulmonary diffusing capacity estimates by steady state methods theory. *Respir. Physiol.* 13:1–22.

Hyde, R.W., Puy, R.J., Raub, W.F., and Forster, R.E. 1968. Rate of disappearance of labeled carbon dioxide from the lungs of humans during breath holding: a method for studying the dynamics of pulmonary CO_2 exchange. *J. Clin. Invest.* 47:1535–1552.

Klocke, R.A. 1980. Kinctics of pulmonary gas exchange. In *Pulmonary Gas Exchange, Vol. I, Ventilation, Blood Flow, and Diffusion*. West, J.B., ed. New York: Academic Press, pp. 173–218.

Piiper, J. 1981. Blood-gas equilibration in lungs and pulmonary diffusing capacity. *Progr. Resp. Res.* 16:115–125.

Piiper, J. and Scheid, P. 1980. Blood-gas equilibration in lungs. In *Pulmonary Gas Exchange, Vol. I, Ventilation, Blood Flow, and Diffusion*. West, J.B., ed. New York:Academic Press, pp. 131–171.

Piiper, J. and Scheid, P. 1981. Model for capillary-alveolar equilibration with special reference to O_2 uptake in hypoxia. *Respir. Physiol.*, in press.

Piiper, J., Meyer, M., and Scheid, P. 1979. Pulmonary diffusing capacity for O_2 and CO at rest and during exercise. Advantages of rebreathing techniques using stable isotopes. *Bull. Eur. Physiopathol. Respir.* 15:145–152.

Piiper, J., Meyer, M., Marconi, C., and Scheid, P. 1980. Alveolar-capillary equilibration kinetics of $^{13}CO_2$ in human lungs studied by rebreathing. *Respir. Physiol.* 42:29–41.

Savoy, J., Michoud, M.-C., Robert, M., Geiser, J., Haab, P., and Piiper, J. 1980. Comparison of steady state pulmonary diffusing capacity estimates for O_2 and CO in dogs. *Respir. Physiol.* 42:43–59.

J.A. Loeppky and M.L. Riedesel, editors
OXYGEN TRANSPORT TO HUMAN TISSUES

Diffusion and Its Limitations

Gail H. Gurtner, J.T. Sylvester, and E. Honig

In gas exchange organs such as the lung and placenta in which blood or gas can be sampled at both input and output sides of the organ, useful information can be gained by comparing the properties of O_2 exchange with those of inert gases. In this communication, we will present two examples of such an analysis; one considering pulmonary gas exchange and the other considering placental exchange. It would have been both scientifically and esthetically pleasing if exactly the same method of analysis could be applied to both organs, however the dissimilar properties of gas exchange between the two organs precludes this. The dissimilarities in rate limiting steps in gas exchange will be emphasized.

A Comparison of Pulmonary O_2 and Inert Gas Exchange

The use of inert gas exchange to describe the properties of the lung was initiated by Farhi and coworkers (Farhi, 1967; Farhi and Yokoyama, 1967) and Wagner et al. (1974) who developed a method to quantitatively estimate the distribution of ventilation and perfusion (V/Q) in the lung using inert gases of different solubility; the method involved sophisticated computer techniques to estimate the V/Q distribution from which arterial PO_2 could be predicted. Although this method is very useful in determining the V/Q distribution, it is possible to compare inert gas and O_2 exchange directly under conditions of hypoxia where O_2 has a quasi-linear dissociation curve and, therefore, can be treated as an inert gas.

Wagner's technique consists of infusing a solution of 6 inert gases of widely varying solubilities (SF6, ethane, cyclopropane, halothane, diethyl ether, and acetone) intravenously at a constant rate and measuring their steady state concentrations in the arterial and mixed venous blood and in the mixed expired air by gas chromatography. In the steady state, this exchange can be expressed by equations which define retention (R) as:

$$R=\frac{Pa-PI}{Pv-PI}=\sum_{i=1}^{n}(\dot{Q}_i/\dot{Q}_T)(1+\dot{V}_i/\dot{Q}_i\lambda)^{-1} \tag{7.1}$$

and excretion (E) as:

$$E=\frac{PE-PI}{Pv-PI}=\sum_{i=1}^{n}(\dot{V}_i/\dot{V}_E)(1+\dot{V}_i/\dot{Q}_i\lambda)^{-1} \tag{7.2}$$

where Pa, Pv, PI and PE denote partial pressures in the arterial and mixed venous blood and in inspired and mixed expired air, respectively; $\dot{Q}_T$ is total blood flow, $\dot{V}_E$ is total ventilation, $\dot{Q}_i$ is the blood flow of the ith compartment, $\dot{V}_i$ is its ventilation and λ is the Ostwald partition coefficient of the inert gas in question. It is assumed that in any given compartment the retention or excretion of a gas is determined solely by the $\dot{V}/\dot{Q}$ ratio of the compartment and the blood solubility (λ) of the gas; although there is some question about diffusion limitation in the gas phase, the assumption seems valid for alveolar capillary inert gas exchange in the normal lung.

We have applied the multiple inert gas technique to two physiological investigations using dogs; the first involves partitioning the A-a gradient and measuring O_2 diffusing capacity during exercise at high altitude. These investigations were carried out by Dr. Jimmie Sylvester and coworkers at the Army Medical Research Institute in Natick, Massachusetts (Sylvester et al., 1981). The second application involves an attempt to demonstrate O_2 tension-related changes in O_2 diffusing capacity (DLCO) which might be due to saturable O_2 transport due to facilitation by a carrier. Such concentration-related changes in DLCO have been demonstrated (Mendoza et al., 1977; Gurtner, 1980). This work was carried out by Dr. Eric Honig in this laboratory supported by a Pulmonary Faculty Training Award.

We used the 3-compartment model originally proposed by Riley and Cournand (1949) to analyze inert gas and O_2 exchange. In this model, the lung is comprised of a shunt compartment which has blood flow ($\dot{Q}_s$) but no ventilation, a dead space compartment having ventilation ($\dot{V}_D$) but no blood flow, and an alveolar compartment having ventilation ($\dot{V}_A$) and blood flow ($\dot{Q}_A$). Using the model, expressions for retention and excretion can be derived:

$$R=\frac{Pa-PI}{Pv-PI}=(\dot{Q}_s/\dot{Q}_T)+(1-\dot{Q}_s/\dot{Q}_T)(1+\dot{V}_A/\dot{Q}_A\lambda)^{-1} \tag{7.3}$$

$$E=\frac{PE-PI}{Pv-PI}=(1-\dot{V}_D/\dot{V}_E)(1+\dot{V}_A/\dot{Q}_A\lambda)^{-1} \tag{7.4}$$

From Equation (7.3), it is seen that as λ approaches zero, retention approaches the shunt fraction, $\dot{Q}_s/\dot{Q}_T$. Thus, in the experiments to be described, we measured shunt fraction as the retention of SF6, the least soluble of the 6 inert gases we used. From Equation (7.4), it is seen that as λ approaches infinity, excretion approaches 1.0 minus the dead space fraction, $\dot{V}_D/\dot{V}_E$. Thus, we measured dead space as 1.0 minus the excretion of acetone, the most soluble of the 6 inert gases. In a similar manner, an expression can be derived for the difference between the partial pressure of the inert gas in the end-capillary blood (Pc′) and that in the alveolar air (PA):

$$\frac{Pc'-PA}{Pv-PI}=(R-\dot{Q}_s/\dot{Q}_T)(1-\dot{Q}_s/\dot{Q}_T)^{-1}-E(1-\dot{V}_D/\dot{V}_E)^{-1} \quad (7.5)$$

In the 3-compartment lung, this gradient will equal zero, since there is only one gas exchanging compartment. In the real lung, however, it will have some finite value, the magnitude of which will be proportional to the degree of V/Q nonhomogeneity (Hlastala and Robertson, 1978; Neufeld et al., 1978). Thus, we measured this gradient as an index of V/Q nonhomogeneity where R and E were measured directly, the shunt fraction was estimated from the retention of SF6 and dead space was estimated from 1.0 minus the excretion of acetone.

Under conditions in which the O_2 dissociation curve can be linearly approximated, it is possible to use the inert gas results to partition the A-a gradient for O_2 into portions related to the shunt, V/Q distribution and diffusion limitation. The portion due to shunt and V/Q distribution can be predicted by Equation (7.5) using the R and E for the inert gas with a λ close to the virtual value for O_2. On the linear part of the O_2 dissociation curve, the effective λ for O_2 can be calculated as: $(CaO_2-CvO_2)(P_B-P_W)/(PaO_2-PvO_2)$, where CaO_2 and CvO_2 are the O_2 contents, and PaO_2 and PvO_2, the O_2 partial pressures in the arterial and mixed venous blood, respectively; P_B is barometric pressure, and P_W is the water vapor pressure at body temperature. The value of λ for O_2 is obviously dependent on hemoglobin levels and tends to vary in different experiments, however λ for O_2 was often very similar to λ for halothane (3.16). Under these circumstances, R and E for halothane could be used in Equation (7.5) to predict the portion of the gradient related to shunt and V/Q distribution. In the other experiments, the effective R and E for O_2 could be estimated by interpolation.

The residual gradient, (Δ PO_2 diff), which remains after subtraction of the shunt and V/Q portions is the diffusion component and can be used to calculate O_2 diffusing capacity by Equation (7.6) which has been derived elsewhere (Piiper, 1962; Piiper et al., 1971).

$$DLO_2=\ln\frac{(PAO_2-PvO_2)}{(\Delta PO_{2\,diff})}\,\frac{\dot{Q}_A\lambda_{O_2}}{K} \quad (7.6)$$

where K relates the volume and pressure units used in DLO_2 from STPD and mm Hg to BTPS and atm, and where, from considerations of mass balance, PAO_2 is calculated by:

$$PAO_2=\frac{PEO_2-PIO_2(\dot{V}_D/\dot{V}_E)}{1-\dot{V}_D/\dot{V}_E} \quad (7.7)$$

Gas Exchange at High Altitude

The subjects for our first set of experiments were 5 awake dogs trained to run on a treadmill. Two months before the experiments, tracheostomies and unilateral carotid loops were created surgically. Each dog was studied twice in a hypobaric chamber, first at an altitude of 6,096 m and then, on a separate day, at sea level. Resting measurements were made after 1 hr at altitude. Exercise measurements were made after 15 to 20 min of treadmill exercise.

At sea level, the mean shunt fraction was very small (0.9%). It did not change significantly during exercise, nor was it altered by exposure to high altitude. Mean dead space fraction was relatively large (39.7%). Perhaps this is explained by the intermittent panting typical of awake dogs. No statistically significant changes were seen in dead space either at sea level or at high altitude. The end-capillary to alveolar inert gas gradients, normalized by the difference between mixed venous and inspired partial pressures, were measured as an index of V/Q nonhomogeneity (Figure 1). Since exercise had no effect on these gradients, only the effect of high altitude is shown. It is easily appreciated that the gradients were significantly smaller at high altitude, indicating an improvement in ventilation-perfusion relationships.

Our next goal was to use these inert gas results to determine how high altitude altered the exchange of oxygen. We therefore measured the A-a gradient for O_2($AaDO_2$) and, as Riley had done before, attempted to de-

Figure 1. Inert gas end-capillary to alveolar (Pć − PA) partial pressure gradients in dogs, normalized by the difference between mixed venous (Pv) and inspired (PI) tensions, as a function of the Ostwald partition coefficient (λ).

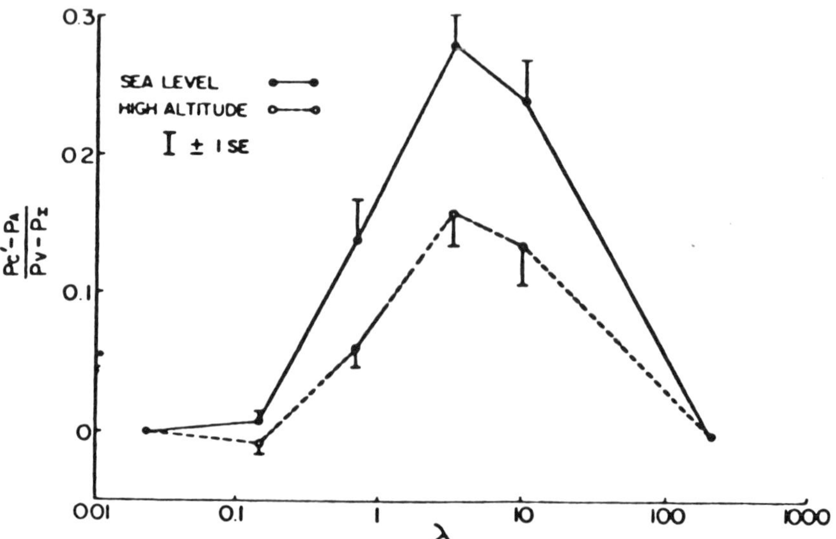

termine how much of this gradient was due to shunt, $\dot{V}/\dot{Q}$ inequality, and diffusion limitation. The first step in this fractionation was to measure the end-capillary O_2 gradient due to diffusion limitation at high altitude. This required the assumption that the relationship between blood O_2 content and tension was linear. Since at 6096 m the dogs were working on the steep, nearly linear portion of the oxyhemoglobin dissociation curve, this assumption was reasonable. The effective Ostwald coefficient for O_2 could then be calculated. Figure 2 shows the partition of $AaDO_2$ at sea level and high altitude. The resting A-a gradient at sea level was about 35 mm Hg; 88% of this gradient was due to V/Q inequality and 12% was due to shunt. Diffusion limitation was assumed to play no role. Exercise had no effect on either the magnitude or composition of $AaDO_2$. At high altitude, resting $AaDO_2$ decreased to about 12 mm Hg. This decrease was caused by a significant reduction in the contribution of V/Q inequality. In addition, the contribution of shunt virtually disappeared. The decrease was not as large as it might have been because diffusion limitation now contributed about 50% of the total. Surprisingly, exercise again had little effect. We had expected the gradient, or at least its diffusion component, to increase under these conditions. The expected increase

Figure 2. A-a gradient for O_2 ($AaDO_2$) and its composition in dogs from inert gas data. (Note: $\dot{V}/\dot{Q}$=V/Q inequality, $\dot{Q}_s/\dot{Q}_T$=shunt, D=diffusion limitation.)

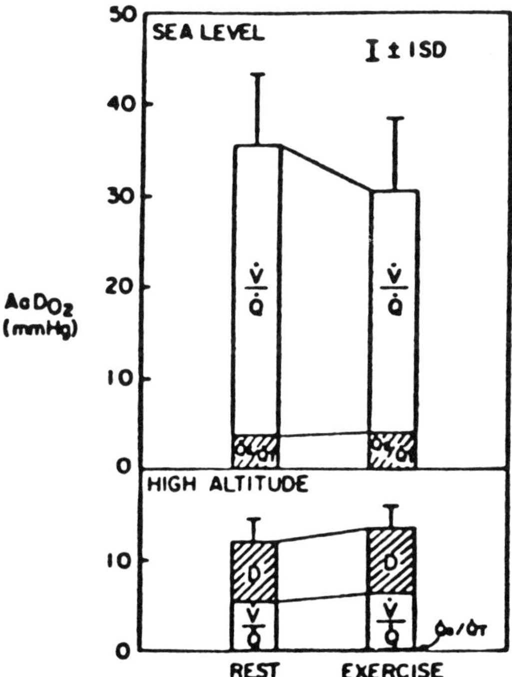

was prevented, however, by a nearly 2-fold increase in O_2 diffusing capacity (from 20.8 to 35.3 ml/min/mm Hg), which we were also able to estimate.

While striking, our observations of diffusion gradients were not nearly as surprising as our measurements of O_2 consumption ($\dot{V}O_2$). At sea level, 20 min of treadmill exercise caused a 3-fold elevation in $\dot{V}O_2$ (188 to 568 ml/min). At high altitude, the same exercise caused only a 2-fold elevation (162 to 346 ml/min). This difference between sea level and high altitude was highly significant. Its mechanism is unknown. Cerretelli (1980) has suggested that the work of breathing makes up a substantial portion of total $\dot{V}O_2$ in the dog. Perhaps this proportion decreased at high altitude because of the decrease in air density. Another possibility is that a steady state $\dot{V}O_2$ may not have been achieved during exercise at high altitude. Whatever the mechanism, a decrease in the amount of O_2 required to perform a given amount of work would constitute a significant adaptation to the stress of high altitude.

In summary, the results suggest that in the awake resting dog at sea level, $AaDO_2$ was due mainly to V/Q nonhomogeneity. Only a small portion was due to shunt. After acute exposure to an altitude of 6,096 m, the contribution of shunt virtually disappeared and that of V/Q nonhomogeneity was diminished. These improvements were partially offset, however, by the appearance of a gradient due to diffusion limitation. Mild exercise had no significant effect on $AaDO_2$ or any of its components, either at sea level or at high altitude.

O_2 Concentration Dependence of DLO_2

One of the phenomena which support the existance of a specific transport mechanism is that of saturation kinetics (Gurtner, 1980). In the lung, this phenomenon is manifested by a concentration dependent change in diffusing capacity. We have worked this out most clearly using DLCO. In both dog and man, there is an inverse correlation between DLCO and end-tidal CO concentration over the range of 500 ppm to 100 ppm (Mendoza et al., 1977; Ayash et al., 1978). Since we found a CO concentration related change in DLCO, we undertook experiments in which DLO_2 was measured at different levels of hypoxia in anesthetized and artifically ventilated dogs. The animals were ventilated with 8, 10, and 12% O_2 in N_2. Steady state DLCO was also measured simultaneously using the method described by Mendoza et al., (1977) at an inspired CO level of 300 ppm. Cardiac output ($\dot{Q}$) was measured by the weighted inert gas Fick method described by Evans and Wagner (1977) and $\dot{V}O_2$ was measured directly. The data reflects 67 separate measurements. The $PACO_2$ varied in these animals from 25 to 35 mm Hg and pH from 7.40 to 7.55. Body temperatures ranged from 34 to 39°C. Venous oxygen saturations ranged from 10 to 60% and arterial oxygen saturations from 15 to 75%. Hemoglobin concentrations varied from 8 to 15 g/100 ml in the animals studied. Because of differences in V/Q ratios, shunt and dead space fractions, similar inspired oxygen tensions produced different alveolar O_2 tensions. The results in Figure 3 are therefore displayed as a function of PAO_2, which was calculated using Equation (7.7). All of the variables in Figure 3 were increased with hypoxia but the greatest increases were seen in DLO_2. Changes in $\dot{Q}$ and $\dot{V}O_2$ with hypoxia have been described previously and may be due to catacholamine release. Changes in DLCO may be explained on the basis of increased pulmonary blood flow and pulmonary artery pressure.

According to the schema of Roughton and Forster (1957), the pulmonary diffusing capacity can be described as the sum of the influences of membrane diffusing capacity (D_m), red cell diffusing capacity (θ) and capillary volume (Vc) as follows:

$$\frac{1}{DL} = \frac{1}{D_m} + \frac{1}{\theta \cdot V_c} \tag{7.8}$$

If θ were to increase as PAO_2 fell in hypoxia, DLO_2 would increase, but θ appears to be constant below a saturation of 75% (Staub et al., 1962). In the present experiments, the largest change in DLO_2 was seen at blood PO_2 values below 50% saturation of hemoglobin so this explanation seems unlikely. An increase in Vc during hypoxia could increase DLO_2. Wagner and Latham (1975) used thoracic windows and a microscope to study pulmonary capillary morphology in hypoxic dogs. They observed a 4-fold increase in the length of perfused capillary per alveolar surface area as PAO_2 fell from 70 to 30 mm Hg. An increase in Vc should also produce an increase in DLCO. The magnitude of changes in DLCO and DLO_2 are related to changes in Vc and to the θ values for the two gases. There is a descrepancy in θ values for O_2 which may be perhaps related to methodology. According to Holland (1981), measurement techniques which use the O_2 electrode give larger values than optical techniques due to the presence of unstirred layers next to the electrode membrane. If this is true, the value measured using optical techniques should be correct. In our calculations, we use a value for O_2 of 1.5 and 0.9 for CO (Piiper and Scheid, 1980; Holland, 1981). These represent the maximum values present under conditions of hemoglobin desaturation. The D_m for CO was assumed to be 40. The D_m for O_2 was calculated to be 1.23 times D_m for CO using the ratio of Krogh's diffusion coefficient for each gas in water or tissue with control Vc being taken to be 22 ml, the value measured by Wanner et al. (1978). The effect of doubling and tripling Vc was calculated. Control DLO_2 was 19.8; DLO_2 at 44 ml Vc was 28.1; DLO_2 at 66 ml Vc was 32.8. The respective values for DLCO were 13.2, 19.9, and 23.9. Note that the predicted control DLO_2 was substantially larger than DLCO and the ratio of DLO_2/DLCO actually decreased as Vc was increased. These latter predictions are different from our experimental results (Figure 3) which cannot be explained by this simple model. We obviously cannot rule out changes in Vc acting in concert with *nonhomogeneity* of DL to Vc as causing the measured relationship between DLO_2 and DLCO at the different PAO_2 levels. This hypothesis could be tested using isolated lungs from animals which do not have marked intrinsic hypoxic vasoconstriction.

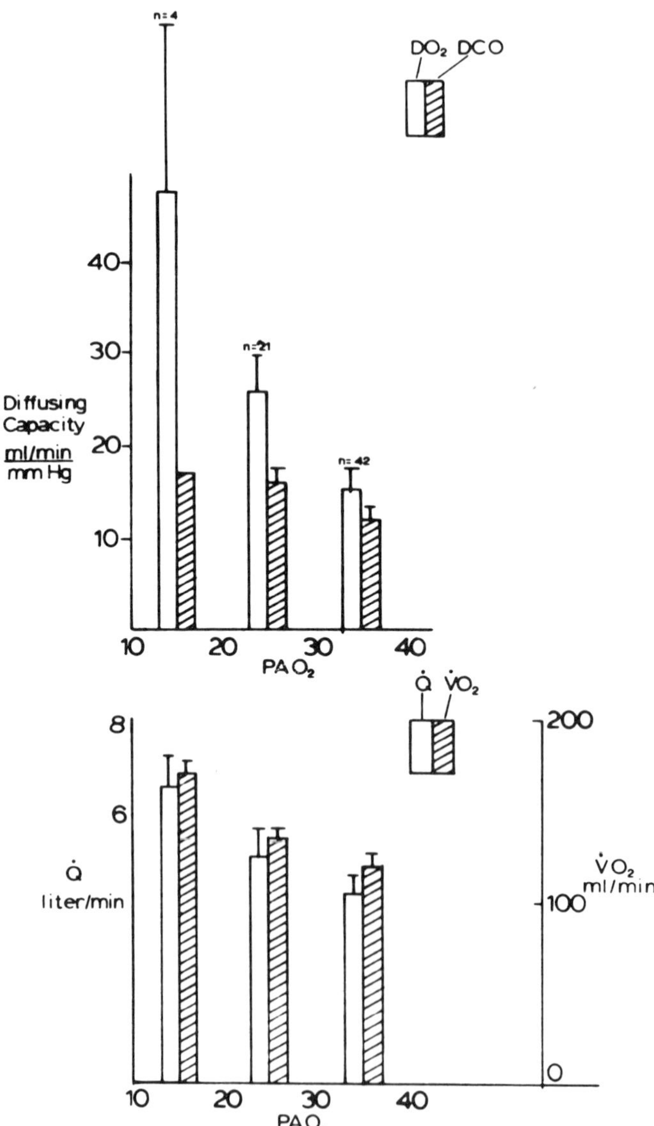

Figure 3. (Top) Pulmonary diffusing capacity for O_2 and CO measured at different alveolar PO_2 levels. DCO increases almost 50% as PAO_2 is decreased, while DO_2 increases more than 200%. (Bottom) Cardiac output and oxygen consumption both increase during progressive hypoxia.

The disproportionate increase in DLO_2 when compared to DLCO observed during progressive hypoxia could be a manifestation of saturation kenetics due to the presence of a specific O_2 carrier (perhaps cytochrome p-450) in the alveolar capillary membrane. If so, the (P_{50}) of the carrier for O_2 would most likely be below 15 mm Hg, but high enough so that changes could occur in DLO_2 at 25 mm Hg.

In other experiments carried out using isolated perfused rabbit lungs, we indirectly estimated the O_2 and CO affinity of pulmonary cytochrome p-450 by measuring the effect of hypoxia or CO on the rate of a cytochrome p-450 mediated reaction (Knoblauch et al., 1981). We found that the reaction was inhibited 50% at a mean tissue PO_2 of 4 mm Hg. According to the schema given in the paper of Mendoza et al. (1977), an O_2 carrier with a PO_2 of 4 mm Hg could explain the PO_2 dependent changes of DLO_2 observed in the present experiments.

A Comparison of Placental O_2 and Inert Gas Exchange

There are several reasons why the useful techniques described above cannot be applied to placental gas exchange. Although the mass balance equations would be identical, several practical and theoretical differences exist between pulmonary and placental gas exchange which do not fulfill the conditions necessary for the method to be valid. First, the O_2 consumption of the placenta is not negligible when compared with the amount of gas transferred. This could cause gradients between maternal and fetal capillaries, if the distribution of metabolism were asymmetric with respect to maternal or fetal capillary flow. Second, the arrangement of maternal and fetal vessels is not known. If the arrangement were counter- or crosscurrent, it is possible that fetal end-capillary gas tension may be higher than maternal end-capillary gas tension. We have some evidence that this might be the case. In experiments reported elsewhere, we found during artificial perfusion of the fetal side of the sheep placenta using a closed recirculation system, that steady-state PO_2 (during no gas exchange) on the fetal side of the placenta was consistently higher than the PO_2 in the uterine vein (Gurtner et al., 1978). During gas exchange, such a PO_2 relationship was not present. However, the presence of counter- or crosscurrent circulation could obscure gradients due to distribution effects or diffusion limitation.

Finally, inert gas transfer in the placenta may not be completely limited by distribution of maternal and fetal blood flow but may be diffusion limited. As described below, the placenta is a more formidable barrier for diffusion processes than the lung and appears to contain a specific O_2 carrier for facilitation of O_2 transport.

Our interest in physiological O_2 carriers began with an incidental observation made in the course of an experiment designed to measure the placental permeability to inert gases with different physical properties (Bissonnette and

Gurtner, 1972). We had initially studied the transfer of inert gases across the sheep placenta. Our experimental procedure was to artificially perfuse the fetal side of the placenta with dextran solutions or blood that was equilibrated with various gas mixtures and to measure inflow and outflow partial pressures of gases on both fetal and maternal sides of the placenta. In a few of the early experiments, we had observed that the PO_2 of the uterine venous and umbilical venous bloods was the same, indicating that O_2 had reached equilibrium between maternal and fetal capillaries (Gurtner and Burns, 1971). This phenomenon never occurred for inert gases, even those with physical properties similar to O_2 such as N_2 or argon. These observations led us to suspect the presence of a specific O_2 carrier in the placenta. Our first experiment, designed to test the carrier hypothesis, involved acute administration of drugs that were known to bind to hepatic cytochrome p-450. We found that these compounds markedly reduced transplacental O_2 flux without systematically affecting inert gas transfer (Gurtner and Burns, 1972, 1975; Gurtner, 1980).

In our early work, we emphasized the drug inhibition studies, which might possibly have alternative explanations. We reasoned that our evidence would be stronger if we could confirm these early experiments by demonstrating substantial differences in placental diffusing capacity for O_2 and argon, the magnitude of which decreased with the administration of the inhibitor. The next series of experiments was performed to attempt to confirm these observations.

In some of these experiments, we perfused the fetal side of the placenta with a fluorocarbon emulsion and partially exchange-transfused the ewe with the same emulsion. The fluorocarbon emulsion was used because, unlike blood plasma, it exhibited a large physical solubility for argon, which was increased 7-fold in the fluorocarbon emulsion in comparison to blood. By perfusing the placenta with fluids having different physical solubilities for oxygen and inert gases, we hoped to gain further information on the rate limiting factor in the transfer of each gas, i.e., was transfer normally "diffusion" or "perfusion" limited. If these gases were reaching equilibrium by diffusion on the two sides of the placental barrier, then the transfer would be perfusion limited and an increase in the amount of gas in solution in the perfusion fluid would increase the flux and the apparent diffusing capacity. If, on the other hand, these gases were diffusion limited, increasing their concentration in the perfusion fluid would not alter the diffusing capacity.

If the argon diffusing capacity did not increase in the presence of fluorocarbon on both sides of the placenta, we could conclude that the rate limiting process in argon and N_2 transfer was the rate of diffusion across the placenta. If equilibrium for O_2 occurred between maternal and fetal veins or if the diffusing capacity for O_2 increased in proportion to the O_2-carrying capacity of the perfusion fluids, we could conclude that the rate limiting process in O_2 transfer was the rate of delivery and removal of the gas since the permeability of the membrane was large for oxygen because of facilitated diffusion. This theory would be supported further if oxygen became diffusion limited after the postulated carrier (cytochrome p-450) was inactivated.

When we first attempted to perform blood perfusion of the fetal side of the placenta, we were unable to achieve high flows without very high perfusion pressures. This caused rapid deterioration of the preparation. In one of the early experiments, we found that administration of a small amount of the α-adrenergic blocker, phenoxybenzamine (Dibenzyline, 10 mg), caused a marked decrease in perfusion pressure and an increase in the O_2 flux. Subsequently we have routinely used phenoxybenzamine at this dosage in the blood and fluorocarbon experiments.

Since we wanted to compare the relative permeability of the placenta to O_2 with the permeability for argon, we chose to calculate an index of diffusing capacity for each gas. In a steady state, the amount of argon entering or leaving the fetal circulation must be equal to the amount leaving or entering the maternal circulation. For this gas, the net flux is equal to the difference in partial pressures between fetal artery and fetal vein multiplied by the solubility and the fetal perfusion rate. When fluorocarbon was used, the solubility was calculated according to the proportion of fluorocarbon to blood. For example, if a 33% emulsion of fluorocarbon was used, the solubility was 0.33 (solubility in fluorocarbon) and 0.67 (solubility in saline). The physical solubility coefficients used in calculating the indices of diffusing capacity were given in our 1975 paper (Gurtner and Burns, 1975). For O_2, the transplacental flux was calculated by multiplying the fetal arteriovenous content difference, which included physically dissolved O_2 as well as chemically bound O_2, by the fetal perfusion rate. As the index of diffusing capacity, we chose the transplacental flux of gas (J) divided by the partial pressure difference between maternal and fetal venous blood, P(MV−FV) or P(FV−MV), depending on the direction of flow of the gas.

This index of diffusing capacity differs from the conventional definition because the venous partial pressure is used rather than the mean capillary difference. It is possible to calculate the mean capillary difference, however, then one would be required to assume a deterministic model for the arrangement of maternal and fetal blood vessels in the placenta. Since it is not known whether the vascular flow arrangement is countercurrent, crosscurrent, pooled, or a combination of these, we chose to present the data in the above manner. The absolute value of diffusing capacity would differ with each model; however, the relationship between the diffusing capacity for each gas would remain the same.

In Figure 4, we have plotted $J_{argon}/\Delta P_{argon}$ against the solubility of argon in the fetal perfusion fluid. In these experiments, it was possible to increase the solubility of argon in the fetal perfusion medium about 7-fold, however $J_{argon}/\Delta P_{argon}$ did not change significantly. It was also possible to increase the solubility of argon in the maternal perfusion fluid more than 4-fold. This increase in solubility was similarly not associated with a significant increase in

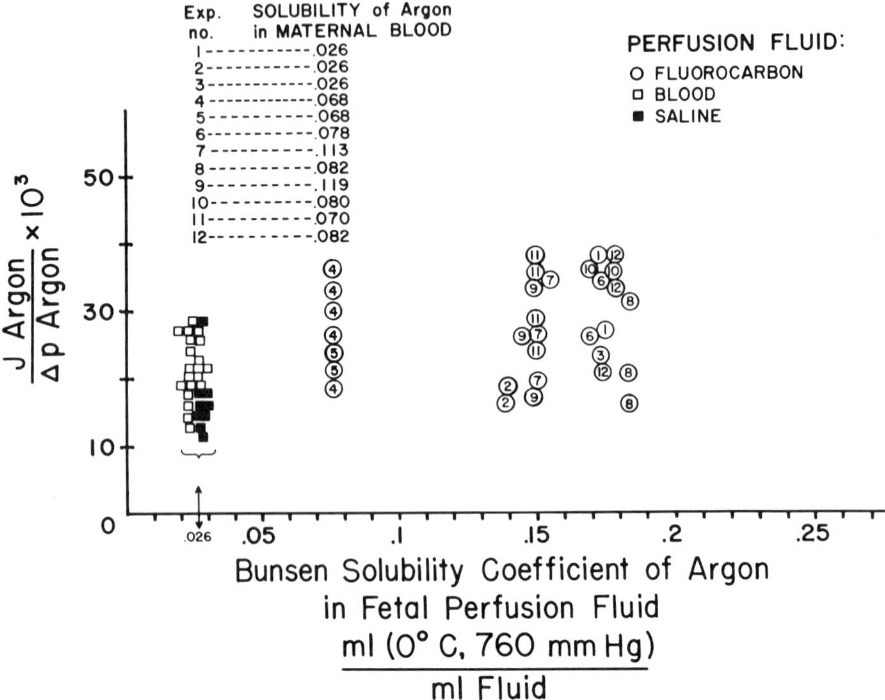

Figure 4. Index of placental diffusing capacity for argon, expressed as the flux of argon in ml/min, (J_{argon}) divided by the partial pressure difference between the venous blood leaving both sides of the placenta (ΔP_{argon}), is plotted against the physical solubility of argon in the perfusion medium on the fetal side of the placenta. Experiments were performed in which argon moved from maternal to fetal and fetal to maternal sides of the placenta. Points clustered about the solubility of 0.026 are the blood and dextran perfusions. Other points represent the fluorocarbon experiments, with the solubility of argon in the maternal blood also indicated, as most of these ewes received partial exchange transfusion with a fluorocarbon emulsion.

$J_{argon}/\Delta P_{argon}$. Thus, the index of diffusing capacity for argon is not affected by increases in solubility for the gas on both sides of the membrane.

Figure 5 shows $J_{O_2}/\Delta PO_2$ plotted against the O_2 capacity of the fetal perfusion fluid at a partial pressure (36 mm Hg) which would cause 50% saturation of adult sheep hemoglobin (Gurtner and Burns, 1975). We chose this arbitrary means of expressing the solubility (physical + chemical) of O_2 because this value of PO_2 and saturation was often found in our experiments. The meaning of the results is not in any way changed if the O_2 content at a different blood PO_2 within the physiological range is chosen.

The results show that sometimes O_2 comes to equilibrium between fetal and maternal veins. This is indicated by the value of infinity for $J_{O_2}/\Delta PO_2$. This

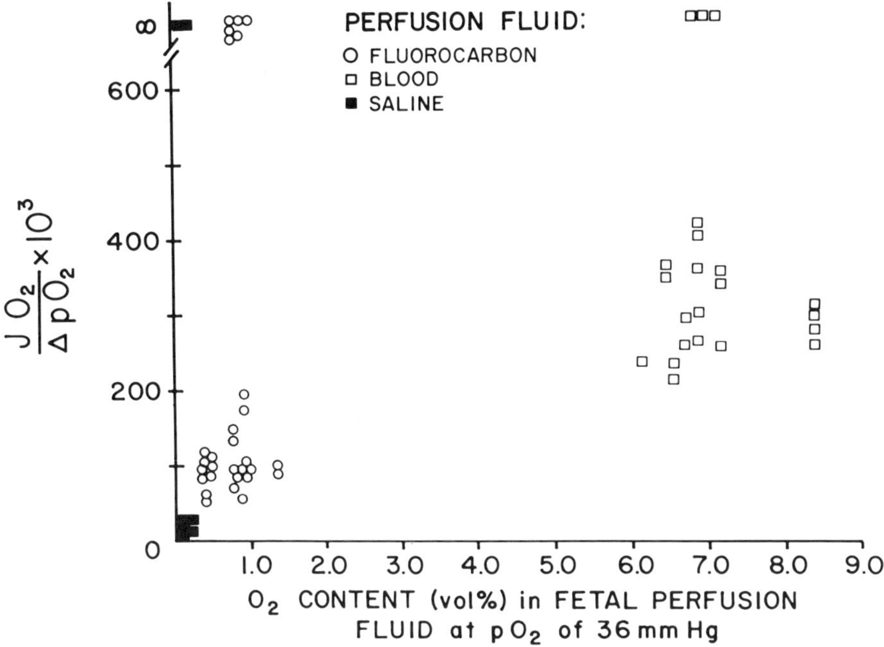

Figure 5. Index of O_2 diffusing capacity $J_{O_2}/\Delta PO_2(MV-FV)$ is plotted against the O_2 capacity of the fetal perfusion medium at 36 mm Hg, which is the P_{50} for adult sheep hemoglobin.

phenomenon appears to occur as frequently under conditions in which the O_2 capacity is high as under the conditions in which the O_2 capacity is low. When there were differences in PO_2 between maternal and fetal veins, $J_{O_2}/\Delta PO_2$ increased markedly as the O_2 capacity of the perfusion fluid increased. The change in $J_{O_2}/\Delta PO_2$ in proportion to the O_2 carrying capacity of the perfusion medium contrasts with the lack of any relationship between $J_{argon}/\Delta P_{argon}$ and the solubility of this gas in the perfusion medium. Thus O_2 transfer appears to be perfusion limited and argon transfer appears to be diffusion limited, thereby indicating the existence of a specific O_2 transport mechanism in the placenta.

The effect of one of the drugs, diphenhydramine, which interacts with cytochrome p-450, is shown in Figure 6. Initially in this experiment $\Delta PO_2(MV-FV)$ was zero. After two doses of the drug, there was a large decrease in $J_{O_2}/\Delta PO_2$ but no change was observed in $J_{argon}/\Delta P_{argon}$. Further doses of the drug did affect argon transfer slightly but decreased O_2 flux even more. The doses that affected inert gas transfer also caused increases in fetal perfusion pressure. After 160 mg of the drug, the O_2 and argon diffusing capacities were nearly equal. This drug, especially in high doses, affected inert gas transfer as

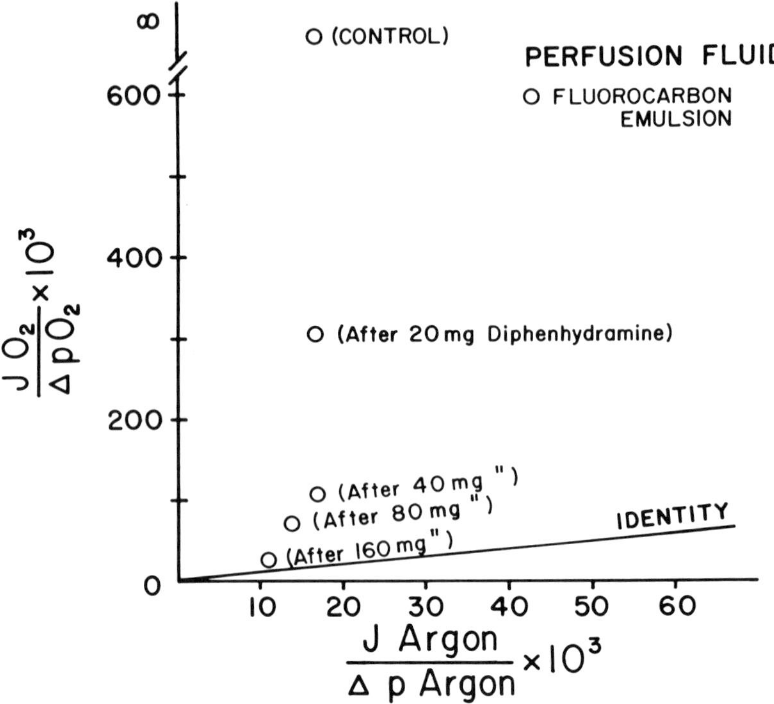

Figure 6. Effect of diphenhydramine, which interacts with cytochrome p-450, on the indices of oxygen and argon diffusing capacity.

well as O_2 transfer. However, in all instances the ratio $(J_{O_2}/\Delta PO_2)/(J_{argon}/\Delta P_{argon})$ decreased after administration of the drug.

In some experiments, we administered some other drugs that interact with cytochrome p-450. These compounds (SKF 525-A, metyrapone, and morphine) decreased $J_{O_2}/\Delta PO_2$ without affecting $J_{argon}/\Delta P_{argon}$. These results in blood perfusion experiments confirm our earlier results obtained during dextran perfusion.

In our previous work, we found that the administration of compounds that interact with cytochrome p-450 selectively decreased transplacental flux of O_2, but did not affect the transplacental flux of the inert gas argon. These results are certainly consistent with the presence of a specific O_2 carrier in the placenta, but can be explained by another mechanism as follows. Let us assume that normally the transfer of argon and O_2 was perfusion limited (i.e., both gases reached equilibrium between maternal and fetal capillaries in one transit time through the placenta). Since the capacity for O_2 in blood is so much greater than that for argon, a generalized decrease in the permeability of the placenta, such as might be caused by administration of a noxious agent, would be manifested initially by a decrease in O_2 transfer. The transfer of argon would be affected only with more severe decreases in permeability. Although it seemed unlikely that such a condition could exist in reality, we could not rule it out by our previous experiments.

The present experiments seem to eliminate this possibility. If the transfer of argon were perfusion limited, we should have observed that $J_{argon}/\Delta P_{argon}$ increased as the solubility of the gas increased in the fetal and maternal blood, and that equilibrium might be reached between maternal and fetal venous blood. The experimental results showed that this did not occur for argon, but did occur for O_2.

The transfer of argon did not change as the solubility for the gas increased in the maternal and fetal perfusion fluids. Thus, the rate limiting step in argon transfer appears to be the relatively small permeability of the placenta to this gas. If the transfer of inert gases is diffusion limited, any generalized decrease in permeability would have caused decreases in inert gas transfer as well as O_2 transfer.

In contrast to argon, the transfer of O_2 appears to be perfusion limited. In 11 instances, PO_2 was the same in maternal and fetal venous blood. This is reflected in Figure 6 as a value of infinity for $J_{O_2}/\Delta PO_2$. This never occurred for argon and probably means that O_2 comes to equilibrium between fetal and maternal capillaries in one pass through the placenta whereas argon does not. Venous equilibrium can only occur when there is a negligible shunt or variation in $\dot{Q}_M/\dot{Q}_F$ ratios throughout the placenta. This appeared to occur fairly frequently and may be related to the use of Dibenzyline in the fetal perfusion fluid. As described above, this drug caused a marked decrease in perfusion pressure at constant flow.

In the remaining experiments, the other factors could cause $\Delta PO_2(MV-FV)$ to be different from zero; however, $J_{O_2}/\Delta PO_2(MV-FV)$ increased as the O_2 carrying capacity of the perfusion fluid increased, indicating that the rate limiting process was the delivery and removal of O_2 and not transplacental diffusion of the gas.

The observation that PO_2 was sometimes the same in umbilical and uterine veins appears to disagree with the observations made by other investigators, who measured the relationship in intact fetal lambs. They found that the PO_2 in the umbilical vein was always lower than in the uterine vein (Meschia, 1972). These observations appear to be species related since there are no such venous PO_2 differences in the fetal foal (Silver and Comline, 1972). There is evidence that normally there is a considerable amount of shunted blood in the sheep placenta. As mentioned above, we found that administration of the α-adrenergic blocker caused large decreases in perfusion pressure at constant fetal blood flow rate. It seems possible that administration of the drug caused a physiologically abnormal state in which there was a substantial decrease in shunt flow and a similar decrease in the nonuniformity of the distribution of maternal and fetal blood flow. At any rate, it is difficult to ascertain if there really is a discordance of experimental results since the experimental situations are different.

The effect of a drug that interacts with cytochrome p-450 is most clearly shown in the experiment depicted in Figure 6. Initially, there was equilibrium for O_2 between maternal and fetal venous blood. The first two doses caused a marked decrease in $J_{O_2}/\Delta PO_2$ while not affecting $J_{argon}/\Delta P_{argon}$. Further doses affected argon transfer, but always brought the indices of diffusing capacity closer to one another. We believe that this type of experiment demonstrates the specific effect on O_2 transfer of compounds that interact with liver cytochrome p-450. Since argon transfer appears to be diffusion limited, nonspecific effects of the drug on membrane permeability would have affected argon transfer as well.

ACKNOWLEDGMENTS
The authors acknowledge the expert technical assistance of Mr. A.M. Sciuto and the assistance of Mrs. Brenda Jordan in the preparation of the manuscript.

References

Ayash, R., Sybert, A., and Gurtner, G.H. 1978. Saturation kinetics for steady state pulmonary CO transfer in man. *Am. Rev. Respir. Dis.* 117:310.

Bissonnette, J.M. and Gurtner, G. 1972. The transfer of inert gases and tritiated water across the sheep placenta. *J. Appl. Physiol.* 32:64–69.

Cerretelli, P. 1980. *Exercise Bioenergetics and Gas Exchange.* Cerretelli, P. and Whipp, B.J., eds. Amsterdam: Elsevier North Holland.

Evans, J.W. and Wagner, P.D. 1977. Limits on $\dot{V}A/\dot{Q}$ distributions from analysis of experimental inert gas elimination. *J. Appl. Physiol.* 42:889–898.

Farhi, L.E. 1967. Elimination of inert gas by the lung. *Respir. Physiol.* 3:1–11.

Farhi, L.E. and Yokoyama, T. 1967. Effects of ventilation-perfusion inequality on elimination of inert gases. *Respir. Physiol.* 3:12–20.

Gurtner, G. 1980. Evidence for facilitated transport of oxygen and carbon dioxide. In *Pulmonary Gas Exchange. Vol. II. Organism and Environment.* West, J., ed. New York: Academic Press. pp. 205–239.

Gurtner, G.H. and Burns, B. 1971. A possible facilitated transport of O_2 and CO_2 across the sheep placenta. *Physiologist* 14:155.

Gurtner, G.H. and Burns, B. 1972. Possible facilitated transport of oxygen across the placenta. *Nature* 240:473–475.

Gurtner, G.H. and Burns, B. 1975. Physiological evidence consistent with the presence of specific O_2 carrier in the placenta. *J. Appl. Physiol.* 39:728–734.

Gurtner, G., Burns, B., Peavy, H., Mendoza, C.J., Summer, W., Sciuto, A.M., and Traystman, R.J. 1978. Specific mechanisms for O_2 and CO transport in the lung and placenta. In *Regulation of Ventilation and Gas Exchange. Research Topics in Physiology. Vol. 1.* Davies, D.J. and Barnes, C.J., eds. New York: Academic Press. pp. 197–215.

Hlastala, M.P. and Robertson, H.T. 1978. Inert gas elimination characteristics of the normal and abnormal lung. *J. Appl. Physiol.* 44:258–266.

Holland, R.A. 1981. Kinetics of O_2 and CO reactions in blood. *Prog. Respir. Res.* 16:152–157.

Knoblauch, A., Sybert, A., Brennan, N.J., Sylvester, J.T., and Gurtner, G. 1981. The effect of hypoxia and CO on a cytochrome p-450 mediated reaction in the lung. *J. Appl. Physiol.*, in press.

Mendoza, C., Peavy, H., Burns, B., and Gurtner, G. 1977. Saturation kinetics for steady-state pulmonary CO transfer. *J. Appl. Physiol.* 43:880–884.

Meschia, G. 1972. Normal exchange of respiratory gases across the sheep placenta. In *Respiratory Gas Exchange and Blood Flow in the Placenta*. Longo, L. and Bartels, H., eds. DHEW Publ. NIH-73-361. Bethesda, Maryland: National Institutes of Health. pp. 229–242.

Neufeld, G.R., Williams, J.J., Klineberg, P.L., and Marshall, B.E. 1978. Inert gas a-A differences: A direct reflection of $\dot{V}/\dot{Q}$ distribution. *J. Appl. Physiol.* 44:277–283.

Piiper, J. 1962. O_2-exchange of the isolated dog lung in the hypoxic region with changes in erythrocyte concentration and circulation. *Pflügers Arch.* 275:193–214.

Piiper, J., Cerretelli, P., Rennie, D.W., and Di Prampero, P.E. 1971. Estimation of the pulmonary diffusing capacity for O_2 by a rebreathing procedure. *Resp. Physiol.* 12:157–162.

Piiper, J. and Scheid, P. 1980. Blood gas equilibration in lungs. In *Pulmonary Gas Exchange. Vol. 1. Ventilation, Blood Flow, and Diffusion*. West, J.B., ed. New York: Academic Press. pp. 131–171.

Riley, R.L. and Cournand, A. 1949. Ideal alveolar air and the analysis of ventilation-perfusion relationships in lungs. *J. Appl. Physiol.* 1:825–847.

Roughton, F.J. and Forster, R.E. 1957. Relative importance of diffusion and chemical reaction rates of gases in determining rate of exchange of gases in the human lung, with special reference to true diffusing capacity of pulmonary membrane and volume of blood in the lung capillaries. *J. Appl. Physiol.* 11:290–302.

Silver, M. and Comline, R.S. 1972. Some observations on the umbilical circulation of the foal compared with the ruminant. In *Respiratory Gas Exchange and Blood Flow in the Placenta*. Longo, L. and Bartels, H., eds. DHEW Publ. NIH-73-361. Bethesda, Maryland: National Institutes of Health. pp. 113–120.

Staub, N.C., Bishop, J.M., and Forster, R.E. 1962. Importance of diffusion and chemical reaction rates in O_2 uptake in the lung. *J. Appl. Physiol.* 17:21–27.

Sylvester, J.T., Cymerman, A., Gurtner, G., Hottenstein, O., Cotte, M., and Wolfe, D. 1981. Components of the O_2 gradient during rest and exercise at sea level and high altitude. *J. Appl. Physiol.* 50:1129–1139.

Wagner, P.D., Saltzman, H.A., and West, J.B. 1974. Measurement of continuous distributions of ventilation-perfusion ratios: theory. *J. Appl. Physiol.* 36:588–599.

Wagner, W.W., Jr. and Latham, L.P. 1975. Pulmonary capillary recruitment during airway hypoxia in the dog. *J. Appl. Physiol.* 39:900–905.

Wanner, A., Begin, R., Cohn, M., and Sackner, M.A. 1978. Vascular volumes of the pulmonary circulation in intact dogs. *J. Appl. Physiol.* 44:956–963.

J.A. Loeppky and M.L. Riedesel, editors
OXYGEN TRANSPORT TO HUMAN TISSUES

The Mechanism of Hypoxic Pulmonary Vasoconstriction: A Working Hypothesis

Ivan F. McMurtry, Hilary S. Stanbrook, and Sharon Rounds

Introduction

Studies of vasomotor control of the pulmonary circulation by Openchowski (1882) and Bradford and Dean (1894) led to the first observations related, at least circumstantially, to the mechanism of hypoxic pulmonary vasoconstriction. These investigators found that asphyxia in open chest dogs increased pulmonary arterial pressure independently of changes in left atrial and systemic arterial pressures. Later, Plumier (1904) observed an increase in pulmonary arterial pressure when dogs breathed hydrogen instead of air, and published what may be the first recording of an hypoxic pressor response. The report opening the floodgate of research into the mechanism of hypoxic vasoconstriction was of course that of Euler and Liljestrand (1946). Suggesting that effects of blood gases on pulmonary arterial pressure merited special interest because of the gas exchanging function of the lung, they showed in cats that an FIO_2 of 10% caused a pulmonary pressor response without an appreciable change in either left atrial or systemic arterial pressure. They suggested that local hypoxia had opposite effects on systemic and pulmonary vascular tone, but that in each case the respective response, systemic vasodilation, and pulmonary vasoconstriction, was homeostatic in that it helped maintain oxygen transport from atmospheric air to respiring body tissues. The interesting question of whether the opposite effects of local hypoxia on the two circulations is due to differences in vasoactive substances released from the respective parenchyma or to inherent differences in the response of the respective vascular smooth muscle remains unanswered. While it is now agreed that matching of capillary perfusion and alveolar ventilation is a major determinant of the lung's ability to arterialize venous blood and that mismatching of these variables is a common cause of hypoxemia in man with lung disease (West 1977), the importance of local hypoxic vasoconstriction in determining the ventilation/perfusion ratio is controversial. In a recent review, Hughes (1977) has concluded that although the hypoxic mechanism is not used to any significant degree to adjust perfusion to ventilation in normal man, "...the contribution of local vasoconstriction to the improvement of local and overall gas exchange is of some importance..." in cases of lung disease. Further interest in the hypoxic pressor response was generated by the discovery that chronic, generalized airway hypoxia, such as that induced by residence at high altitude or by certain lung diseases, can cause severe pulmonary hypertension, pulmonary vascular thickening, and right heart failure (Grover, 1965; Harris and Heath, 1977). In addition, hypoxic vasoconstriction is a major cause of the high pulmonary vascular resistance and resultant shunting of blood flow from the unventilated fetal lung (Rudolph et al., 1977). Thus, research into the mechanism of hypoxia pulmonary vasoconstriction is relevant to our understanding of the physiology and pathology of pulmonary vascular control, the effects of hypoxia on the physiology of vascular smooth muscle and the biochemistry of tissue oxygen sensing.

Review of Mechanism of Hypoxic Pulmonary Vasoconstriction

Numerous reviews of hypoxic pulmonary vasoconstriction have been published in the past 12 years (Staub, 1969; Hauge, 1970; Barer, 1976; Fishman, 1976; Severinghaus, 1977; Bergofsky, 1979; Reeves et al., 1979). Hypoxic vasoconstriction exists to one degree or another in every mammalian and avian species that has been tested. There is also evidence that it occurs in some reptiles and amphibians (Johansen, 1979). Although the magnitude of the pressor response is influenced in intact animals by cardiac output, left atrial pressure, and neural and humoral signals of systemic origin, the basic mechanism relating the oxygen sensor-transduction process and effector is intrapulmonary since hypoxic vasoconstriction occurs in isolated lungs perfused with cell-free perfusates. Although there is little doubt that smooth muscle of peripheral pulmonary arteries or arterioles is the effector, the site and nature of the oxygen sensor and the series of events which converts sensing of hypoxia into contraction of vascular smooth muscle are unknown. There is no conclusive evidence, but general opinion is that vasoconstriction is caused either by a direct excitatory effect of hypoxia on the vascular smooth muscle or by an hypoxia-induced release of a chemical mediator from extravascular lung tissue, e.g., from mast cells, neuroepithelial bodies, autonomic nerve endings, or other parenchymal cells (or possibly from the vascular endothelium as proposed by Singer et al., 1981). In addition to these possibilities, it has recently been suggested that perhaps the constriction should be viewed as being allowed by an hypoxia-induced decrease in release or activity of a vasodilator, rather than caused by elaboration of a vasoconstrictor (Weir, 1978). Furthermore, it has been proposed that the pressor response is due to contraction of alveolar septal cells rather than of vascular smooth muscle (Kapanci et al., 1974). Regardless of the cellular locus of the oxygen sensor, there is indirect evidence that the underlying action of hypoxia is to decrease the rate of oxidative phosphorylation, i.e., cytochrome oxidase of some lung cell is the molecular oxygen sensor (Lloyd, 1964, 1965; Fishman, 1976). On the other hand, it is also possible that an extra-mitochondrial, oxygen-sensitive molecule or biochemical reaction acts as the sensor (Jobsis, 1977; Sylvester and McGowan, 1978). Even though the site and nature of the oxygen sensor are unknown, it is likely that an increased level of cytosolic calcium is a necessary component of the transduction process between sensor and effector, i.e., increased cytosolic calcium is an integral event in both excitation-secretion and excitation-contraction coupling (Rasmussen and Goodman, 1977). An increased level of free calcium could be due to release from intracellular pools, to decreased sequestration and extrusion by the cell, or to an increased influx across the plasma membrane that might be associated with depolarization.

Working Hypothesis for Mechanism of Hypoxic Vasoconstriction

We have formulated the working hypothesis shown in Figure 1 to study the mechanism of hypoxic pulmonary vasoconstriction. The rationale is based primarily on the following evidence. Despite examination of numerous candidates, e.g., catecholamines, histamine, serotonin, angiotensin II, bradykinin, acetylcholine, vasopressin, prostaglandins, lactic acid, and ATP, there is no convincing support for involvement of a unique chemical mediator (Fishman, 1976; Bergofsky, 1979). An extravascular oxygen sensor is apparently not necessary since oxygenation of the peripheral pulmonary arterial wall is determined by airway oxygen tension (Conhaim and Staub, 1980). Although hypoxia generally has no effect on or relaxes isolated vascular smooth muscle, it causes contraction under some *in vitro* conditions (Paul, 1980). The chemical inhibitors of oxidative phosphorylation, cyanide, and 2,4-dinitrophenol, mimic hypoxia by eliciting pulmonary vasoconstriction (Lloyd, 1964, 1965). It is possible that hypoxic depression of mitochondrial oxidative phosphorylation alters concentrations of various metabolites, e.g., lowers the ratio (ATP/ADP$\cdot$ P_i), without decreasing the supply of ATP to the contractile machinery of vascular smooth muscle (Honig, 1968; Wilson et al., 1979). Alterations in concentrations of metabolites other than ATP might influence plasma membrane ion permeability or pump activity (Horn, 1978). A low degree of $K+$ conductance activation in the plasma membrane might allow such changes to lead to depolarization, calcium influx, and contraction (Harder and Sperelakis, 1978). We have begun to test this working hypothesis (Figure 1) by examining the questions: (1) is hypoxic pulmonary vasoconstriction dependent on increased influx of extracellular calcium, (2) is the underlying action of hypoxia

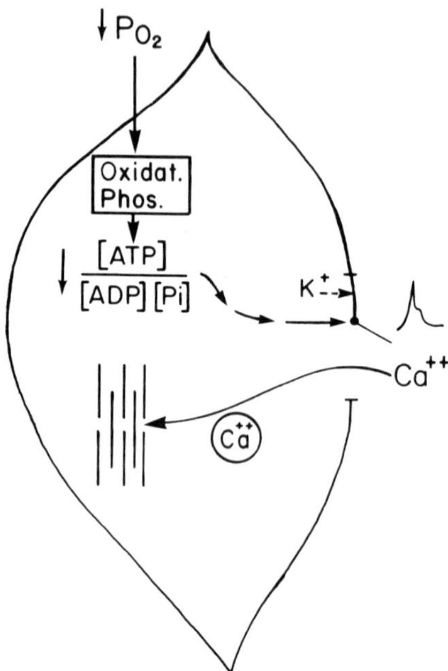

Figure 1. A working hypothesis for mechanism of hypoxic pulmonary vasoconstriction. It is proposed that hypoxia acts directly on smooth muscle of small, peripheral arteries reducing the rate of mitochondrial oxidative phosphorylation and the cytosolic [ATP]/[ADP][Pi] ratio. The decrease in phosphate potential (or change in level of some other metabolite) then leads to membrane depolarization, calcium influx, and contraction. Depolarization and calcium influx are allowed to reach a regenerative level because of a low degree of K+ conductance activation in the plasma membrane.

to depress the rate of oxidative phosphorylation, and (3) is the hypoxic contraction of vascular smooth muscle in the presence of inhibitors of K+ conductance an acceptable *in vitro* model of hypoxic pulmonary vasoconstriction?

Dependence of Hypoxic Vasoconstriction on Calcium Influx

To test the idea that hypoxic vasoconstriction is dependent on influx of extracellular calcium, we have examined the effect of the so-called calcium antagonist or slow channel blocker, verapamil (Nayler and Poole-Wilson, 1981), on pressor responses to hypoxia, angiotensin II, and prostaglandin $F_{2\alpha}$ in isolated rat lungs (McMurtry et al., 1976). Since neither saralasin, an antagonist of angiotensin II, nor meclofenamate, an inhibitor of prostaglandin synthesis, prevented hypoxic vasoconstriction, we reasoned that neither angiotensin II nor prostaglandin $F_{2\alpha}$ was a mediator of the hypoxic mechanism and that they could be used as reference agonists to judge relative susceptibility to inhibition by verapamil. The results showed that verapamil inhibited pressor responses to hypoxia more readily than responses to the pharmacologicical stimuli. Suggett et al. (1980) reported similar findings with lungs from both rats and ferrets, and Tucker et al. (1976) found in dogs that verapamil reduced the pulmonary pressor response to hypoxia, but not that to prostaglandin $F_{2\alpha}$. We have also observed that increasing the level of calcium in the perfusate of rat lungs inhibits subsequent pressor responses to hypoxia more severely than those to angiotensin II (McMurtry et al., 1980; Rounds and McMurtry, 1981). In addition, a bolus injection of either verapamil or calcium into the arterial line during an hypoxic response causes immediate reversal of the vasoconstriction, i.e., there is rapid relaxation of the vascular smooth muscle despite continued exposure to hypoxia (Figure 2). Other studies show that treatment with verapamil decreases development of right ventricular hypertrophy in rats exposed chronically to simulated high altitude (Davidson et al., 1978; Kentera et al., 1979). In summary, since both verapamil and high extracellular calcium are thought to "stabilize" the membrane and reduce influx of extracellular calcium, these results suggest that the hypoxic mechanism is critically dependent on an increased rate of calcium influx, i.e., calcium influx is a necessary component of the transduction process which couples sensing of hypoxia to contraction of vascular smooth muscle. This finding is consistent with our working hypothesis (Figure 1), but does not indicate whether calcium influx is mediating release of a vasoconstrictor or a direct action of hypoxia on the smooth muscle.

Figure 2. Hypoxic ($FIO_2 = 3\%$) vasoconstriction in blood-perfused rat lung is rapidly reversed by return to normoxic ventilation (top tracing) or by injection of verapamil into arterial line (bottom tracing). Since verapamil acts primarily by inhibiting calcium influx, the rapid relaxation suggests that hypoxia leads to increased membrane permeability, rather than to decreased intracellular sequestration or extrusion.

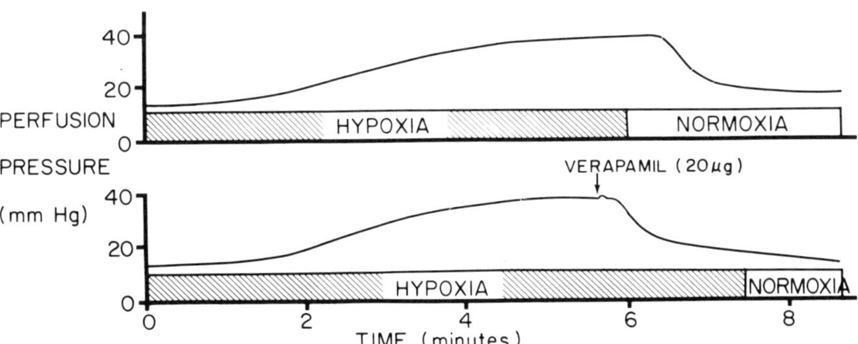

Initiation of Hypoxic Vasoconstriction by Depression of Oxidative Phosphorylation

The possibility that hypoxic vasoconstriction is initiated by a decreased rate of mitochondrial oxidative phosphorylation stems largely from the fact that reduction of molecular oxygen by cytochrome oxidase accounts for the majority of total cellular oxygen use, and from Lloyd's (1964, and 1965) finding that cyanide and 2,4-dinitrophenol cause vasoconstriction in dog lungs. To test this possibility further, we reasoned that if several, chemically different inhibitors all elicited pulmonary pressor responses, then it would be more likely that depression of oxidative phosphorylation, and not other actions of the chemicals, accounted for the vasoconstriction (Rounds and McMurtry, 1981). We found in isolated rat lungs that each of four inhibitors of electron transport, antimycin A, azide, cyanide, and rotenone, and one uncoupler of electron transport from phosphorylation, 2,4-dinitrophenol, caused a transient pressor response that was readily blocked by verapamil or high extracellular calcium (Figure 3). The metabolic inhibitors also led, in time, to blunting of vascular reactivity. Severe airway hypoxia has also been observed to elicit transient pressor responses and to reduce reactivity to other agonists (Harabin et al., 1981). Lower concentrations of cyanide and dinitrophenol than those used in our study caused sustained pressor responses and did not reduce reactivity to other vasoconstrictors in Lloyd's (1964, 1965) studies. Assuming that the one

Figure 3. Pressor responses (mean ± S.E.) in blood-perfused rat lungs following addition of antimycin (ATM, 5 to 10 μM), azide (AZ, 10 mM), cyanide (CN, 1 mM), dinitrophenol (DNP, 1 mM), or rotenone (ROT, 0.5 μM) to the perfusate reservior. Responses to airway hypoxia (HYP, 0 to 3% O_2) and to intraarterial angiotensin II (A-II, 0.5 μg) are also shown. Open bars are responses in control lungs and solid bars are those in lungs perfused with blood to which either verapamil (22 μM) or high calcium (10 mM) was added. Verapamil and calcium were added to an equal number of lungs in each group. Number in parentheses under each bar is sample size.

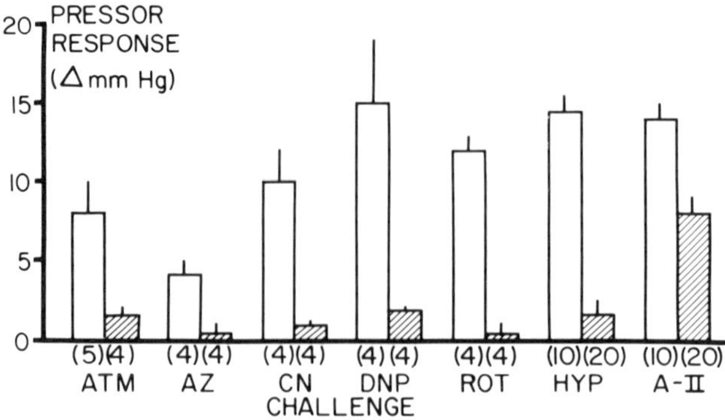

action shared by hypoxia, antimycin, azide, cyanide, rotenone, and dinitrophenol is to reduce mitochondrial oxidative phosphorylation, a possible interpretation of these findings is that while moderate depression signals vasoconstriction, severe inhibition lends to vasodilation. However, since chemical inhibitors are rarely, if ever, specific, further experiments involving direct measurements of tissue energy and redox states are required to substantiate this concept.

In many tissues, an increased rate of anaerobic glycolysis buffers the metabolic effects of decreased mitochondrial oxidative phosphorylation. Therefore, if a functional response is initiated by depression of oxidative phosphorylation, then one might expect the response to be attenuated by increased glycolysis. This reasoning led us to propose that if hypoxic vasoconstriction was signaled by depression of oxidative phosphorylation, then pressor sensitivity to airway hypoxia might be increased by inhibition of glycolysis (Stanbrook and McMurtry, 1981). We measured hypoxic dose-response curves in rat lungs perfused with blood that had been preequilibrated with an inhibitor of glycolysis, iodoacetate, or 2-deoxyglucose. Lungs exposed to either inhibitor showed greater responses to less severe hypoxia than did their respective controls. Additional experiments have shown that lungs perfused with a glucose-free, salt-albumin solution containing meclofenamate are more sensitive to airway hypoxia than are those perfused with the same solution containing glucose (Figure 4). The dose-pressor response curve to angiotensin II was not similarly affected. Since perfusate lactate accumulation was less in inhibitor-treated than in control lungs (Stanbrook and McMurtry, 1981) and since glucose-free perfusion reduces glycolysis in isolated rat lungs (Kerr et al., 1979), these results indicate that inhibition of glycolysis increases pressor sensitivity to hypoxia. This finding provides further indirect support for the idea that depression of mitochondrial oxidative phosphorylation is the initiating signal for hypoxic vasoconstriction.

The above results are consistent with our working hypothesis (Figure 1), but they do not differentiate between a direct effect of hypoxia on the vascular smooth muscle or on some other lung tissue. Since smooth muscle contraction is ATP-dependent, it could be argued that the postulated decrease in oxidative phosphorylation would likely occur in an extravascular, highly oxygen-dependent tissue and be linked to vasoconstriction by release of a mediator. However, Wilson et al. (1979) have found that hypoxia within the physiological range of oxygen tension reduces the rate of mitochondrial oxidative phosphorylation and leads to decreases in intramitochondrial [NAD+]/[NADH] and cytosolic [ATP]/[ADP] [Pi], but not in cellular [ATP]. This observation makes it possible to argue that some metabolic effect of an hypoxic depression of oxidative phosphorylation in the smooth muscle of the peripheral pulmonary arteries might lead to excitation of the cell without limiting energy supply to the contractile machinery.

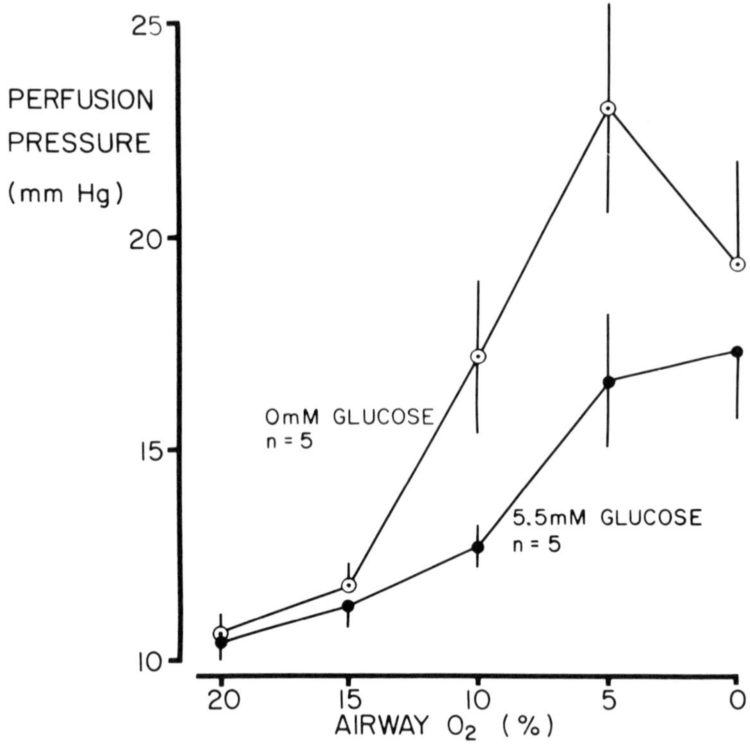

Figure 4. Successive pressor responses (mean ±S.E.) to increasing airway hypoxia are greater in rat lungs perfused with glucose-free perfusate than in those perfused with the same solution containing 5.5 mM glucose.

Development of *In Vitro* Model of Hypoxic Vasoconstriction

Elucidation of the mechanism of hypoxic pulmonary vasoconstriction will require studies of intact animals, isolated lungs, and *in vitro* preparations. The physiology and pharmacology of the first two preparations are fairly well-understood, but a reasonable *in vitro* model of hypoxic vasoconstriction has not been established. If the hypoxic pressor response is due either to direct excitation of the vascular smooth muscle or to release of a constrictor from the parenchyma, then it should be theoretically possible to elicit hypoxic contraction in a segment of pulmonary artery isolated either with or without an adherent layer of lung tissue. The level of the pulmonary arterial bed undergoing hypoxic constriction has not been identified precisely, but the response is apparently located somewhere between major lobar arteries and capillaries (Kato and Staub, 1966; Dawson et al., 1979; Allison and Stanbrook, 1980). Although the pharmacologic reactivity of small, distal pulmonary arteries has been examined *in vitro* (Su et al., 1978), there are no reports as to whether vascular segments distal to the lobar artery show hypoxic contraction either with or without adherent parenchyma. This deficiency is due to the technical difficulty of isolating small arterial branches in a physiological manner, and it may be necessary to establish an *in vitro* model with vascular smooth muscle other than that undergoing hypoxic contraction in the lung. Lloyd (1968) observed that strips of rabbit lobar artery with adherent parenchyma showed hypoxic contractions after more than 60 min of incubation in a substrate-free fluorochemical and subsequent exposure to hypoxia in a mixture of plasma and physiological salt solution. He also found that exposing the tissue to procaine facilitated development of the hypoxic contractions. The enthusiasm for this preparation as a model of hypoxic pulmonary vasoconstriction was dampened by latter findings that parenchyma-free strips in a humid-gas environment also showed increases in isometric tension when made hypoxic (Lloyd, 1970), and by reports that the hypoxia-induced increase in isometric tension of substrate-free smooth muscle is probably caused by formation of rigor linkages, rather than by a calcium-triggered interaction of the myofilaments (Bose, 1976). However, the facilitation by procaine may provide a clue to the problem of developing a valid *in vitro* model.

Hypoxia generally either does not alter or reduce the tone of isolated vascular smooth muscle, but it causes contraction under certain *in vitro* conditions. For instance, Shepherd and Vanhoutte (1975) reported that hypoxia contracted dog cutaneous veins in the presence of $BaCl_2$, and, as mentioned above, Lloyd (1968) found that procaine enhanced development of hypoxic contractions in rabbit pulmonary artery-parechyma strips. Since both barium and procaine inhibit membrane $K+$ conductance (Harder and Sperelakis, 1978; Horn, 1978; Keatinge, 1978), we investigated whether tetraethylammonium (TEA), a widely used inhibitor of the outward $K+$ current (Harder and Sperelakis, 1978; Horn, 1978), would also allow hypoxic contractions by isolated vascular smooth muscle (McMurtry and Keatinge, 1980). Rings of rat thoracic aorta and sheep carotid artery were studied in a physiologic salt solution (Hansen and Bohr, 1975) aerated by 95% O_2 and 5% CO_2 at 37°C. Hypoxia (aeration by 95% N_2 and 5% CO_2) did not alter resting tension and reduced the active tension induced by 20 mM $K+$ or by 10^{-8} M norepinephrine. However, after 1 to 5 mM TEA was added to the muscle bath, hypoxia caused contractions of both the aortic and carotid artery rings (Figure 5). Antimycin, cyanide, and rotenone also elicited contractions after, but not before, addition of TEA to the salt solution aerated with 95% O_2 and 5% CO_2. The contractions were not blocked by the α-adrenergic antagonist, phentolamine, but were inhibited by verapamil. Similar hypoxic contractions were also observed occasionally with rings of rat main pulmonary artery in the presence of TEA. These preliminary results suggest that inhibition of plasma membrane $K+$ conductance alters the excitability of vascular smooth muscle in some manner that allows expression of a calcium-dependent contractile response to

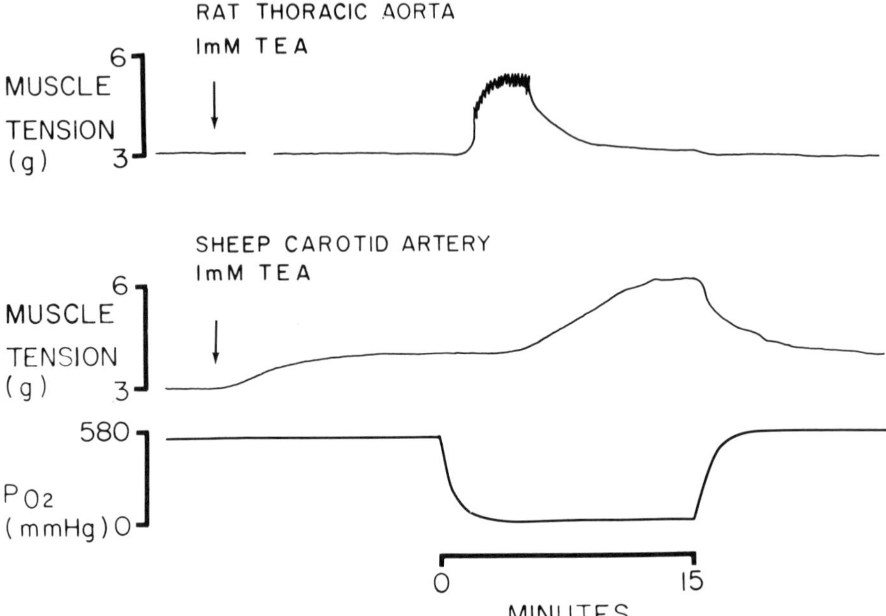

Figure 5. After addition of tetraethylammonium (TEA) to physiologic salt solution, hypoxia (aeration with 95% N_2 and 5% CO_2 instead of with 95% O_2 and 5% CO_2, bottom tracing) elicits transient, rhythmic contraction of rat thoracic aorta (top tracing) and more sustained, less rhythmic contraction of sheep carotid artery (middle tracing). Tracings of muscle tension are from separate experiments.

hypoxia. Further experiments are required to determine if hypoxic contraction is due to a direct effect on the smooth muscle or is mediated by release of a constrictor from the endothelium (Singer et al., 1981).

To be considered a valid *in vitro* model of hypoxic pulmonary vasoconstriction, vascular smooth muscle treated with an inhibitor of K+ conductance should behave much like the isolated lung. It should undergo a moderately rapid, well-sustained, readily reversible contractile response to hypoxia. Contraction should be elicited by hypoxia, rather than only by anoxia, and, ideally muscle tone would be inversely related to oxygen tension over a certain range. Chemical inhibitors of oxidative phosphorylation would also be expected to elicit contraction, and inhibition of glycolysis should potentiate the hypoxic response. The hypoxic contraction should be readily inhibited by verapamil and by a moderate decrease in temperature. It should not be mediated, but possibly modulated, by catecholamines, histamine, serotonin, acetylcholine, angiotensin II, and prostaglandins. The finding of strong similarity between hypoxic vasoconstriction in isolated lungs and hypoxic contraction of vascular smooth muscle exposed to inhibitors of K+ conductance will clearly not prove the identity of the two mechanisms, but it will provide a reasonable *in vitro* model with which to determine if and how hypoxia alters the interactions among energy metabolism, membrane potential, calcium kinetics, and tone.

Summary

The mechanism by which airway hypoxia causes pulmonary arterial constriction is unknown. General opinion is that hypoxia either stimulates directly the smooth muscle or peripheral pulmonary arteries or elicits release of a constrictor from the parenchyma. We are testing the working hypothesis that hypoxia acts directly on the vascular smooth muscle depressing mitochondrial oxidative phosphorylation and causing shifts in cytosolic metabolite concentrations which lead to membrane depolarization, calcium influx, and contraction. The results of studies in isolated lungs with pharmacologic inhibitors of oxidative phosphorylation, glycolysis, and calcium influx are consistent with this hypothesis, but a preparation allowing direct measurements of energy metabolism, calcium kinetics, and electrical activity is needed. Inhibitors of K+ conductance allow hypoxic contractions by isolated vascular smooth muscle, and such preparations may be valid *in vitro* models of hypoxic pulmonary vasoconstriction.

ACKNOWLEDGMENTS
We thank Sharon Barrett, Michele Jones, and Eva Toyos for their help in preparing this manuscript. Our work has been supported intellectually and technically by the faculty and staff of the CVP Research Laboratory and financially by USPHS Grants HL14985 and F32HL05036, and by Grants from the Burroughs Wellcome Fund and the Parker B. Francis Foundation.

References

Allison, D.J. and Stanbrook, H.S. 1980. A radiologic and physiologic investigation into hypoxic pulmonary vasoconstriction in the dog. *Invest. Radiol.* 15:178–190.

Barer, G.R. 1976. The physiology of the pulmonary circulation and methods of study. *Pharmacol. Ther. B.* 2:247–273.

Bergofsky, E.H. 1979. Active control of the normal pulmonary circulation. In *Pulmonary Vascular Diseases.* Moser, K.M., ed. New York: Marcel Dekker.

Bose, D. 1976. Increase in resting tension of tracheal muscle due to rigor during metabolic inhibition. *Am. J. Physiol.* 231:1470–1475.

Bradford, J.R. and Dean, H.P. 1894. The pulmonary circulation. *J. Physiol. (London).* 16:34–96.

Conhaim, R.L. and Staub, N.C. 1980. Reflection spectrophotometric measurement of O_2 uptake in pulmonary arterioles of cats. *J. Appl. Physiol.* 48:848–856.

Davidson, A., McMurtry, I.F., and Reeves, J.T. 1978. Pulmonary vascular effects of verapamil. *Am. Heart J.* 95:810–811.

Dawson, C.A., Grimm, D.J., and Linehan, J.H. 1979. Lung inflation and longitudinal distribution of pulmonary vascular resistance during hypoxia. *J. Appl. Physiol.* 47:532–536.

Euler, U.S.v. and Liljestrand, G. 1946. Observations on the pulmonary arterial blood pressure in the cat. *Acta Physiol. Scand.* 12:301–320.

Fishman, A.P. 1976. Hypoxia on the pulmonary circulation. How and where it acts. *Circ. Res.* 38:221–231.

Grover, R.F. 1965. Pulmonary circulation in animals and man at high altitude. *Ann. N.Y. Acad. Sci.* 127:632–639.

Hansen, T.R. and Bohr, D.F. 1975. Hypertension, transmural pressure, and vascular smooth muscle response in rats. *Circ. Res.* 36:590–598.

Harabin, A.L., Peake, M.D., and Sylvester, J.T. 1981. Effect of severe hypoxia on the pulmonary vascular response to vasoconstrictor agents. *J. Appl. Physiol.* 50:561–565.

Harder, D.R. and Sperelakis, N. 1978. Membrane electrical properties of vascular smooth muscle from guinea pig superior mesenteric artery. *Pflügers Arch.* 378:111–119.

Harris, P. and Heath, D. 1977. *The Human Pulmonary Circulation. Second Edition.* Edinburgh: Churchill Livingstone.

Hauge, A. 1970. The pulmonary vasconstrictor response to acute hypoxia. Studies on mechanism and site of action. *Progr. Respir. Res.* 5:145–155.

Honig, C.R. 1968. Control of smooth muscle actomyosin by phosphate and 5′AMP: Possible role in metabolic autoregulation. *Microvasc. Res.* 1:133–146.

Horn, L. 1978. Electrophysiology of vascular smooth muscle. In *Microcirculation.* Vol. II. Kaley, G. and Altura, B.M., eds. Baltimore: University Park Press. pp. 119–157.

Hughes, J.M.B. 1977. Local control of blood flow and ventilation. In *Regional Differences in the Lung.* West, J.B., ed. New York: Academic Press. pp. 420–450.

Jobsis, F.F. 1977. What is a molecular oxygen sensor? What is a transduction process? *Adv. Exp. Med. Biol.* 78:3–18.

Johansen, K. 1979. Cardiovascular support of metabolic functions in vertebrates. In *Evolution of Respiratory Processes. A Comparative Approach.* Vol. 13. Wood, S.C. and Lenfant, C., eds. New York: Marcel Dekker. pp. 107–192.

Kapanci, Y., Assimacopoulos, A., Irle, C., Zwahlen, A., and Gabbiani, G. 1974. "Contractile interstitial cells" in pulmonary alveolar septa: a possible regulator of ventilation-perfusion ratio? Ultrastructural immunofluorescence and *in vitro* studies. *J. Cell Biol.* 60:375–392.

Kato, M. and Staub, N.C. 1966. Response of small pulmonary arteries to unilobar hypoxia and hypercapnia. *Circ. Res.* 19:426–440.

Keatinge, W.R. 1978. Mechanism of slow discharges of sheep carotid artery. *J. Physiol. (London).* 279:275–289.

Kentera, D., Susic, D., and Zdravkovic, M. 1979. Effects of verapamil and aspirin on experimental chronic hypoxic pulmonary hypertension and right ventricular hypertrophy in rats. *Respiration* 37:192–196.

Kerr, J.S., Baker, N.J., Bassett, D.J., and Fisher, A.B. 1979. Effect of perfusate glucose concentration on rat lung glycolysis. *Am. J. Physiol.* 236:E229–E233.

Lloyd, T.C., Jr. 1964. Effect of alveolar hypoxia upon pulmonary vascular resistance. *J. Appl. Physiol.* 19:1086–1094.

Lloyd, T.C., Jr. 1965. Pulmonary vasoconstriction during histotoxic hypoxia. *J. Appl. Physiol.* 20:488–490.

Lloyd, T.C., Jr. 1968. Hypoxic pulmonary vasoconstriction: role of perivascular tissue. *J. Appl. Physiol.* 25:560–565.

Lloyd, T.C., Jr. 1970. Responses to hypoxia of pulmonary arterial strips in nonaqueous baths. *J. Appl. Physiol.* 28:566–569.

McMurtry, I.F. Davidson, A.B., Reeves, J.T., and Grover, R.F. 1976. Inhibition of hypoxic pulmonary vasoconstriction by calcium antagonists in isolated rat lungs. *Circ. Res.* 38:99–104.

McMurtry, I.F. and Keatinge, W.R. 1980. Hypoxia contracts vascular smooth muscle treated with tetraethylammonium. *Physiologist* 23:61.

McMurtry, I.F., Morris, K.G., and Petrun, M.D. 1980. Blunted hypoxic vasoconstriction in lungs from short-term high altitude rats. *Am. J. Physiol.* 238:H849–H857.

Nayler, W.R. and Poole-Wilson, P.H. 1981. Calcium antagonists: definition and mode of action. *Basic Res. Cardiol.* 76:1–15.

Openchowski, T. 1882. Über die druckverhaltnisse im kleinen kreislaufe. *Pflügers Arch. Physiol.* 27:233–266.

Paul, R.J. 1980. Chemical energetics of vascular smooth muscle. In *Handbook of Physiology, Sec. 2: The Cardiovascular System, Vol. II. Vascular Smooth Muscle.* Bohr, D.F., Somlyo, A. P., and Sparks, H.V., Jr., eds. Baltimore: Williams and Wilkens. pp. 201–235.

Plumier, L. 1904. La circulation pulmonaire chez le chein. *Arch. Int. Physiol.* 1:176–213.

Rasmussen, H. and Goodman, D.B.P. 1977. Relationships between calcium and cyclic nucleotides in cell activation. *Physiol. Rev.* 57:421–509.

Reeves, J.T., Wagner, W.W., Jr., McMurtry, I.F., and Grover, R.F. 1979. Physiological effects of high altitude on the pulmonary circulation. *Int. Rev. Physiol.* 20:289–310.

Rounds, S. and McMurtry, I.F. 1981. Inhibitors of oxidative ATP production cause transient vasoconstriction and block subsequent pressor responses in rat lungs. *Circ. Res.* 48:393–400.

Rudolph, A.M., Heymann, M.A. and Lewis, A.B. 1977. Physiology and pharmacology of the pulmonary circulation in the fetus and newborn. In *Development of the Lung.* Hodson, W.A., ed. New York: Marcel Dekker.

Severinghaus, J.W. 1977. Pulmonary vascular function. *Am. Rev. Respir. Dis.* 115:149–158.

Shepherd, J.T. and Vanhoutte, P.M. 1975. *Veins and Their Control.* Philadelphia: W.B. Saunders.

Singer, H.A., Wagner, J.D., Duling, B. and Peach, M.J. 1981. Endothelial-smooth muscle interactions in rabbit thoracic aorta: muscarinic relaxation and hypoxia-induced contraction. *Fed. Proc.* 40:689.

Stanbrook, H.S. and McMurtry, I.F. 1981. Inhibitors of glycolysis potentiate the hypoxic pressor response in isolated rat lungs. *Fed. Proc.* 40:504.

Staub, N.C. 1969. Respiration. *Ann. Rev. Physiol.* 31:173–202.

Su, C., Bevan, R.D., Duckles, S.P., and Bevan, J.A. 1978. Functional studies of the small pulmonary arteries. *Microvasc. Res.* 15:37–44.

Suggett, A.J., Mohammed, F.H., and Barer, G.R. 1980. Angiotensin, hypoxia, verapamil, and pulmonary vessels. *Clin. Exp. Pharmacol. Physiol.* 7:263–274.

Sylvester, J.T. and McGowan, C. 1978. The effects of agents that bind to cytochrome p-450 on hypoxic pulmonary vasoconstriction. *Circ. Res.* 43:429–437.

Tucker, A., McMurtry, I.F., Grover, R.F., and Reeves, J.T. 1976. Attenuation of hypoxic pulmonary vasoconstriction by verapamil in intact dogs. *Proc. Soc. Exp. Biol. Med.* 151:611–614.

Weir, E.K. 1978. Does normoxic pulmonary vasodilatation rather than hypoxic vasoconstriction account for the pulmonary pressor response to hypoxia? Hypothesis. *Lancet.* 232:476–477.

West, J.B. 1977. Ventilation-perfusion relationships. *Am. Rev. Respir. Dis.* 116:919–943.

Wilson, D.F., Erecinska, M., Drown, C., and Silver, I.A. 1979. The oxygen dependence of cellular energy metabolism. *Arch. Biochem. Biophys.* 195:485–493.

J.A. Loeppky and M.L. Riedesel, editors
OXYGEN TRANSPORT TO HUMAN TISSUES

Oxygen and Carbon Dioxide Interactions in Blood

Michael P. Hlastala

Oxygen and carbon dioxide interactions are important at many different levels in the gas exchange of man. This is the case in blood, not only from the point of view of O_2 and CO_2 transport, but also from the point of view of facilitating gas exchange at the lung and at the systemic tissue.

The position of the hemoglobin oxygen dissociation curve (ODC) for human blood is defined in terms of the P_{50}, the pressure at which the hemoglobin is 50% saturated, which for standard blood is 27 Torr. Many years ago, Hill (1910) pointed out that the ODC could be partially linearized with a simple transformation (Figure 1). To the left of the standard curve (solid curve) is a dashed curve for blood with increased oxygen affinity, or decreased P_{50}, and to the right is a dashed curve with decreased oxygen affinity, or increased P_{50}. As the hemoglobin oxygen affinity is decreased, relatively less oxygen is bound to hemoglobin at a given PO_2; or alternately, a greater PO_2 is needed to bind the same amount of oxygen. Several ligands of hemoglobin affect oxygen-hemoglobin affinity and, hence, shift the ODC. For example, the curve is shifted to the right with elevated H^+, CO_2, 2,3-diphosphoglycerate (DPG), and temperature. The effect of CO_2 on oxygen-hemoglobin affinity was first described by Bohr, Hasselbalch, and Krogh (1904) and is now called the Bohr effect. However, it was not until thirty years later that it was pointed out by Margaria and Green (1933) that only part of the Bohr effect is due to CO_2, with part of the effect being due to the presence of H^+ formed by the hydration of CO_2 and subsequent dissociation of carbonic acid. More recently, the effects have been explained in terms of structural changes in the hemoglobin molecule.

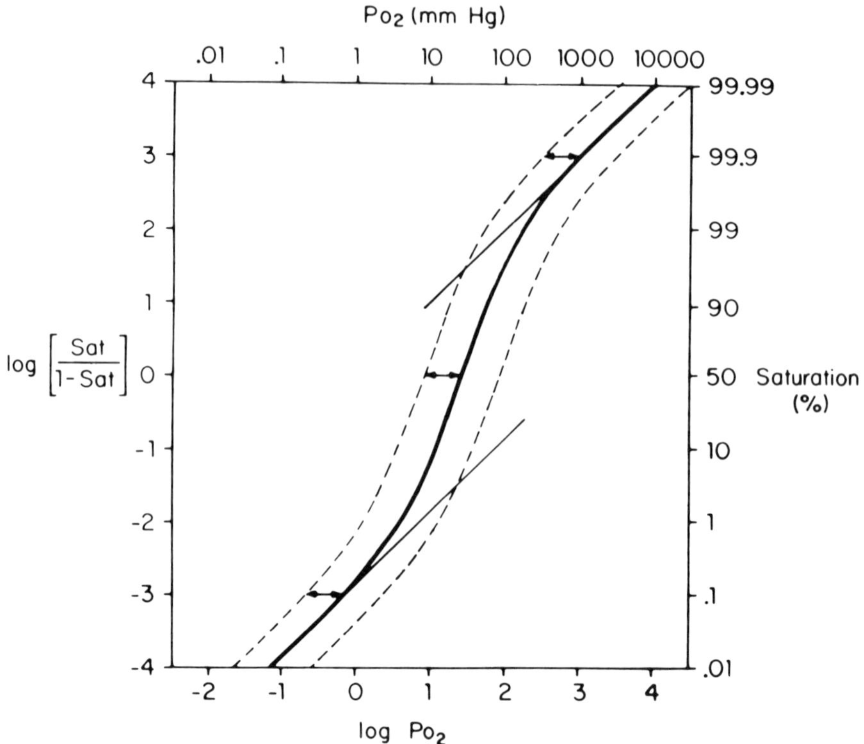

Figure 1. Hill plot of the oxygen-hemoglobin dissociation curve. The normal curve with a P_{50} of 27 Torr is indicated by the solid curve. One curve with increased affinity (left) and one curve with decreased affinity (right) are indicated by the dashed lines.

The shape of the ODC and the shifts in position of the curve are thought to be physiologically significant. At the high end of the curve where oxygen is loaded in the lung at sea level, the curve is quite flat. Therefore, as PO_2 is reduced, either by lung disease or by slight increases in altitude, there is very little loss of hemoglobin saturation. As oxygen is extracted and saturation is reduced, the PO_2 falls to the venous value. Here again, the S-shaped nature of the curve is thought to be an advantage. Diffusion of oxygen from the capillary to the metabolizing cell depends on an adequate partial pressure difference. The shape of the curve is an advantage because oxygen can be extracted while the pressure is maintained. The Bohr effect is thought to play a role in helping to shift the curve to the right in systemic tissue allowing sufficient oxygen to be delivered at a high enough pressure for diffusion to the cells. This important role for the Bohr effect has been known for a long time, but only recently have we begun to realize that the effects of CO_2, H^+, and DPG are strongly interrelated and also dependent on temperature.

Hemoglobin-Ligand Interactions

The CO_2 Bohr effect represents the shift in the ODC when pH is changed by altering PCO_2, leading to a change in both hydrogen ion and CO_2 content. As explained below, the CO_2 Bohr factor is greater at low saturations than in the intermediate range, and decreases at higher saturations (Garby et al., 1972; Meier et al., 1974; Hlastala and Woodson, 1975; Teisseire et al., 1975). Therefore, as PCO_2 changes, there is a slight change in the shape of the ODC. This, in itself, may be a significant physiological advantage. As the blood gets to a critically low PO_2 and saturation at the venous end of the capillary, the greater CO_2 Bohr effect will result in a more rightward shift of the curve which may provide the needed extra boost in PO_2 for diffusion.

The fixed acid Bohr effect is determined when the pH is changed by addition of fixed acid or base alone. In this case, for normal DPG levels in blood, there is a marked decrease in the Bohr factor at very low saturations. The values for the fixed acid Bohr factors at intermediate and high saturations are not significantly different from the CO_2 Bohr factor (Garby et al., 1972; Hlastala and Woodson, 1975). Since we know the magnitude of the CO_2 Bohr factor obtained when we change CO_2 and hydrogen ion and can compare that with the fixed acid Bohr factor, which is obtained with shifts in hydrogen ion alone, it is possible to calculate the effect of CO_2 alone on the ODC.

The effect of molecular CO_2 on O_2 affinity is strongly oxygen saturation dependent. At high saturations, there is no significant difference between the fixed acid and the CO_2 Bohr effects and, therefore, there is essentially no effect of molecular CO_2. However, at very low saturation there is a large effect of molecular CO_2, which is thought to be explained by the sequencing of oxygen binding. Oxygen binds first to the heme units attached to the two alpha chains of hemoglobin, then to the two beta chains; the alpha chains are bound at low saturation and the beta chains are bound at high saturation. The DPG competitively binds at the N-terminal valine site of the beta chains to prevent the interaction of CO_2 at high oxygen saturation where the beta chain is oxygenating. Thus, the ODC responds differently whether subjected to respiratory or metabolic changes. Because of the high CO_2 effect at low oxygen saturation, this difference is greatest for low oxygen saturations.

One other important variable is temperature. Because oxygen binding is accompanied by the release of DPG from hemoglobin and because the binding of DPG to hemoglobin is an exothermic process, one might expect a profound influence of temperature on these ligand interaction. Certainly, the binding of oxygen should be temperature dependent and because it has been shown that ligands interact differently at different saturations, it seems reasonable to expect that the effect of temperature would vary with saturation. In fact, the direct temperature effect on the ODC ($\Delta \log P_{O_2}/\Delta T$) increases only slightly from 0.021 at 90% O_2 saturation to 0.024 at 10% O_2 saturation (Hlastala et al., 1977). For low DPG blood, this saturation dependence is accentuated.

Temperature also influences the ligand interaction with hemoglobin. The CO_2 Bohr factor increases with increasing temperature. The fixed acid Bohr factor decreases slightly with increasing Bohr factor (Hlastala et al., 1977; Oeseburg, 1979). The difference between the two shows a marked increase in the direct effect of CO_2 on oxygen affinity with increasing temperature (Figure 2). This increase in CO_2 effect is most important for low O_2 saturation and low DPG concentration.

Figure 2. Effect of molecular CO_2 (carbamino) on oxygen affinity at constant pH ($\Delta \log P_{O_2}/\Delta \log P_{CO_2}$) vs oxygen saturation in normal and DPG-depleted blood at four different experimental temperatures.

SOURCE: *Hlastala et al., 1977.*

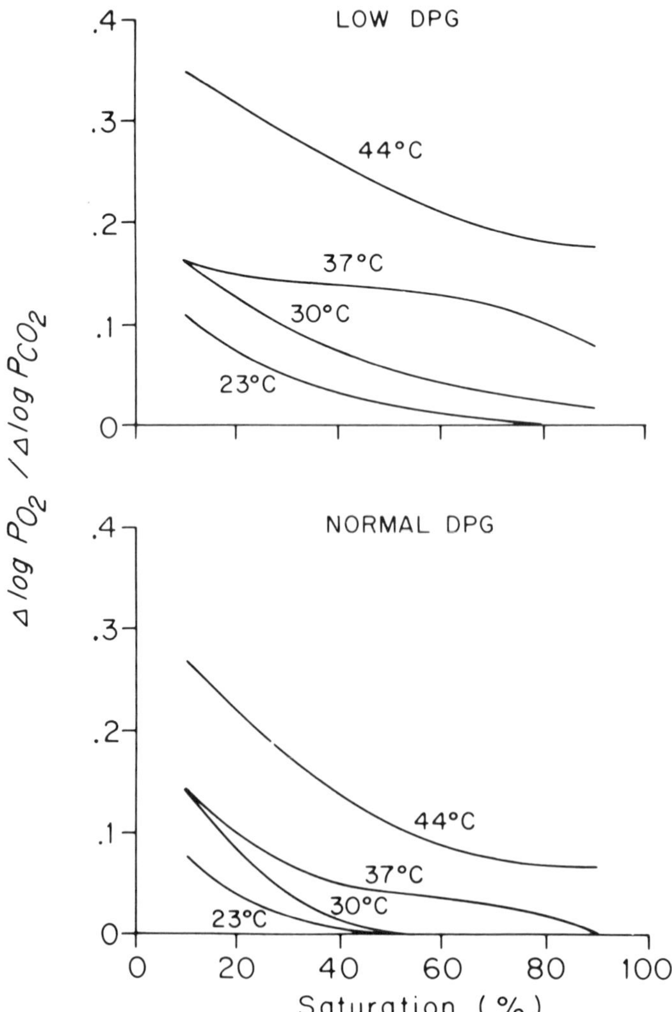

The direct binding of DPG to the hemoglobin molecule and, therefore, the effect of DPG on the position of the ODC decreases with increasing temperature (Figure 3). The direct DPG effect is O_2 saturation dependent, decreasing at both very high and very low saturation. It is probable that part of the effect of temperature on the ODC is mediated directly by decreasing oxygen-hemoglobin binding while part of the effect is mediated through a reduction in DPG binding and consequent effects on ligand interaction.

Another important ligand is the ever present carbon monoxide. Chronic levels of 10 to 15% carboxyhemoglobin are not unusual and acute levels of over 50% are often seen. Carbon monoxide competitively binds at the heme site, thus reducing the total oxygen capacity. In addition, because of the interaction of the heme sites, binding of carbon monoxide affects the ability of the remaining heme sites to bind oxygen (Roughton, 1970). The binding of oxygen to one heme site also affects the ability of the remaining heme sites to bind oxygen. However, the effect of carbon monoxide on heme–heme interaction is

Figure 3. Effect of DPG on oxygen affinity at pH 7.4 vs oxygen saturation.
SOURCE: *Hlastala et al., 1977.*

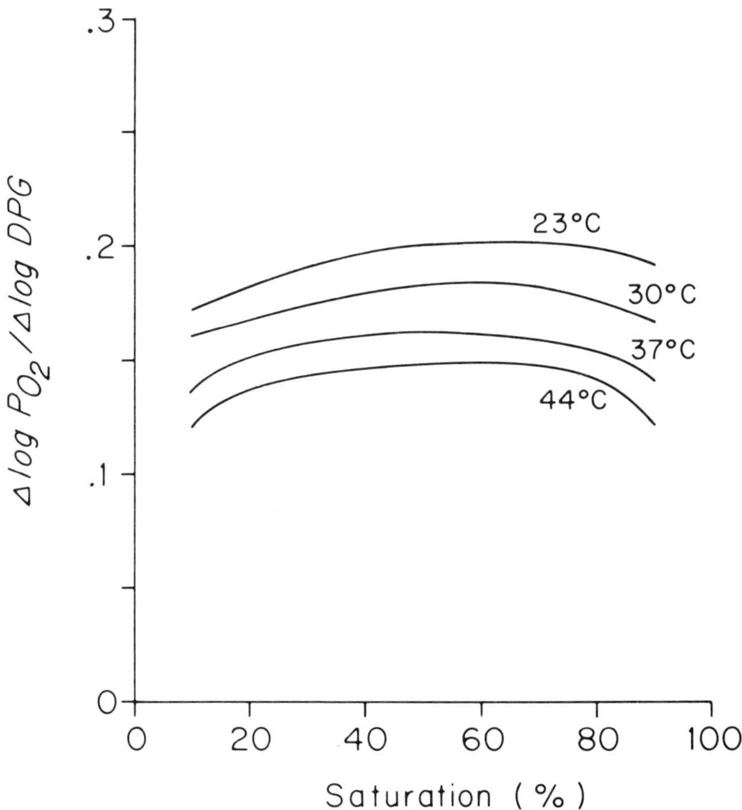

different from the effect of oxygen (Hlastala et al., 1976). Up to a saturation of 40%, oxygen actually lowers the P_{50} more than carbon monoxide indicating a greater influence of oxygen on heme–heme interaction. At higher saturations, the shift for carbon monoxide is greater than for oxygen.

There seems to be a separate physiological protective mechanism at high carboxyhemoglobin levels mediated though an enhancement of the Bohr effect with the presence of carbon monoxide. As the initial carboxyhemoglobin level increases, the interaction of hydrogen ion with oxygen affinity increases dramatically at the lower oxygen saturations (Figure 4). This means there is a greater Bohr factor at low oxygen saturations where it is needed. When the same analysis is performed for the CO_2 Bohr factor, it is virtually identical to the fixed acid Bohr factor for carboxyhemoglobin levels above 50%. Therefore, there is no direct interaction of molecular CO_2 with oxygen affinity at high carboxyhemoglobin levels.

The schematic representation shown in Figure 5 summarizes the ligand interrelationships in a qualitative fashion. Elevation of hydrogen ion decreases the relative presence of oxyhemoglobin through the fixed acid Bohr effect. This is indicated as a negative influence of HbO_2. Carbon dioxide has a negative effect on HbO_2 independent of the hydrogen ion effect. The combination of the two is the CO_2 Bohr effect. Because of the binding of DPG to hemoglobin in all but the most oxygenated form, DPG has several forms of action. It has a

Figure 4. Fixed acid Bohr factor vs total hemoglobin saturation ($CO + O_2$) for initial carboxyhemoglobin concentrations of 2, 25, 50, or 75%.
SOURCE: *Hlastala et al., 1976.*

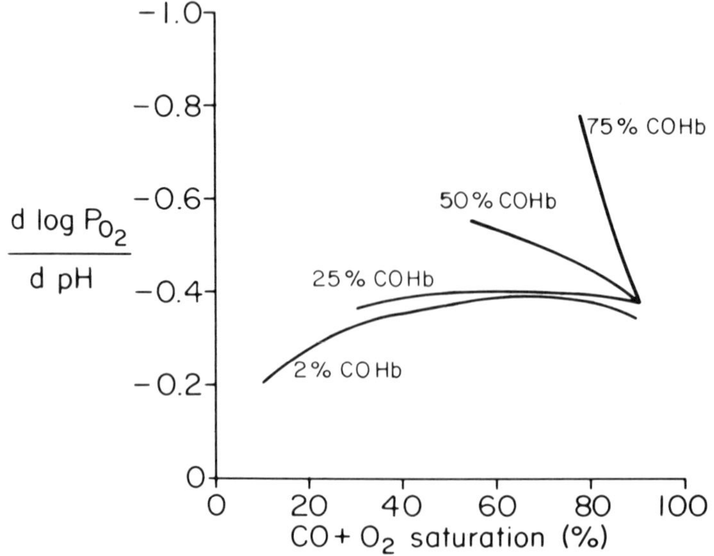

direct effect on hemoglobin; the binding of DPG to hemoglobin reduces the affinity to oxygen. In addition, because of the binding of DPG to the N-terminal valine of the beta chains, the presence of DPG decreases the effect of CO_2. Increased temperature has a direct effect on hemoglobin, reducing its affinity for oxygen. It also decreases the fixed acid Bohr effect and increases the effect of molecular CO_2. Increased temperature also decreases the binding of DPG to hemoglobin.

Altitude

From knowledge of the different effects of fixed acid and CO_2 on the ODC, it is possible to describe the *in vivo* response of the ODC to altitude. At sea level, the dissociation curve has a P_{50} of 27 Torr at a PCO_2 of 40 Torr and a pH of 7.4. With rapid exposure to hypoxia, respiratory alkalosis occurs, resulting in a change in P_{50} due to the CO_2 Bohr effect. If the pH changes to 7.6, then the P_{50} will shift to a value of 21 Torr. Gradually, after acclimatization and metabolic compensation for the respiratory alkalosis, the curve shifts via the fixed acid Bohr factor toward a 7.4 pH. Because of differences between these two Bohr factors, the *in vivo* P_{50} returns to 24.5 Torr. The net result in an adapted man at an altitude of approximately 6000 meters would be a P_{50} lowered by 2.5 Torr at a pH of around 7.4 and a lowered PCO_2. At this point, if a man were to ascend acutely to a higher altitude, then the superimposed respiratory alkalosis would drive the P_{50} even lower via the CO_2 Bohr effect. A left-shifted ODC is thought to be a particular advantage at extreme altitude because of increased oxygen loading by the blood in the lung.

Figure 5. Schematic diagram showing ligand and temperature effects on oxygen-hemoglobin affinity.

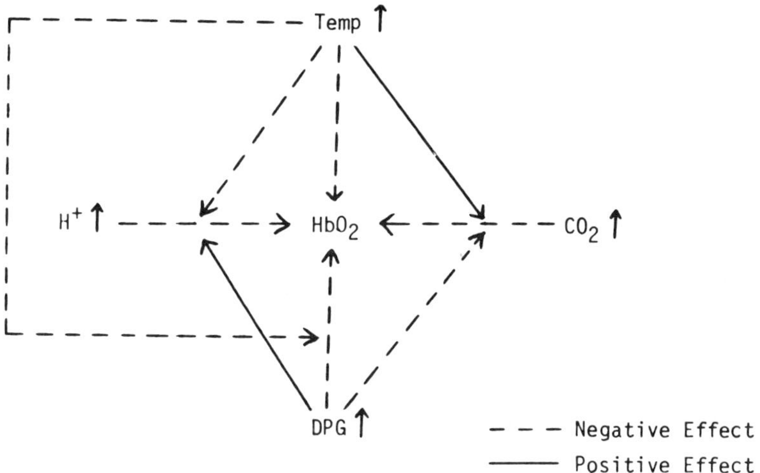

Another factor is the increase in 2,3-DPG associated with altitude. There is some controversy in the literature over the exact amount of increase in DPG after adaptation to altitude. If one takes an average increase in DPG of 20%, the increase in P_{50} would be a little over 1 Torr, and the effect on *in vivo* P_{50} would be minimal.

As pointed out above, the magnitude of the decrease in P_{50} by decreasing CO_2 is much greater at lower oxygen saturation and equivalent to a P_{50} of 20 to 21 Torr at very low saturations. Theoretically, it is possible that this shift is important to certain tissues with low critical PO_2, but this has yet to be determined.

Pulmonary Capillary Oxygen Exchange

What is the relative importance of shifts in the ODC? Many of these shifts behave in a dynamic fashion. Specifically, the Bohr shift takes place during the transit through systemic and pulmonary capillaries. As blood is traversing the systemic tissue capillary, oxygen is being delivered by diffusion to the peripheral cells as CO_2 is being taken up by the blood. Therefore, the physiological point in blood is shifting down the curve as oxygen is being unloaded, and the curve is also shifting to the right as CO_2 is being taken up. The dynamics of this shift are complex because of the time-dependent interactions of CO_2 within the erythrocyte. Carbon dioxide not only binds directly, but also is stored in the form of bicarbonate which must diffuse through the erythrocyte membrane. The point is that the dynamics of this shift in the ODC and, therefore, the change in oxygen delivery, is affected by the interaction of CO_2 within the erythrocyte.

A theoretical calculation for the uptake of oxygen as blood traverses the pulmonary capillary during hypoxia in Figure 6 shows that under resting conditions blood stays in the pulmonary capillary for approximately 0.75 sec. The conditions shown are for a mixed venous PO_2 of 28 Torr and an alveolar PO_2 of 43 Torr. The upper curve shows the expected profile of PO_2 when there is no change in CO_2 (an unphysiological condition shown for illustrative purposes). The lower curve shows the physiological situation where CO_2 is changing while O_2 is being taken up. As oxygen comes into the blood from the alveolus, CO_2 is going in the opposite direction causing the ODC to shift toward the left which results in a lower PO_2 at any given time during this transit. This lower PO_2 results in a larger gradient between the blood and the alveolus and, hence, a slightly greater flux of oxygen. At the systemic tissue level, the same kind of interaction goes on with oxygen delivery facilitated by the Bohr effect mechanism and by the uptake of CO_2; the same principle is acting but in the opposite direction. Quantitatively, this effect is of limited importance as the Bohr effect results in only a 2% enhancement of oxygen exchange. However, it has also been shown that O_2 enhances CO_2 exchange through the analogous Haldane effect of O_2 on the CO_2 dissociation curve

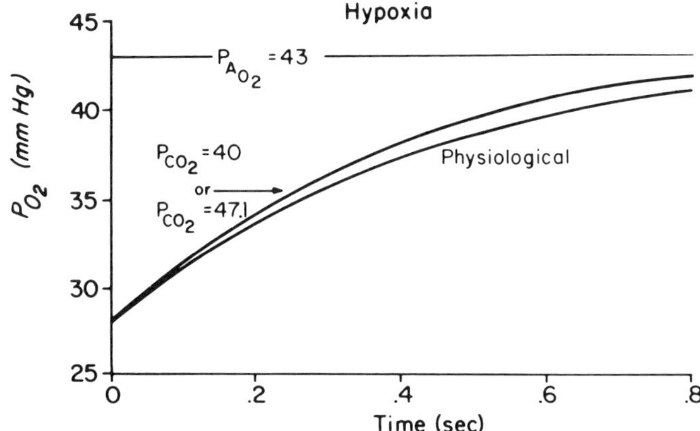

Figure 6. The PO_2 in blood vs time during passage through the pulmonary capillary in hypoxia. Top curve represents profile with PCO_2 held constant. Lower curve represents the physiological situation with simultaneous CO_2 exchange.

SOURCE: *Hlastala, 1973.*

(Christiansen et al., 1914). As O_2 increases, the carbon dioxide curve shifts to the right; approximately 50% of the CO_2 exchange is a result of the simultaneous O_2 exchange, thus demonstrating the importance of the interaction between O_2 and CO_2 exchange.

Summary

The oxygen delivery system has remarkable capabilities to adapt to environmental stress to maximize oxygen delivery. This is facilitated by various ligands interacting with the hemoglobin molecule. The Bohr effect is mediated through independent effects of hydrogen ion and carbon dioxide which are dependent on oxygen saturation. These interactions are affected by 2,3-diphosphoglycerate, carbon monoxide, and temperature in a way which enhances oxygen delivery under stress. These ligand interactions also act to enhance oxygen exchange in the lung and in the systemic tissue. The separate effects of metabolic and respiratory acid-base changes in the ODC should be taken into account when determining *in vivo* P_{50}, particularly at altitude.

References

Bohr, C., Hasselbalch, K., and Krogh, A. 1904. Ueber einen in biologischer Beziehung wichtigen Einfluss, den die Kohlensaurespannung des Blutes auf dessen Sauerstroffbindung übt. *Skand. Arch. Physiol.* 16:402–412.

Christiansen, J., Douglas, C.C., and Haldane, J.S. 1914. The absorption and dissociation of carbon dioxide by human blood. *J. Physiol.* (*London*) 48:244–277.

Garby, L., Robert, M., and Zaar, B. 1972. Proton and carbamino linked oxygen affinity of normal human blood. *Acta Physiol. Scand.* 84:482–492.

Hill, A.V. 1910. The possible effects of the aggregation of the molecules of hemoglobin on its dissociation curve. *J. Physiol.* (*London*) 40:4–7.

Hlastala, M.P. 1973. Significance of the Bohr and Haldane effects in the pulmonary capillary. *Respir. Physiol.* 17:81–92.

Hlastala, M.P., McKenna, H.P., Franada, R.L., and Detter, J.C. 1976. Influence of carbon monoxide on hemoglobin-oxygen binding. *J. Appl. Physiol.* 41:893–899.

Hlastala, M.P. and Woodson, R.D. 1975. Saturation dependency of the Bohr effect: interactions among H^+, CO_2, and DPG. *J. Appl. Physiol.* 38:1126–1131.

Hlastala, M.P., Woodson, R.D., and Wranne, B. 1977. Influence of temperature on hemoglobin-ligand interaction in whole blood. *J. Appl. Physiol.* 43:545–550.

Margaria, R. and Green, A.A. 1933. The first dissociation constant, pK_1, of carbonic acid in hemoglobin solutions and its relation to the existence of a combination of hemoglobin with carbon dioxide. *J. Biol. Chem.* 102:611–634.

Meier, U., Boning, D., and Rubenstein, H.J. 1974. Oxygenation dependent variations of the Bohr coefficient related to whole blood and erythrocytic pH: effect of lactic and carbonated acid. *Pflügers Arch.* 349:203–213.

Oeseburg, B. 1979. Determination of O_2 affinity of hemoglobin by independent continuous measurement of S_{O_2}, P_{O_2}, and pH, with control of pH, P_{CO_2}, and temperature. *Crit. Care Med.* 7:396–398.

Roughton, F.J.W. 1970. The equilibrium of carbon monoxide with human hemoglobin in whole blood. *Ann. N.Y. Acad. Sci.* 174:177–187.

Teisseire, B., Teisseire, L., Herigault, R., and Soulard, C. 1975. Methode d'enrigistrement en continu sur micro-enchantillons de la courbe d'association $Hb\text{-}O_2$. II. Etude de l'effet Bohr et de la carbamino-formation. *Bull. Physiopathol. Respir.* 11:853–862.

SECTION III:

Cardiovascular Adjustments, Oxygen Delivery, and Metabolic Needs

J.A. Loeppky and M.L. Riedesel, editors
OXYGEN TRANSPORT TO HUMAN TISSUES

Biophysics of Gas and Blood Flow

Richard L. Riley

Two remarkable papers were presented back to back at the spring meetings of the American Physiological Society in Atlantic City in 1954. The first, by Stanley Sarnoff (1955), dealt with the Frank-Starling law of the heart. Sarnoff showed that the ventricular function curve is in fact a whole family of curves, giving the heart enormous versatility. The next paper was by Arthur Guyton (1955), who presented the case for mean circulatory pressure, measured under static conditions, as the upstream pressure for venous return. He showed venous return and cardiac response curves with right atrial pressure at the point of intersection. Both of these papers are now classics. However, Sarnoff's reinforced the prevailing belief that the heart alone controls blood flow. Guyton's deviated sharply by arguing that cardiac output is determined by the interaction of cardiac and peripheral vascular factors. In the years following the 1954 symposium, feelings in the cardiovascular community ran high. Guyton was ridiculed, and he fought back. Few who lionize him now remember the early years.

As a respiratory physiologist, it was easy to be one of Guyton's early supporters. He made blood vessels seem like lungs. My discussion of blood flow begins with an analogy to air flow.

Consider a model in which both the lung-airway system and the peripheral vascular system are represented as elastic balloons that are filled and emptied through collapsible tubes (Figure 1). The airways have one tube for bidirectional flow, and the blood vessels have two tubes for arterial and venous flow. The elastic elements are lumped in the alveoli and the small veins—a liberty that does but slight injustice to the facts. The lungs are held open from without by the chest wall, while the vascular system is held open from within by the

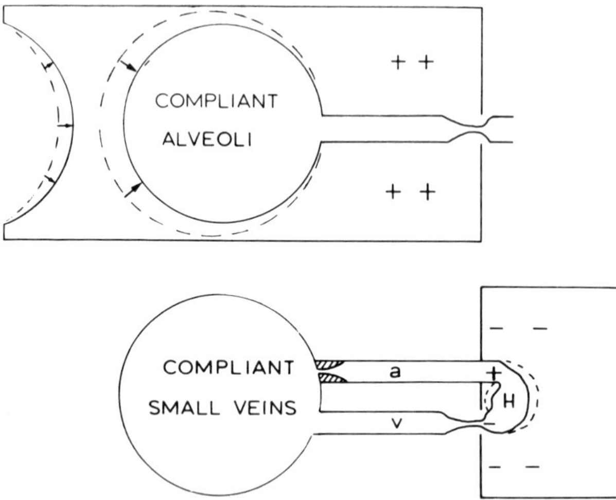

Figure 1. Model showing similarities between breathing and blood flow. Narrowed segments of airways and vessels represent partial collapse as in a Starling resistor. H: heart; a: arteries; v: veins. ++: positive intrathoracic pressure; − −: negative intrathoracic pressure.

blood. The pump that further distends the lungs in inspiration is predominantly the diaphragm, and the pump that ejects blood through the arteries and into the capacitance vessels is the heart. The force that empties the lungs in expiration is the elasticity of the lungs and chest wall and in the absence of skeletal muscle activity, the force that returns the blood to the heart is the elasticity of the capacitance vessels. The muscles of respiration cannot appreciably speed up expiration because of airway collapse, and the heart cannot appreciably speed up venous return because the veins collapse on entering the thorax. Airways collapse when intrapleural pressure is positive as in forced expiration, and veins collapse when intrapleural pressure is negative. This is vintage Guyton, although venous collapse had been described earlier by Holt (1941). The collapse phenomena, which mimic Starling resistors, are now generally understood. Less well-understood is a putative arteriolar collapse mechanism where smooth muscle tone acts like the surrounding pressure in a Starling resistor.

In 1963, Permutt and Riley suggested that vascular smooth muscle could act like a surrounding pressure and that arteriolar critical closing pressure, described by Burton (1951), serves as the effective downstream pressure for arterial flow. Burton never accepted this extension of his critical closure concept even though Permutt and I had some entertaining correspondence with him on the subject. In any case, Burton's concept of a sudden closure at a critical pressure is inconsistent with the Starling resistor hypothesis, which holds that the surrounding pressure causes continuous partial closure (the collapse phenomenon) and maintains constant pressure regardless of flow. The fact that arterial pressure-flow curves have a positive intercept at zero flow has long been known (Jackman and Green, 1977). More recently, arterial pressure-flow curves determined during a single prolonged diastole, with readings at 50 msec intervals, have carried the curves to zero flow so quickly that reflex changes in vascular tone cannot have occurred. Such studies by Ehrlich et al. (1975), Bellamy (1978), J.F. Green (personal communication) have provided curves for the femoral, coronary, and renal arteries, as well as for the body as a whole.

The zero flow intercepts for the different vascular beds occur at widely different pressures, being very high in the femoral artery and as low as 20 mm Hg in the renal artery (Figure 2). For the body as a whole, the average value is about 50 mm Hg. In every case, the pressure-flow curve is almost perfectly straight. There can no longer be any doubt that the slope of this line is inversely related to arterial resistance and that the zero flow intercept represents the effective downstream pressure for arterial flow. This pressure is a function of arteriolar tone.

If arteriolar tone is equivalent to the pressure surrounding a Starling resistor, then, when arteriolar pressure exceeds capillary pressure, there is every reason to expect an abrupt pressure drop or "vascular waterfall," to use the term coined by Permutt (Permutt and Riley, 1963). The pressure must drop abruptly from an arteriolar value of about 50 mm Hg to the value at the upstream end of the capillaries. Even if one takes an upstream capillary pressure of 35 mm Hg, as given in many texts but which I consider much too high, there still remains a sizable gap between arteriolar and capillary pressures. This gap is

Figure 2. Arterial pressure-flow curves from several vascular beds. Femoral artery before 30 sec occlusion (extreme right) could be studied accurately.
SOURCE: *W. Ehrlich, personal communication.*

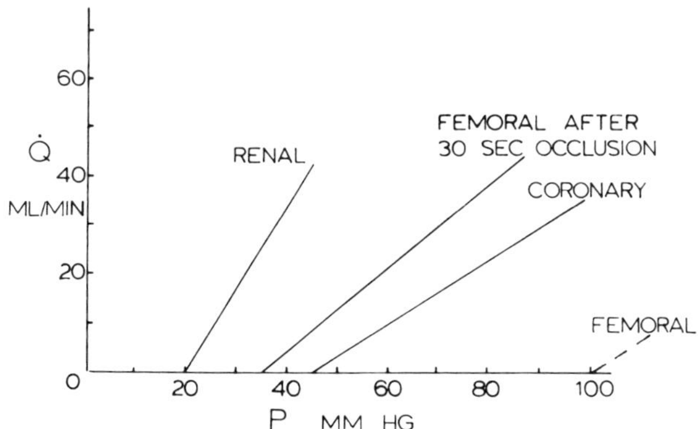

precisely where one would expect a vascular waterfall. Obviously these remarks apply only to the peripheral vascular bed.

The venous side of the peripheral circulation was studied in dogs by Caldini, Permutt, Waddell, and Riley (1974). These authors used a right heart bypass preparation and observed the characteristics of venous drainage after a step decrease in right atrial pressure at constant blood flow. The data could not be explained by assuming a simple elastic system but were satisfactorily accounted for by postulating two vascular compartments with slow and fast time constants of drainage, respectively. Such a model is shown in Figure 3.

I have extended the analysis given in Tables 1 and 2 and Figures 5 and 6 of Caldini et al. (1974). Using total flows ($\dot{Q}_{max}$) from Table 1 and fractional flows ($F_1 : F_2$) from Table 2, I first calculated the individual flows through each compartment ($F_1\dot{Q}_{max}$: $F_2\dot{Q}_{max}$) and then, using venous resistance values from Table 2, the individual upstream pressures for venous return ($Ps_1 = Rv_1 F_1 \dot{Q}_{max}$; $Ps_2 = Rv_1 F_2 \dot{Q}_{max}$). Because the calculated upstream pressure for dog number 6 was unreasonably high during epinephrine infusion (52 mm Hg) and because of other inconsistencies in this experiment, these data were not included in the average values. This deletion had no significant effect on the findings under control conditions to be discussed now.

Guyton-type venous return curves for slow and fast compartments were drawn by connecting average upstream pressures at zero flow with average flows at zero pressure (Figure 4). The upstream pressure for venous return was 7.2 mm Hg for the fast compartment and 15.6 mm Hg for the slow compart-

Figure 3. Two-compartment model of the circulation. S: slow compartment; F: fast compartment; H-L: heart and lungs; a: arteries; v: veins.
SOURCE: *Caldini et al., 1974.*

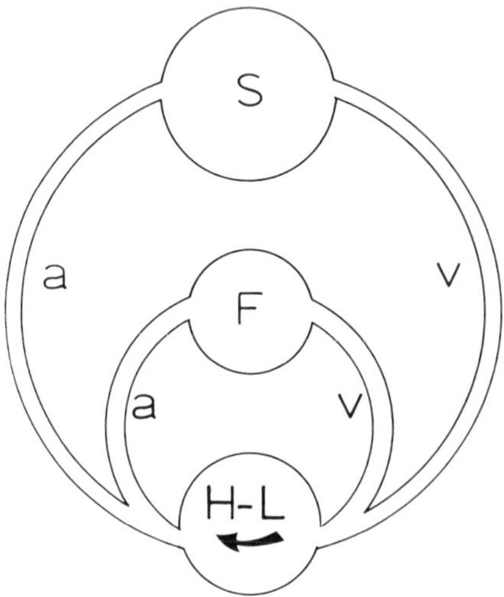

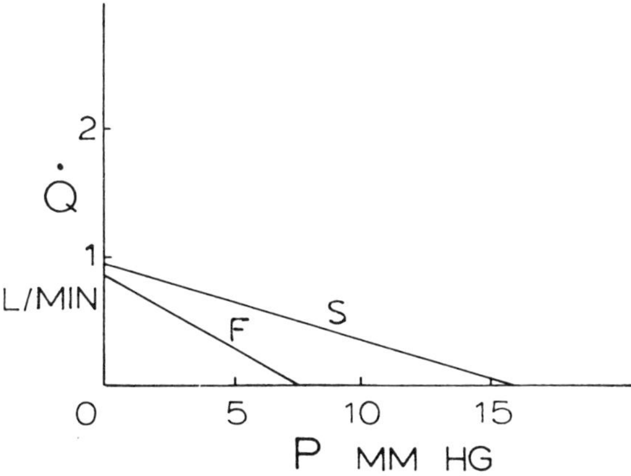

Figure 4. Venous return curves for slow and fast compartments, calculated from data of Caldini et al., 1974. The pressures at zero flow represent the upstream pressures for venous return. The flows at zero pressure represent flows when downstream pressure, i.e., right atrial pressure, was zero. S: slow compartment; F: fast compartment.

ment. The fast compartment had a little less flow than the slow compartment when the downstream pressure, i.e., the right atrial pressure, was zero.

Figure 5 has the same format as the familiar diagram appearing in most texts, showing the pressures in different parts of the systemic circulation. The arteriolar pressures, 60 and 40 mm Hg, are in the range of zero flow intercepts for arterial pressure-flow curves but were not determined simultaneously with the venous curves. The upstream pressures for venous return are from Figure 4. The gradients between aortic and arteriolar pressures are the driving pressures for arterial flow in the fast and slow compartments. The gradients between venular and vena caval pressure are the driving pressures for venous return. The shapes of the arterial and venous pressure curves are arbitrary. The differences between arteriolar and venular pressures are attributed to vascular waterfalls.

Where in this scheme of things is capillary pressure? In my opinion, capillary pressure and venular pressure are, for practical purposes, the same. It seems to me unlikely that capillaries, with an average length of less than 1 mm and a total cross section 700 times that of the aorta (Guyton, 1961, p. 353), can interpose any significant resistance to the flow of blood. Calculations based on resistance being inversely proportional to the fourth power of the radius, though not strictly applicable to compliant tubes, suggest that the pressure drop along the capillaries is the same order of magnitude as the pressure drop along a 50 cm length of aorta. I infer, therefore, that the pressure gradient along the course of the capillaries is small. I infer also that the gradient between capillary and venular pressure is small, so that the absolute value of

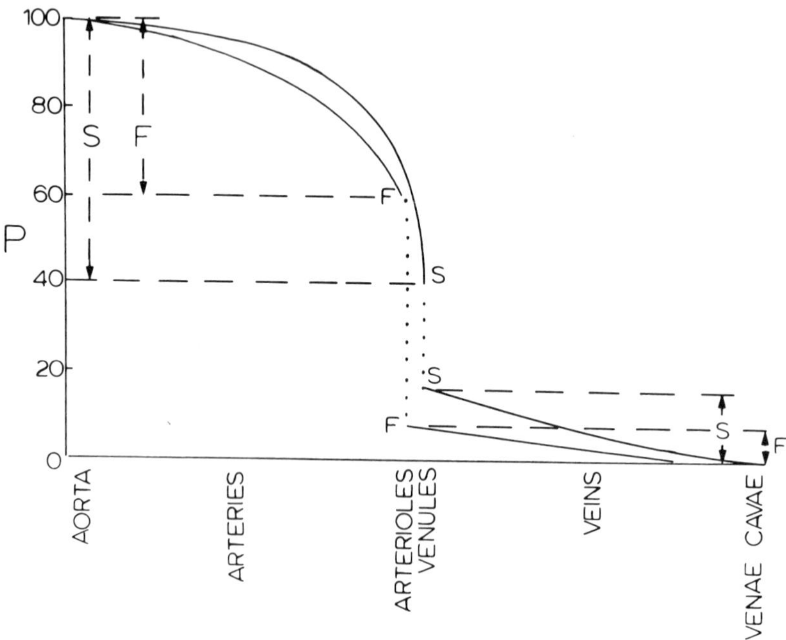

Figure 5. Pressures in different parts of the systemic circulation, showing driving pressures for arterial and venous flow. Vertical dotted lines indicate vascular waterfalls between arteriolar and venular pressures. Capillary pressure assumed to be approximately equal to venular pressure, i.e., the pressure in the capacitance vessels. S and F: compartments with slow and fast drainage, respectively.

capillary pressure is close to, and determined by, the capacitance vessels into which they drain.

If, in the experiments of Caldini et al. (1974), the capillary pressure in the fast compartment were indeed 7.2 mm Hg, like the pressure in the capacitance vessels, the balance between osmotic and hydrostatic forces would require that interstitial fluid pressure be in the vicinity of −17 mm Hg. This is not impossible for resting muscle with minimal blood flow, but it may also be possible that with minimal capillary flow there is minimal fluid exchange and that interstitial fluid pressure is not reduced so drastically. In the much larger slow compartment, a capillary pressure of 15.6 mm Hg would be associated with an interstitial fluid pressure of about −8 mm Hg, which, according to Guyton (1961, p. 446), is about average (Figure 6).

After administration of epinephrine, the pressure in the capacitance vessels of both compartments rose to 21.5 mm Hg in the experiments of Caldini et al. (1974). If capillary pressures in both compartments had this same value, interstitial fluid pressure would be only slightly negative and thus close to

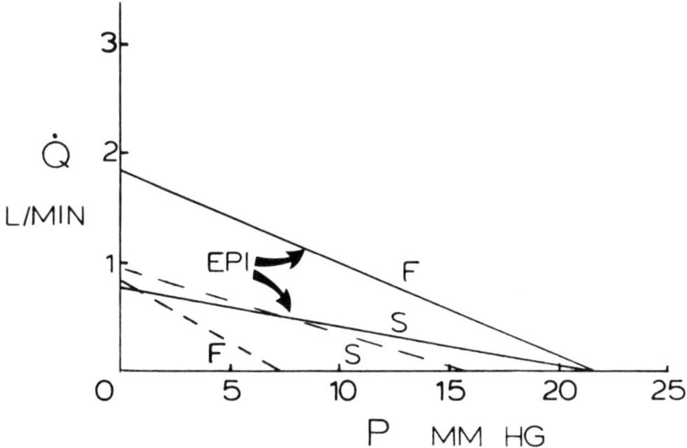

Figure 6. Venous return curves for slow and fast compartments after administration of epinephrine calculated from data of Caldini et al., 1974. Broken lines show control findings before epinephrine and are identical to circles along ordinate show total flow before and after epinephrine. S: slow compartment; F: fast compartment; EPI: epinephrine.

edema level. Since capillary pressure could not be lower than 21.5 mm Hg, which was the pressure in the capacitance vessels downstream, and could not be much higher without causing edema, the capillary pressure must have been about the same as that in the capacitance vessels.

I am aware that my arguments are indirect and oversimplified. However, since direct measurement of capillary pressure may interfere with the dynamic requirements of the vascular waterfall, an indirect approach that is consistent with basic principles has much to recommend it.

If, as this indirect evidence indicates, capillary pressure is determined by the pressure in the capacitance vessels, then an important physiological dividend accrues: the amount of blood in the vascular system is automatically adjusted to the size and compliance of the system. If blood volume is too small, the pressure distending the capacitance vessels drops, capillary pressure drops, and interstitial fluid is drawn into the capillaries to balance the hydrostatic and osmotic forces. Conversely, an overfilled vascular bed will have a high capillary pressure and will lose fluid to the interstitium. This capillary fluid shift has been discussed by Guyton in connection with mean circulatory pressure. However, Guyton (1961, p. 446) found mean circulatory pressure in dogs to be 7 mm Hg, which is considerably below capillary pressure in most tissues and implies a pressure drop between capillaries and capacitance vessels. From the experiments of Caldini et al. (1974), the pressure in the capacitance vessels appears to be close to, if not virtually the same as, capillary pressure.

With the advent of the two-compartment model, mean circulatory or mean systemic pressure can no longer be considered the upstream pressure for venous return since the pressures in the capacitance vessels of the fast and slow compartments differ. These pressures still depend, as Guyton saw, on the elastic properties of the capacitance vessels, and their pressures still provide the force that drives the blood back to the heart. However, the quantitative estimation of the upstream pressures in fast and slow compartments requires an indirect approach such as that of Caldini et al. (1974).

We return to the 1954 controversy between those who believed that the heart alone controls blood flow and those who believed that cardiac output is determined by the interaction of cardiac and peripheral factors. If the heart cannot appreciably speed up venous return because the veins collapse on entering the thorax, what is the mechanism by which venous return and hence cardiac output is speeded? If the discussion is limited to the experimental animal in the horizontal posture with inactive skeletal muscles, then according to Guyton's original model the options were limited: mean circulatory pressure could increase and resistance to venous return could decrease. This proved inadequate to explain the effects of epinephrine. The two-compartment model added a third important option: more of the arterial outflow can be diverted from the slow compartment to the fast compartment. This redistribution of flow is determined by the smooth muscle tone of the arterioles and precapillary sphincters. More blood is directed from the high pressure arterial system to the capacitance vessels of the fast compartment. Upstream pressure for venous return from this compartment is increased, and flow is augmented. The normal heart pumps the increased venous return back into the arterial system without an increase in right atrial pressure by shifting to a new ventricular function curve, as described by Sarnoff (1955). The increased arterial flow increases arterial blood pressure.

Figure 7 shows arterial and venous pressure-flow curves and cardiac response curves before and after administration of epinephrine. These are curves for total flow in which fast and slow compartments are combined. The broken lines for the arterial curves indicate that they are estimates. The horizontal dots represent vascular waterfalls. While pulling together many of the points that have been discussed, these curves conceal the important differences between fast and slow compartments. On the left are intersecting venous return and cardiac response curves, reminding us, as did Guyton in 1954, that blood flow is determined by the interaction between cardiac and peripheral vascular factors.

Summary

1. Breathing and blood flow have comparable active phases; inspiration and cardiac ejection, and comparable passive phases; expiration and venous return. The tubes in both systems are collapsible and, under appropriate conditions, act like Starling resistors.

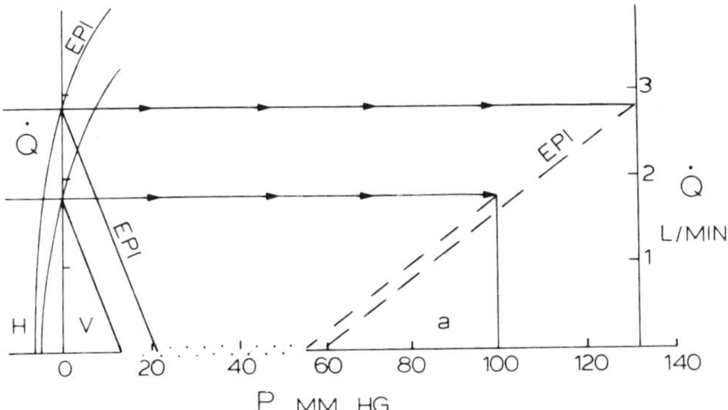

Figure 7. Combined response of fast and slow compartments to epinephrine. On left: venous return and cardiac response curves. Broken lines: estimated arterial pressure-flow curves. Horizontal dots: vascular waterfalls. EPI: epinephrine; a: arteries; v: veins; H: heart. Arrows link venous return and cardiac output with arterial flow.

2. Arterial pressure-flow curves have a positive pressure intercept at zero flow. This arterial downstream pressure is determined by arteriolar tone and differs widely in different tissues.
3. Venous pressure-flow curves calculated from the data of Caldini et al. (1974) have upstream pressures that represent the pressures in the capacitance vessels. These pressures can differ widely between compartments with fast and slow drainage but are usually far below arteriolar pressure. The pressure gap between arterioles and venules is believed to be accounted for by a vascular waterfall.
4. Capillary pressure in most beds is believed to be determined by the pressure in the capacitance vessels into which capillaries drain. This assures that capillary fluid shifts keep blood volume adjusted to the size and compliance of the vascular bed.
5. Cardiac output is increased primarily by diverting blood from slow to fast time constant beds. This redistribution is accomplished by relaxing the smooth muscle tone of the arterioles and precapillary sphincters leading to the fast compartment. Other vascular adjustments, including changes in resistance and compliance, play lesser roles. The heart pumps away the increased venous return without an increase in right atrial pressure by shifting to a new ventricular function curve.

References

Bellamy, R.F. 1978. Diastolic coronary artery pressure-flow relations in the dog. *Circ. Res.* 43:92–101.

Burton, A.C. 1951. On the physical equilibrium of small blood vessels. *Am. J. Physiol.* 164:319–329.

Caldini, P., Permutt, S., Waddell, J.A., and Riley, R.L. 1974. Effect of epinephrine on pressure, flow, and volume relationships in the systemic circulation of dogs. *Circ. Res.* 34:606–623.

Ehrlich, W., Schrijen, F.V., Solomon, T.A., Rodriguez-Lopez, E. and Riley, R.L. 1975. Arterial pressure-flow relations in the awake standing dog. *Am. J. Physiol.* 229:1261–1267.

Guyton, A.C. 1955. Determination of cardiac output by equating venous return curves with cardiac response curves. *Physiol. Rev.* 35:123–129.

Guyton, A.C. 1961. *Textbook of Medical Physiology*. Second edition. Philadelphia: W.B. Saunders.

Holt, J.P. 1941. The collapse factor in the measurement of venous pressure: the flow of fluid through collapsible tubes. *Am. J. Physiol.* 134:292–299.

Jackman, A.P. and Green, J.F. 1977. Arterial pressure-flow relationships in the anesthetized dog. *Ann. Biomed. Eng.* 5:384–394.

Permutt, S. and Riley, R.L. 1963. Hemodynamics of collapsible vessels with tone: vascular waterfall. *J. Appl. Physiol.* 18:924–932.

Sarnoff, S.J. 1955. Myocardial contractility as described by ventricular function curves; observations on Starling's law of the heart. *Physiol. Res.* 35:107–122.

J.A. Loeppky and M.L. Riedesel, editors
OXYGEN TRANSPORT TO HUMAN TISSUES

The Distribution of Blood Flow and Its Regulation in Humans

Loring B. Rowell

It is well-established that diseases which comprise cardiac performance during rest or exercise are associated with a redistribution of cardiac output when adequate vasomotor control is present (Wade and Bishop, 1962). In this way, the distribution of cardiac output is optimized so that adequate perfusion of vital organs is maintained. In addition, regional vasoconstriction helps to maintain arterial blood pressure and it also permits optimal distribution of blood volume.

The importance of a neurogenically mediated redistribution of cardiac output in *normal* humans was disputed for some time because similar patterns of response are not observed in dogs under stress. Some took the position that the techniques for measuring regional blood flow in humans might be deficient and thus a source of apparent discrepancies (Vatner, 1975).

The methods applied to humans for measurement of regional blood flow yield the same results as those made by electromagnetic flow probes or by direct measurements of flow (see Figure 8-2, Rowell, 1975). Measurements by dye clearance and flowmeter do not agree, however, when dye extracting mechanisms have been damaged by local ischemia (Selkurt, 1946) and comparison of methods under these conditions is clearly inappropriate. In short, the apparent discrepancies cited above are not attributable to the techniques of measuring regional blood flow, but rather are due to what are now well-established and important species differences in control of the peripheral circulation (Zelis, 1975). In this presentation, I will describe 5 conditions in which regional vasoconstriction and redistribution of blood flow are important homeostatic mechanism for humans. The conditions are: (1) upright posture, (2) hemorrhage, (3) heat stress, (4) exercise, and (5) combined heat stress and exercise.

Upright Posture

In the upright posture, humans are confronted with unique regulatory problems (Amberson, 1943). Seventy percent of total blood volume is below the heart in upright man and 70% of this volume is in compliant veins. The dependent veins are subjected to the full hydrostatic effect of a continuous column of blood between them and the heart once they have filled and their valves are open. The volume shifted into the legs alone is estimated to be 600 to 700 ml (Sjöstrand, 1952). The regulatory problems result from the shift in blood volume away from the thorax and a consequent reduction in cardiac filling pressure and stroke volume. In contrast to man, 75% of the dog's blood volume is at or above heart level so that hydrostatically-induced volume shifts are negligible.

Few would question the need for regional vasoconstriction to maintain blood pressure and adequate blood flow to vital organs in upright posture. Its loss in patients with certain lesions of the central nervous system and peripheral neuropathies leads to severe orthostatic intolerance (Johnson and Spalding, 1974). An important question is whether or not the venous system participates in orthostatic reflexes. Although peripheral venoconstriction would, transiently at least, translocate blood volume from the deep veins back to the thorax and restore ventricular filling pressure, venoconstriction does not normally attend upright posture (Shepherd and Vanhoutte, 1975). (Veins in skin and skeletal muscle, wherein venous tone can readily be measured, do not participate in orthostatic reflexes. Veins in the splanchnic system might, however, constrict but we have no evidence from humans.) Instead humans rely on *vasoconstriction* which accomplishes two things. First, it reduces the rate at which dependent veins fill. Of course, they will eventually fill and reach a volume depending upon the hydrostatic pressure head, their compliance, and the extent to which their transmural pressure is reduced by tension in surrounding muscle (Amberson, 1943; Gauer and Thron, 1965). Second, vasoconstriction regulates the distribution of blood volume by redistributing blood flow between compliant and noncompliant circuits. To grasp the importance of this second effect of vasoconstriction, we must go back to an old idea first put forward by Krogh (1912) and recently expanded by others (Caldini et al., 1974).

Krogh divided the circulation into two parallel circuits, one compliant and one noncompliant. He saw the distribution of blood volume as being changed by shifting blood flow between these two compartments. Krogh's ideas are expressed in a hydraulic model shown in Figure 1, where muscle is an example of a noncompliant circuit and the skin and splanchnic regions are compliant circuits. A rise in blood flow to skeletal muscle does not translocate blood volume from the thorax, but an increase in blood flow to compliant cutaneous vessels is associated with a large increase in cutaneous venous volume and a reduction in thoracic blood volume. Figure 1 illustrates that partial compensa-

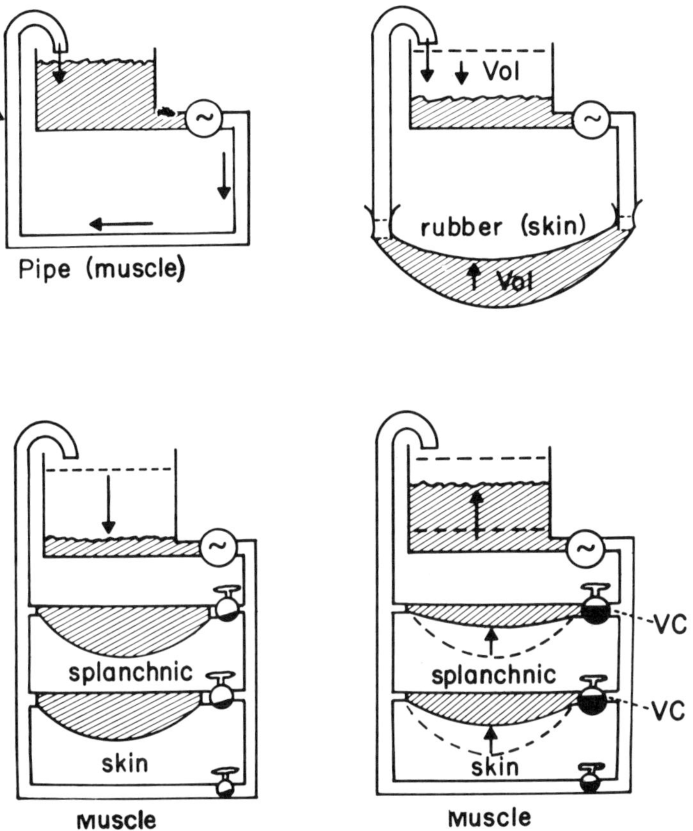

Figure 1. A hydraulic model to contrast effects of increasing blood flow through noncompliant (e.g., muscle, upper left) vs compliant circuits (e.g., skin, upper right) on thoracic blood volume. Vasodilation of compliant circuits (e.g., skin and splanchnic, lower left) will deplete the volume of central "reservoirs" (heart and pulmonary vessels). Vasoconstriction of compliant circuits (lower right) will passively displace their volumes back to the reservoir.

SOURCE: *Rowell, 1981.*

tion for vasodilation of a compliant circuit such as skin can be achieved by vasoconstriction of another large compliant circuit such as the splanchnic region. Arteriolar vasoconstriction reduces downstream venous distending pressure causing veins to empty passively. In this way, the distribution of blood *flow* can determine the distribution of blood *volume* between different organs and between thoracic and peripheral venous beds. Stated differently, the redistribution of blood flow can alter what might be called a "weighted effective compliance" of the vasculature without any active venomotor changes. The loss of these adjustments in autonomic insufficiency and peripheral neuropathies leads to severe orthostatic problems. The crucial point here is that the distribution of blood flow is probably the major determinant of distribution of blood volume in humans.

In addition to central activation of vasomotor outflow, a local sympathetic axon reflex (sometimes called a "venoarteriolar reflex") was recently shown by Henriksen (1977) to modify vascular resistance when veins are distended by upright posture. Skin blood flow decreased 40% in a region where vascular transmural pressure was increased 25 Torr. The receptor sites are in the small veins of skin, skeletal muscle, and subcutaneous adipose tissue and the effector cites are in the arterioles of these tissues.

Hemorrhage

In humans, hemorrhage is associated with regional vasoconstriction. In man, we commonly simulate hemorrhage (and upright posture) by means of lower body negative pressure (LBNP). The negative pressure increases vascular transmural pressure and sequesters blood in the legs just as in upright posture. Figure 2 illustrates approximate magnitudes and time-courses of the circulatory changes. As in upright posture, the fall in aortic pulse pressure appears to trigger a powerful baroreflex which in turn raises heart rate (HR) and constricts cutaneous, skeletal muscle, renal, and splanchnic arterioles (Rowell et al., 1972; Wolthius, 1974; Rowell, 1977). The splanchnic circulation, which normally receives 25% of total cardiac output and contains 25% of total blood volume, plays an important role in the cardiovascular adjustment to hemorrhage; its vasoconstriction contributes one-third of the total compensatory decrease in vascular conductance. If skin and muscle vasculature respond over the entire body as they do in the forearm, then 39% of the total change in conductance occurs in these tissues (Rowell et al., 1972). The remaining 28% decrease in total vascular conductance most probably occurs in the kidneys as they are the only remaining tissue in which vasoconstriction can significantly alter total vascular conductance; i.e., they receive approximately 20% of cardiac output. In short, arterial mean pressure is well-maintained during simulated hemorrhage by regional vasoconstriction. If these regions failed to vasoconstrict, then mean pressure would fall from 100 to 58 Torr.

Receptors other than arterial baroreceptors appear to be involved in the redistribution of blood flow during LBNP. Figure 3 shows that if LBNP is applied in a slow ramp of -1 Torr/min, a marked vasoconstriction in the skin and muscle and also some splanchnic vasoconstriction accompany a progressive decline in right atrial pressure (Johnson et al., 1974). Vasoconstriction appears to be elicited by cardiopulmonary baroreceptors, since it occurs before there is any change in aortic mean or pulse pressure or aortic dP/dt. The rise in HR accompanies the first measurable change in arterial pulse pressure; at this time the arterial baroreflex contributes to the regional vasomotor responses. How low pressure baroreceptors could achieve such precise regulation of a pressure they cannot "sense" (they are hydraulically isolated from the arterial system) is still a mystery.

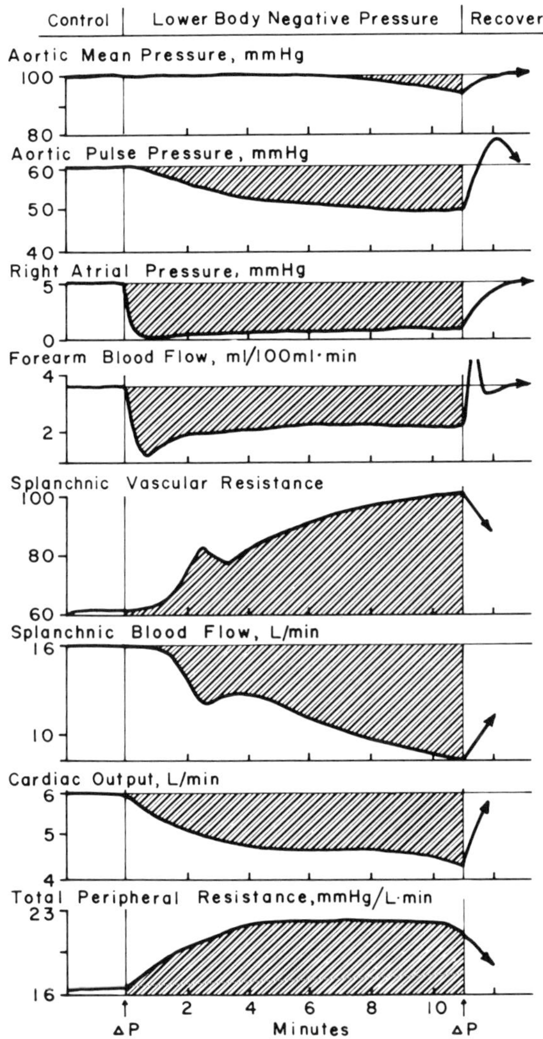

Figure 2. Schematic illustration of cardiovascular responses to LBNP at −50 Torr applied below the iliac crests.

SOURCE: *Rowell, 1973.*

Hyperthermia

Hyperthermia caused by environmental heating is another stress that elicits a marked redistribution of blood flow and blood volume in humans (Rowell, 1974). This is not to be confused with fever which causes quite different responses. Environmental heat stress causes blood volume to shift from central organs to capacious cutaneous veins, a result of some unique features of the human cutaneous circulation. Skin contains a neurogenic vasodilator system

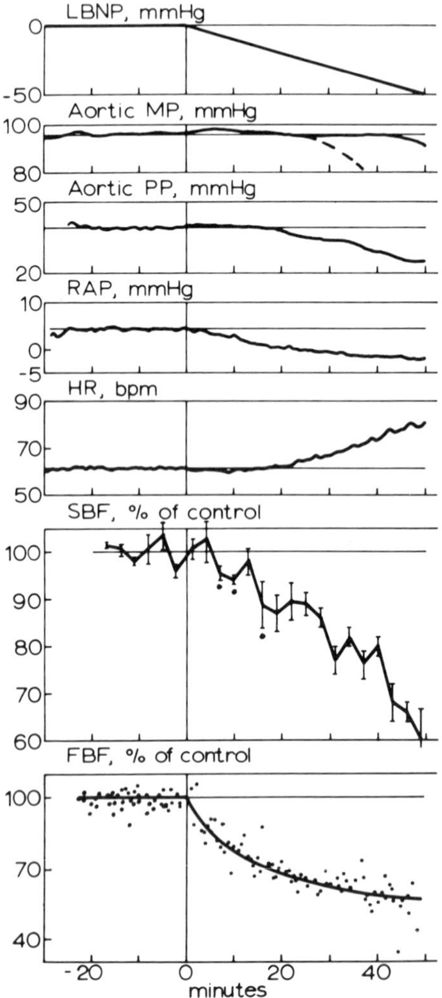

Figure 3. Cardiovascular responses to a ramp of LBNP applied at a rate of −1 Torr/min (average from 9 subjects). Up to −20 Torr of LBNP, no measurable changes in heart rate (HR), aortic mean pressure (MP), pulse pressure (PP), or dP/dt (not shown) occurred, whereas right atrial mean pressure (RAP) declined in a ramp. Note the large changes in forearm blood flow (FBF) associated with decreasing RAP. SBF is splanchnic blood flow.

SOURCE: *Johnson et al., 1974.*

which, when activated, permits very high rates of cutaneous perfusion which in turn fills a capacious and highly distensible cutaneous venous network (Rowell, 1977). Figure 4 shows responses to direct whole-body heating in supine resting subjects. Cardiac output increases markedly along with skin blood flow (SkBF)

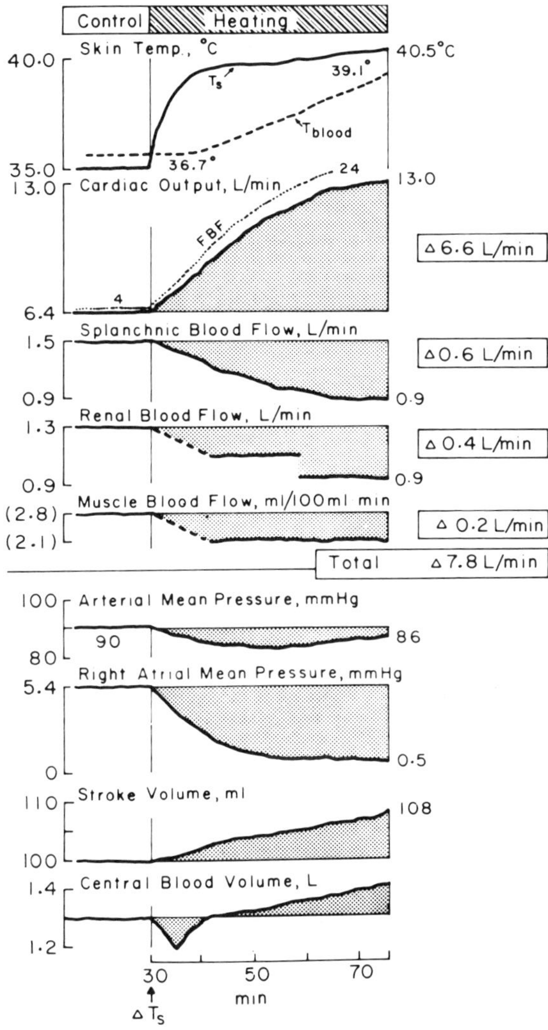

Figure 4. Average circulatory changes in men directly heated by raising body skin temperature to 40 to 41°C by means of water-perfused suits. Boxes on the right show average changes in flow to the specified regions; the sum of these changes (Total Δ) must go to skin. Note the decline in atrial pressure.

SOURCE: *Rowell, 1974.*

as measured in the forearm. Blood flow is redistributed away from splanchnic organs, kidneys, and to a minor degree from skeletal muscle. The large increase in cardiac output is accompanied by a fall in central venous pressure; in this situation, a large pressure gradient develops in the venous systems which is not rhythmically emptied by a muscle pump as it is during exercise.

The importance of splanchnic vasoconstriction during heat stress lies more in the redistribution of blood *volume* than in blood flow. The fall in right atrial pressure establishes a pressure gradient between the right atrium and the hepatic-splanchnic venous system. A fall in venous pressures transmitted through this system must lead to a passive mobilization of splanchnic venous volume to the right heart (Rowell, 1974). Splanchnic vasoconstriction further reduces splanchnic venous pressure and still more volume is mobilized passively. By these mechanisms, blood volume is eventually translocated to cutaneous veins.

Evidence from humans (Rowell, 1974, 1977) and other species (Simon and Riedel, 1975) shows that unloading of arterial baroreceptors is not the cause of the regional vasoconstriction during heat stress. In subhuman species, selective heating of either the hypothalamus or the spinal cord will increase sympathetic vasomotor outflow to visceral organs (Simon and Riedel, 1975). Increased temperature of central thermoreceptors activates the cutaneous vasodilator system in man and probably elicits the redistribution of blood flow away from visceral organs as well (Rowell, 1974, 1977).

Exercise

The most marked redistribution of blood flow from one organ system to another is observed during severe exercise (Clausen, 1977; Rowell, 1974). In contrast to heat stress, it is the redistribution of *flow* rather than volume that is more important here (except when the skin vasodilates as discussed later). The blood volume in active skeletal muscle does not increase along with increased blood flow as is the case in the skin.

The shift of blood volume into the legs with a change to upright posture is rapidly reversed by muscle contraction. Venous blood is forced centrally by muscular compression of the veins, i.e., if venous valves are competent (Gauer and Thron, 1965). With movement, average venous pressure in the legs rapidly decreases and in the lower leg it may decrease from 100 Torr to approximately 20 Torr. The blood forced centrally raises central venous pressure (from 0 to 5 Torr), central blood volume, and stroke volume.

The redistribution of cardiac output permits as much as 80 to 85% of total cardiac output to supply working skeletal muscle. This adjustment becomes increasingly important when the ability to raise cardiac output is limited by disease or by heat stress, for example. Endurance athletes, normal sedentary subjects and patients with "pure" mitral stenosis serve as examples of those having normal resting regional blood flows but very different ranges over which cardiac output can increase in response to exercise (Rowell, 1974). All of these subjects distribute cardiac output in the same way during exercise (Figure 5). For each group, it was calculated that 3 liters of blood or 600 ml of O_2 could be redistributed to working muscle each minute by 80% reductions in blood flow to nonexercising regions (Rowell, 1974). This means that the max

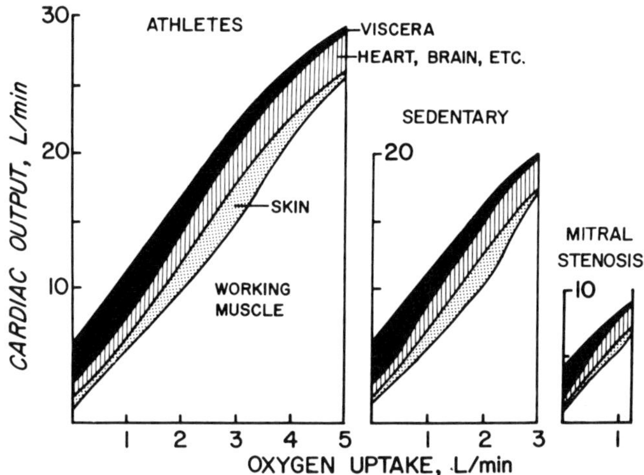

Figure 5. The distribution of cardiac output during upright exercise in endurance athletes with high max $\dot{V}O_2$ (5 liter/min), sedentary men (max $\dot{V}O_2$: 3 liter/min) and patients with pure mitral stenosis (max $\dot{V}O_2$: 1.4 liter/min). All subjects redistribute blood away from visceral organs to the same degree at any given percent of their max $\dot{V}O_2$.

SOURCE: *Rowell, 1974.*

$\dot{V}O_2$ values for each group are about 600 ml/min higher than they would be without this adjustment. Thus, the loss of this regional vasoconstriction would reduce max $\dot{V}O_2$ by nearly 40% in the mitral stenosis patient but only about 10% in the athlete. In essence, the significance of the adjustment in regional blood flow is inversely related to the magnitude of maximal cardiac output and the fraction of it required for muscles during exercise.

For nearly 100 years, physiologists have sought to identify those stimuli that lead to the close matching between blood flow and $\dot{V}O_2$ during exercise. The close inverse proportionality between splanchnic (and renal) blood flows and the percent of max $\dot{V}O_2$ required during exercise signifies that the *relative* demands on the circulation for O_2 delivery are somehow "sensed." One possibility is that chemosensitive nerve fibers in the muscle constitute the afferent arm of a metabolic error signal that can detect any mismatch between blood flow and $\dot{V}O_2$ in working muscle (Longhurst and Mitchell, 1979).

Exercise Plus Heat Stress

The combination of heat stress and exercise presents humans with two severe regulatory problems. The first problem is that a fall in stroke volume limits the extent to which cardiac output can increase. The fall in stroke volume is caused by the shift of blood volume into cutaneous veins when skin vasodilates. This lowers central blood volume and cardiac filling pressure. The muscle pump is still operative, but it is less effective (Gauer and Thron, 1965). Although the cutaneous veins still empty with each muscle contraction, they refill so rapidly that average cutaneous venous pressure and volume are increased substantially. Vasoconstriction of the compliant splanchnic circuit (Figure 1) will passively shift blood volume centrally and partially compensate for the shift of blood volume to the skin.

A second problem is that the cardiovascular system is presented with two large competing demands for blood flow; the heart is called upon to supply both the skin and active skeletal muscle. These are *competing* demands because the need for greater cardiac output is opposed by the reduction in stroke volume; thus, both demands cannot be met simultaneously. During moderate to heavy exercise, cardiac output must be maintained by higher HR (Rowell, 1974). However, as HR approaches maximal values at *submaximal* levels of $\dot{V}O_2$, cardiac output can no longer increase and eventually falls below normal relative to $\dot{V}O_2$ and then both skin and muscle may be underperfused (Rowell, 1974). Hence, reduced work capacity and severe hyperthermia are observed.

The normal pattern of blood flow distribution during exercise is changed by superimposition of heat stress (Figure 6). The limited ability of the normal heart to meet the combined needs for skin and muscle blood flow is partly

Figure 6. The approximate distribution of cardiac output during upright exercise in 6 normal subjects in cool (25°C) and hot (43°C) environments. At 43°C, the reduction in stroke volume (SV) led ultimately to reduced cardiac output and both maximal HR and systemic arteriovenous O_2 difference (AVO_2) were reached at submaximal levels of $\dot{V}O_2$. Note the fall-off in blood flow to skin which was observed by Brengelmann et al. (1977) in the forearm.

SOURCE: *Rowell, 1974.*

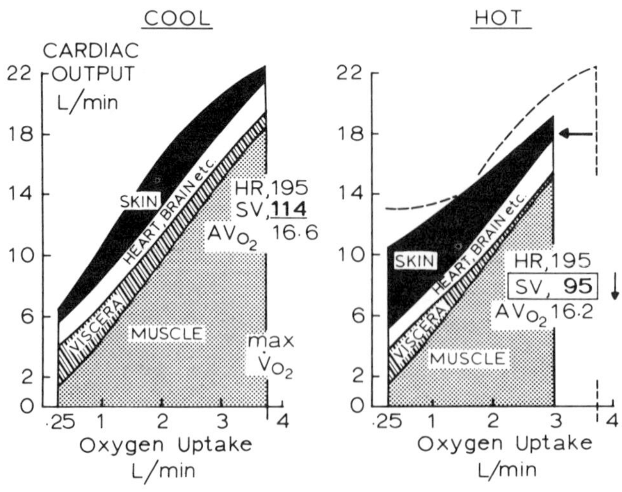

compensated for by augmented redistribution of blood flow away from visceral organs and possibly from working skeletal muscle as well (Rowell, 1974). The normal relationship between splanchnic blood flow (SBF) and $\dot{V}O_2$ at 25°C is shifted leftward in a hot environment so that SBF is much lower at any given $\dot{V}O_2$. Together with similar reductions in renal blood flow, this additional vasoconstriction could redistribute about 600 to 800 additional ml of blood to skin each minute at moderate intensities of exercise.

The adjustments just described would not maintain blood pressure at normal levels were curtaneous vessels not also responsive to the increased sympathetic vasoconstrictor outflow (Rowell, 1977). During exercise, forearm SkBF is reduced below what it would be at the same core temperature (T_c) during rest in hyperthermic subjects. Once T_c exceeds 38°C, the SkBF response tends to saturate at values that are only half of those attainable at rest (Brengelmann et al., 1977). Thus a relative cutaneous vasoconstriction reduces or delays the peripheral displacement of blood volume and helps to compensate for the reduced ability to raise cardiac output so that blood pressure is maintained, but temperature regulation is impeded.

In summary, humans with normal cardiovascular function adjust to large changes in total vascular resistance by changing cardiac output and its distribution. As cardiac function is reduced by disease or other stresses, redistribution of blood flow assumes greater relative importance in the maintenance of blood pressure and blood flow to critical organs. However, humans have difficulty in dealing with shifts in blood volume, especially in upright posture. As we seem to lack adequate venoconstrictor mechanisms, we rely instead on vasoconstriction to minimize rates of peripheral venous filling and to mobilize blood volume passively from compliant regions. When man stands up, suffers blood loss, or dilates the citaneous vessels, regulation of regional vascular resistance and the distribution of blood volume become crucial homeostatic mechanisms. Man's uprightness seems to have favored adjustments not commonly found in other species.

ACKNOWLEDGMENTS

Studies from the author's laboratory were supported by Grants from the National Institutes of Health (HL 09773 and HL 16910) and the Clinical Research Center of the University of Washington supported by National Institutes of Health Grant RR-37.

References

Amberson, W.R. 1943. Physiologic adjustments to the standing posture. *Bull. School Med. Univ. Maryland.* 27:127–145.

Brengelmann, G.L., Johnson, J.M., Hermansen, L., and Rowell, L.B., 1977. Altered control of skin blood flow during exercise at high internal temperature. *J. Appl. Physiol.* 43:790–794.

Caldini, P., Permutt, S., Waddell, J.A., and Riley, R.L., 1974. Effect of epinephrine on pressure, flow, and volume relationships in the systemic circulation of dogs. *Circ. Res.* 34:606–623.

Clausen, J.P. 1977. Effect of physical training on cardiovascular adjustments to exercise in man. *Physiol. Rev.* 57:779–815.

Gauer, O.H. and Thron, J.L. 1965. Postural changes in the circulation. In *Handbook of Physiology, Section 2. Circulation, Vol. III.* Hamilton, W.F. and Dow, P., eds. Washington, D.C.: American Physiological Society. pp. 2409–2439.

Henriksen, O. 1977. Local sympathetic reflex mechanism in regulation of blood flow in human subcutaneous adipose tissue. *Acta. Physiol. Scand.* 450 (suppl.):1–48.

Johnson, J.M., Rowell, L.B., Niederberger, M., and Eisman, M.M. 1974. Human splanchnic and forearm vasoconstrictor responses to reductions of right atrial and aortic pressure. *Circ. Res.* 34:515–524.

Johnson, R.H. and Spalding, J.M. 1974. *Disorders of the Autonomic Nervous System.* Philadelphia: F.A. Davis.

Krogh, A. 1912. The regulation of the supply of blood to the right heart. *Scand. Arch. Physiol.* 27:227–248.

Longhurst, J.C. and Mitchell, J.H., 1979. Reflex control of the circulation by afferents from skeletal muscle. In *International Review of Physiology. Cardiovascular Physiology III.* Guyton, A.C. and Young, D.B., eds. Baltimore: University Park Press. pp. 125–148.

Rowell, L.B. 1973. Regulation of splanchnic blood flow in man. *Physiologist* 16:127–142.

Rowell, L.B. 1974. Human cardiovascular adjustments to exercise and thermal stress. *Physiol. Rev.* 54:75–159.

Rowell, L.B. 1975. The splanchnic circulation. In *The Peripheral Circulations.* Zelis, R., ed. New York: Grune and Stratton. pp. 163–192.

Rowell, L.B. 1977. Reflex control of the cutaneous vasculature. *J. Invest. Dermatol.* 69:154–166.

Rowell, L.B. 1981. Circulatory adjustments to thermal stress. In *Handbook of Physiology: The Cardiovascular System.* Shepherd, J.T. and Abboud, F.M., eds. Bethesda: American Physiological Society. In press.

Rowell, L.B., Detry, J.R., Blackmon, J.R., and Wyss, C. 1972. Importance of the splanchnic vascular bed in human blood pressure regulation. *J. Appl. Physiol.* 32:213–218.

Selkurt, E.E. 1946. Comparison of renal clearances with direct renal blood flow under control of conditions and following renal ischemia. *Am. J. Physiol.* 145:376–386.

Shepherd, J.T. and Vanhoutte, P. 1975. *Veins and Their Control.* Philadelphia: W.B. Saunders.

Simon, E. and Riedel, W. 1975. Diversity of regional sympathetic outflow in integrative cardiovascular control: patterns and mechanisms. *Brain Res.* 87:323–333.

Sjöstrand, T. 1952. The regulation of the blood distribution in man. *Acta Physiol. Scand.* 26:312–327.

Vatner, S.F. 1975. Effects of exercise on distribution of regional blood flows and resistances. In *The Peripheral Circulations.* Zelis, R., ed. New York: Grune and Stratton. pp. 211–233.

Wade, O.L. and Bishop, J.M. 1962. *Cardiac Output and Regional Blood Flow.* Oxford: Blackwell.

Wolthius, R.A., Bergman, S.A., and Nicogossian, A.E. 1975. Physiological effects of locally applied reduced pressure in man. *Physiol. Rev.* 54:566–595.

Zelis, R. 1975. *The Peripheral Circulations.* New York: Grune and Stratton.

J.A. Loeppky and M.L. Riedesel, editors
OXYGEN TRANSPORT TO HUMAN TISSUES

Some Functional Characteristics of the Low Pressure System

Karl A. Kirsch and H. von Ameln

Introduction

Whether or not the low pressure system (LPS), consisting of the systemic veins plus the intrathoraic vascular bed up to the aortic valves, can be looked upon as a passive elastic volume container (Gauer and Thron, 1965) or whether the contractile components within the walls of the peripheral veins play an active role in the control of central blood volume and cardiac filling pressure is still under debate (Shepherd and Vanhoutte, 1975). How the questions arising from this debate are answered depends somewhat upon the models used during experimentation.

Earlier experiments performed by O.H. Gauer and coworkers (Gauer and Henry, 1963; Gauer and Thron, 1965) showed that the functional pecularities of the LPS can best be demonstrated with models involving the changes occurring during orthostasis. Under these conditions, the pressure distribution and hence the volume distribution within the LPS change due to gravitational forces may not be balanced by the active contractile components.

Methods and Results

The problems outlined above can best be described as shown in Figure 1. Here the LPS is simplified and regarded as an elastic tube having (in recumbency) a uniform pressure of 15 cm H_2O, taking into account only the hydrostatic component of the venous pressure. When tilting such a system from the horizontal to upright position, the pressures will fall in the upper parts and will rise in the dependent parts. There necessarily exists a transition zone where the intravascular pressure stays constant. This zone will be referred to as the "Hydrostatic Indifferent Point" (HIP) (Gauer and Sieker, 1956; Gauer and Thron, 1965). At the HIP level, the pressures remain unaffected during changes of body posture and hence no volume changes are expected there. The model is arranged in such a way that the heart is well above the HIP which means that pressures inside the heart must fall during assumption of upright posture (Gauer and Thron, 1965).

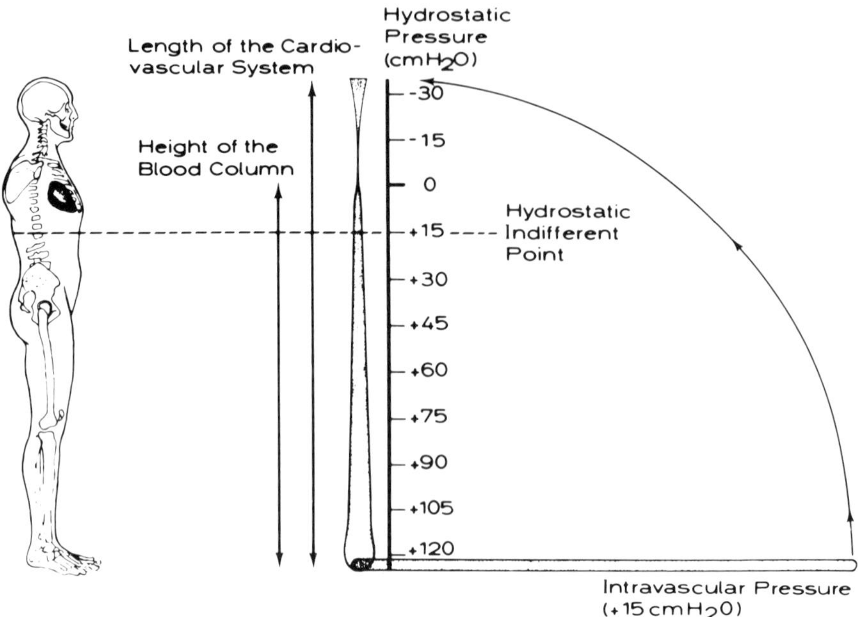

Figure 1. Schematic representation of the effect of orthostasis on the redistribution of pressure within the low pressure system along the body axis. The Hydrostatic Indifferent Point is below the heart. The collapse of the veins in the upper part of the thorax separates the blood column within the low pressure system.

Due to collapse of the veins in the region of the neck, the blood column is divided and the height of the column extending from the heels up to the upper thoracic cavity is not identical with the total length of the cardiovascular system. Despite this simple approach, such a model apparently fits in several ways with the LPS in situ that can be seen in man by X-ray and plethysmographic methods.

The assumption made in Figure 1, that the heart lies above the HIP, was supported up to the present by only a few measurements in man (Gauer and Sieker, 1956; Gauer and Thron, 1965) and therefore needed to be reinvestigated since this fact was challenged by other authors (Greganti and Guyton, 1955). A newly developed sensor which allowed us to trace volume changes within small superficial tissue cylinders was applied to man during tilting maneuvers (Kirsch et al., 1980a, b). An example is given in Figure 2, where the small sensors were attached along the body axis. As expected, during assumption of upright posture, the tissue thickness in the upper part of the body rapidly decreased within 5 sec, which can be taken as an indicator of rapid emptying of the capacitance vessels. This must occur in all locations above the HIP (Figure 1). Below the HIP, the fluid must accumulate and consequently

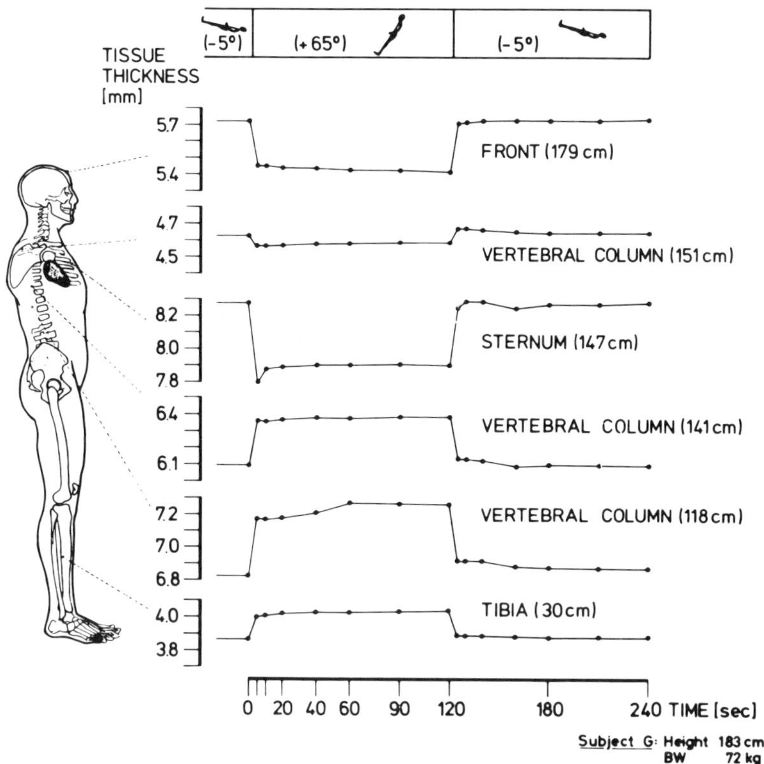

Figure 2. Typical experiment in one subject of the effect of tilting on tissue layer thickness as measured in 6 different locations along the body axis. Above the apex of the heart, the tissue layer thickness decreased. At the vertebral column below the heart, only minor changes were visible. At the tibia, a slow but continuous increase of the tissue layer thickness towards the end of the tilting period was evident.

the tissue thickness must increase. In the upper part of the body after the first rapid phase, the tissue thickness remained unchanged or even increased. This might be due to the collapse of the veins after their rapid emptying which creates a certain resistance so that fluid can accumulate within the vessels. On the other hand, below the HIP a slow but constant increase of tissue thickness was usually found which can be interpreted as a slow outward filtration lasting until the end of the tilting period.

According to these experiments, the HIP was located below the heart, however, its exact localization with this simple noninvasive method was sometimes tedious. In Figure 3, the results are given from experiments when the subjects were tilted in 5-degree steps from $-5°$ to $+5°$ and later in 20-degree steps. One would expect that the further from the HIP the sensor is placed, the greater would be the change in tissue thickness. Figure 3 supports

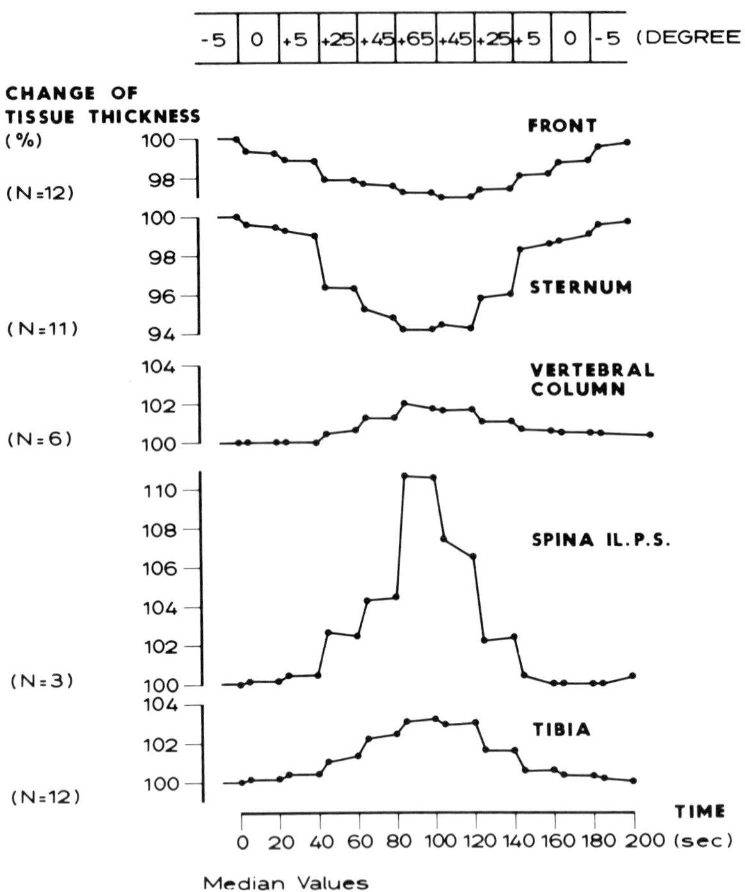

Figure 3. The effect of stepwise tilting on fluid distribution along the body axis. Median values from 12 subjects. The subjects were tilted in 5 steps up to 65° and in return to the resting position. The subjects remained for 20 sec in each position. Resting values are taken at 100%.

this assumption because in the frontal area and in the tibia a change of only 5 degrees induced small decrements or increments of tissue thickness which were statistically significant. In the vertebral column around the HIP, rather large changes of body posture were necessary to induce deviations of tissue volume. This can only be interpreted to mean that close to the HIP only small intravascular pressure changes occur during the tilting maneuvers. All experiments, however, supported the concept that the HIP was located about 10 to 15 cm below the heart.

Further details of the postural behavior pattern of the LPS as a whole were studied in a rubber tube model (length 100 cm), where a pressure/volume

(P/V) relationship was approximated in supine and upright positions as shown in Figure 4 (Brechmann, 1967; Thron and Kirsch, 1978). The supine P/V relationship is characterized by a flat limb (A), which represents the part of the unstressed volume, and a steeply rising part (B), which shows that the tube is distended with each volume increment. The corresponding upright pressure curve ascends almost uniformly throughout the whole range of added volumes. It is remarkable that in part A the upright pressure curve is steeper than supine, whereas in part B it is definitely less steep than the supine curve. In this model, the HIP level is situated just below the point of collapse and moves upward when volume is added. At a level corresponding to about 70% of the total system length from the bottom, with additional volume a definite downward slope ensues which obviously tends to level off finally in the middle region of the model. It needs to be pointed out that changing the volume

Figure 4. The effect of changing filling volume (water) in a thin-walled collapsible rubber tube model of the venous system on the hydrostatic pressure in both the horizontal and the vertical position, on the height of the vertical fluid column in the noncollapsed downward model segment (left side) and on the location of the Hydrostatic Indifferent Point (HIP) along the model axis. A and B on the top of the picture are related to the flat and steeply ascending limbs of the supine pressure/volume diagram, respectively.

SOURCE: *Brechmann, 1967.*

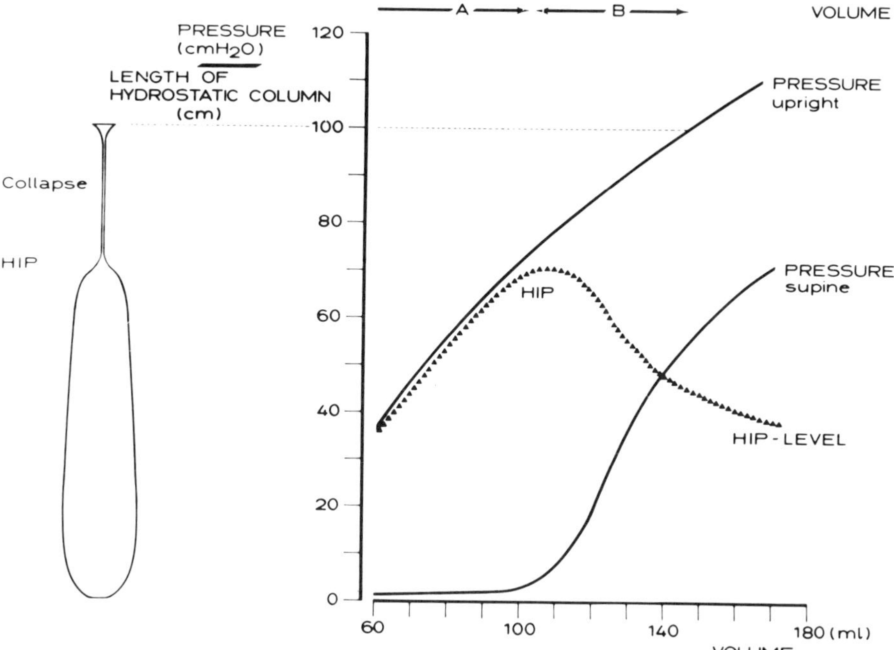

capacity of the system or perfusing the system constantly does not change the basic characteristics of the model.

Transferring these model experiments directly to an animal reveals the results presented in Figure 5. In an anesthetized dog, P/V relationships were worked out in supine and upright positions (dashed lines, lower part). In the upper part, the decrease in the central venous pressure after tilting during the different filling stages is shown. The pressures were determined with a catheter tip manometer in the right atrium. The fact that the pressure decreases in the

Figure 5. Typical experiment in anesthetized dog of the effect of augmentation of intravascular filling volume on central venous pressure in upright and supine position (dashed lines, lower part). Postural changes of central venous pressure in the upper part of the graph.

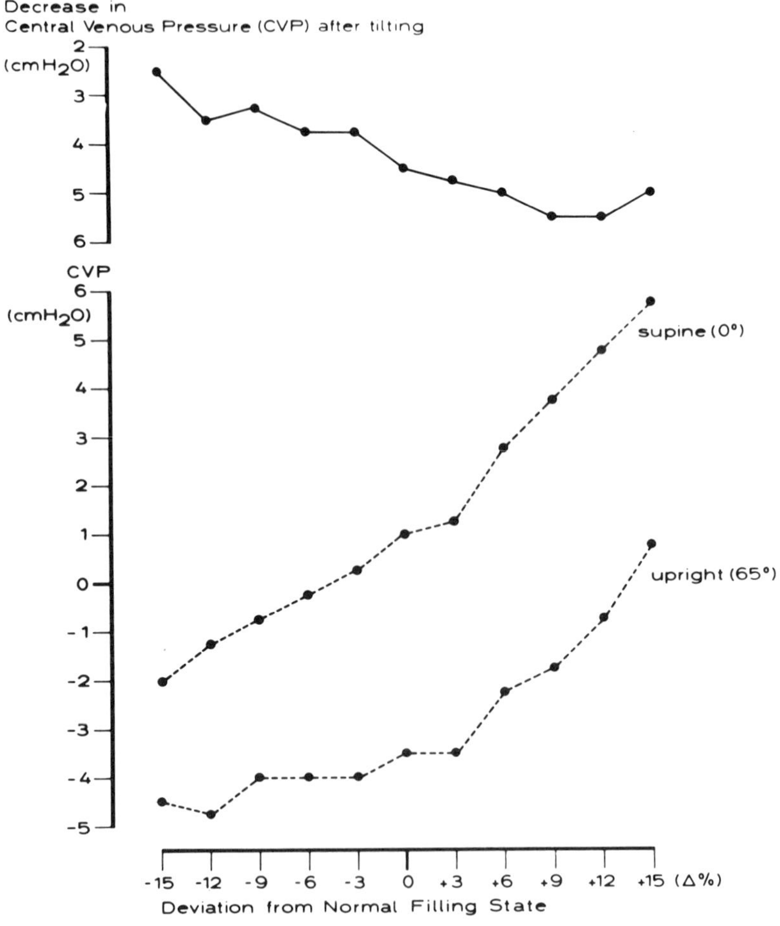

right atrium after tilting is not surprising, but the pressure decrement is more pronounced when more volume is added to the system. With respect to the models in Figure 1 and 4, one can conclude that the animal was in the filling range B (Figure 4) which means that the distance between the HIP in the right atrium increased with higher filling volumes. This assumption is supported by the steep slope derived in the supine position which is generally steeper over the whole range as compared to the slope derived in the upright position.

Now the interesting question remains whether this pattern can be modified by a vasoactive substance such as dihydroergotamine (DHE), known to induce venoconstriction. The results of a typical experiment are given in Figure 6 where the pressures along the vena cava up to the right atrium were determined in supine and upright position with and without DHE. In the supine position, a typical pattern was seen with the characteristic pressure drop of 2.5 mm Hg near the diaphragm and a total pressure gradient of 7 mm Hg from the iliac vein downstream to the right atrium. In the upright position, the straight line covers a pressure decrease of 20 mm Hg. The pressure in the right atrium decreased by 2 mm Hg during the tilt. Per definition, the HIP is at the point where the lines cross, which means the same pressures prevail at this point during both positions. In our case, the HIP was about 3.5 cm below the right atrium. The application of DHE led to an increase of the central venous pressure in the supine position by 3 mm Hg, and the pressure gradient along the vena cava was only 4 mm Hg. One can assume that a volume translocation from peripheral towards central parts of the LPS had taken place induced by precapillary vasoconstriction and venoconstriction. Tilting the animal did not change the shape of the curve as compared to the control. The central venous pressure decreased now by 4 mm Hg, being on the same level as under control conditions. This was due to a downward movement of the HIP by 4.5 cm (see shaded area) and is to be expected from the assumption of the filling state in Figure 4, part B.

Comments

A common question is raised concerning the localization of the HIP in man. According to the results presented here the HIP should be 10 to 15 cm below the heart at the level of the liver. Gauer and Sieker (1956) and Gauer and Thron (1965) have postulated the HIP to be 5 to 10 cm below the diaphragm with the pressure there being about 15 cm H_2O. From the point of view of hydrostatic pressure distribution, the heart is by no means independent of hydrostatic changes as it would be if the heart were at the HIP level. Indeed, during assumption of upright posture, central venous pressure falls and cardiac output decreases (Bevegård et al., 1960), a pattern one would expect from our models (Figure 1 and 4) and shown in the experiments (Figures 5 and 6). Another consequence of the HIP being in this location is that the postcapillary area of the liver and the upper parts of the portal circulation are protected

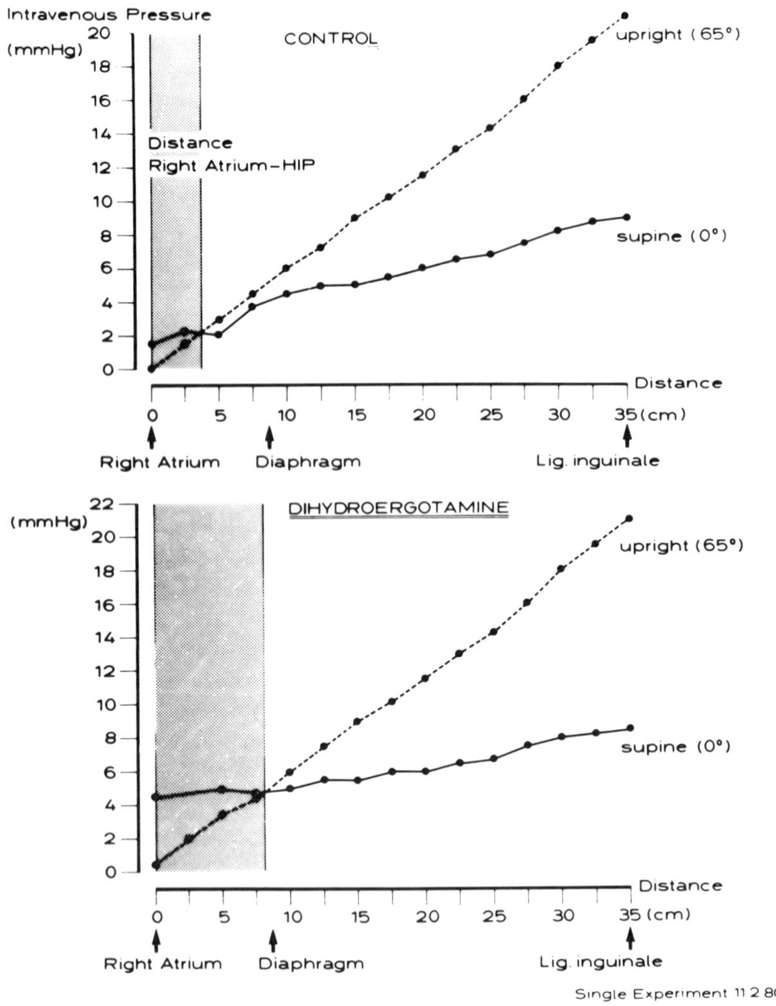

Figure 6. Typical experiment in anesthetized dog of the pressure distribution along vena cava in supine (solid line) and upright (dashed line) position. Upper part shows control values. Shaded area on the left side represents the distance between the right atrium and the HIP at the crossing point of the pressures. Abscissa gives the distance between the right atrium and lig. inguinale in cm. Lower part represents the results under DHE. Note the downward movement of the HIP with DHE and the difference between the central venous pressure in supine and upright position.

against great changes of venous pressure which could lead to an outward filtration and pooling of blood volume in these areas. Just the opposite is probable, with the veins of the portal circulation being well-equipped with muscles and adrenergic fibers that can expel their volume towards the more central parts of the circulation (Shepherd and Vanhoutte, 1975, 1979). This would be impossible if the HIP would be located near the heart. In the latter case, the hydrostatic load on the portal veins would be at such a level that the veins could hardly overcome the burden induced by gravity.

Another remarkable observation was that the HIP was by no means fixed at one particular point along the venous column but moved up or down depending upon the filling state of the system (Figures 4 and 6). In our case, the downward movement of the HIP location with increased filling volume leads finally to progressively larger pressure decrements in the right atrium during tilting than one might anticipate. In practice this means adding volume is followed by a substantial increase of the central venous pressure in the supine position, but does not necessarily mean an increased filling pressure of the heart in the upright position. This pattern cannot be changed by giving vasoactive agents. The LPS as a whole behaves in this case differently than one would expect from studies on isolated segments. This should be taken into consideration in order to understand the role of venomotor tone in orthostatic regulation.

Summary

The location of the Hydrostatic Indifferent Point (HIP) was identified in man, with the help of a noninvasive method, to be 10 to 15 cm below the heart which has important physiological consequences. Furthermore, the Low Pressure System (LPS) as a whole was compared with a rubber tube model simulating orthostasis. The predictions concerning the orthostatic response patterns of the LPS in man and animals as derived from model experiments showed that the LPS behaves in many ways as a passive elastic volume container. Application of vasoactive substances like dihydroergotamine (DHE) have a strong influence on the system in the supine position elevation of central venous pressure), however, they are of minor importance in altering the filling pressure of the heart in upright posture.

ACKNOWLEDGMENT

This study was supported by the Bundesministerium für Forschung und Technologie.

References

Bevegård, S., Holmgren, A., and Jonsson, B., 1960. The effect of body position on the circulation at rest and during exercise, with special reference to the influence on the stroke volume. *Acta Physiol. Scand.* 49:279–298.

Brechmann, W. 1967. *Der Hydrostatische Indifferenzpunkt im Venensystem des Menschen*. Inaug. Dissertation, Medizinische Fakultät der Freien Universität, Berlin.

Gauer, O.H. and Henry, J.P., 1963. Circulatory basis of fluid volume control. *Physiol. Rev.* 43:423–481.

Gauer, O.H. and Sieker, H.O., 1956. The continuous recording of central venous pressure changes from an arm vein. *Circulation Res.* 4:74–78.

Gauer, O.H. and Thron, H.L., 1965. Postural changes in the circulation. *Handbook of Physiology, Section. 2: Circulation. Vol. III.* Hamilton, W.F. and Dow, P., eds. Washington, D.C.: American Physiological Society. pp. 2409–2439.

Greganti, F.P. and Guyton, A.C., 1955. Right ventricle as physiological level for reference of pressures in circulatory system. *Am. J. Physiol.* 183:622.

Kirsch, K., Merke, J., and Hinghofer-Szalkay, H. 1980a. Fluid volume distribution within superficial shell tissues along body axis during changes of body posture in man: the application of new miniature plethysmographic method. *Pflügers Arch.* 383:195–201.

Kirsch, K.A., Merke, J., Hinghofer-Szalkay, H., Barnkow, M., and Wicke, H.J. 1980b. A new miniature plethysmograph to measure volume changes in small circumscribed tissue areas. *Pflügers Arch.* 383:189–194.

Shepherd, J.T. and VanHoutte, P.M., 1975. *Veins and Their Control.* Philadelphia: W.B. Saunders. pp. 171–189.

Shepherd, J.T. and Vanhoutte, P.M., 1979. *The Human Cardiovascular System. Facts and Concepts.* New York: Raven Press.

Thron, H.L. and Kirsch, K. 1978. Active and passive components in the orthostatic behavior of the venous system in man and in animals. *International Symposium on the Regulation of Capacitance Vessels.* Chernukh, A.M. and Tkachenko, B.I., eds. Budapest: Akadémiai Kiadó (Moskva: Akademiia Meditsinskikh nauk SSSR). pp. 197–220.

J.A. Loeppky and M.L. Riedesel, editors
OXYGEN TRANSPORT TO HUMAN TISSUES

Noninvasive Measurement of Blood Flow Using Pulsed Doppler Ultrasound

E. Richard Greene

Introduction

A complete and quantitative characterization of the human cardiovascular system would ideally require a method which could noninvasively, nontraumatically, and dynamically measure vessel geometry, intraluminal pressure, and volumetric blood flow. These anatomical and physiological variables have been previously measured by indirect or invasive methods (Rushmer, 1976, pp. 36–75). The various measurement techniques were restricted by the instrumentation that was available to the researcher. Generally, the evaluation of human cardiovascular physiology (Rowell, 1974) and pathophysiology (Detweiler, 1973) has been based on radiological techniques (anatomy), indwelling catheters (pressures and flows), and sphygmography (indirect pressure). The most difficult but perhaps the most important physiological variable to measure, either invasively or noninvasively, has been volumetric blood flow.

Volumetric blood flow expressed in liter/min or ml/min, generally reflects the oxygen transport capabilities of the cardiovascular system and represents tissue perfusion. When measured concomitantly with blood pressure gradients, vascular blood flow impedance can be determined (McDonald, 1974; Murgo et al., 1980; Murgo et al., 1981). Until recently, neither left ventricular stroke volume (LVSV) nor regional blood flows could be measured specifically and dynamically by a noninvasive and nontraumatic method. Consequently, invasive or indirect measurements of blood flow were limited to animal models or a small number of human volunteers without any emphasis on serial studies. Whenever an invasive study was presented, questions generally surfaced about the measurements being representative of the true, undisturbed physiological state (Rushmer, 1976, pp. 36–75). Clearly, the natural effects of stress, aging, and disease on the oxygen transport capabilities and blood flow in the human cardiovascular system can best be studied by nontraumatic and noninvasive techniques.

Recent technological developments in ultrasonic pulsed Doppler flowmetry have resulted in systems which appear capable of exhibiting more of the characteristics of an ideal blood flowmeter than previously used systems. The purpose of this presentation is to describe the theory and the instrumentation of noninvasive ultrasound pulsed Doppler flowmetry and to demonstrate applications in the human cardiovascular system.

Theory and Instrumentation

Accurate use of Doppler flowmetry requires an appreciation of hemodynamics as well as an understanding of the fundamental Doppler principle and the interaction of acoustic energy with biological tissues and moving blood. A brief summary of these principles will be presented here, but the reader is referred to the literature for a more comprehensive treatment (Baker, 1970; Jorgensen et al., 1973; McDonald, 1974; Wells, 1977).

The term "ultrasound" is used to describe mechanical vibrations at frequencies above the limit of human audibility. Audible sound ranges in frequencies from 16 to 20,000 cycles/sec (Hz). Most nontraumatic ultrasound used in physiological studies is between 1 and 20 megahertz (MHz) and produces energy at less than 5.0 W/cm^2. Ultrasonic energy in the form of waves is generated when a piezoelectric crystal, the transducer, vibrates at its resonant frequency after the application of a controlled burst of electromagnetic energy to its surface. When the vibrating transducer contacts the skin, the ultrasonic energy is transmitted into the tissues. As this acoustic energy propagates through the tissue, it is absorbed which reduces the energy intensity at each point along the beam and the energy is also reflected at points along the beam where the acoustic impedance (Z) changes. If ultrasonic energy from the transducer is delivered in short bursts of energy (pulsed), the same transducer can then be used to receive reflected energy as a result of changes in Z. Impedance depends on the mechanical properties of the tissue and is given by the formula:

$$Z = \rho \cdot C \tag{13.1}$$

where ρ is the tissue density and C is the velocity of sound in the biological tissues which is generally 1500 m/sec in blood and soft body tissues.

If the location of the interface between two tissues with different values of Z is stationary, the frequency of the reflected wave will be approximately the same as the incoming wave and can be received by the same transducer for dynamic structural information, such as cardiac chamber and blood vessel dimensions (Wells, 1977; Feigenbaum, 1981). In contrast, a moving interface will cause the reflected signal frequency to be frequency-shifted by a magnitude which is proportional to the interface velocity in the direction of the sound beam axis (Baker, 1970). In the simplest form, this relationship is given by the classic Doppler equation:

$$\Delta f = \frac{2 \cdot v \cdot f \cdot \cos\theta}{C} \tag{13.2}$$

where Δf represents the Doppler shift (Hz), v is the velocity vector of the interface (cm/sec), f is the frequency of the transmitted ultrasound (Hz), C is the velocity of sound (cm/sec) in the tissue media supporting the acoustic energy, and θ is the Doppler incident angle between the transmitted beam and the velocity vector. If the values of f and C are assumed constant (a reasonable assumption in most applications), one can measure θ and Δf to calculate v.

When the incident sound beam traverses a blood vessel, small amounts of sound energy are absorbed by each red cell. Since the dimensions of the red cells are small compared to the wave length of the acoustic energy, the reflected wave is radiated in all directions (Wells, 1977). This phenomenon is termed "backscatter." If the red cell is moving relative to the transducer, a backscattered Doppler shift can be recorded (Baker, 1970). Since a distribution of blood velocities is present in each segment of a blood vessel (McDonald, 1974, pp. 101–117), a spectrum of Doppler shift frequencies will be present. This spectrum can become quite dynamic and complex in physiological states of blood flow. Analysis of the spectrum of Doppler shift frequencies is further complicated by the inherent motion of the blood vessel (Davis et al., 1979). If the *mean* frequency shift can be electronically extracted from the Doppler shift spectrum, the spatial average velocity (v_{sa}) as a function of time can be measured (Greene and Histand, 1979). Volumetric blood flow ($\dot{Q}$) can then be determined from an independent ultrasonic measurement of lumen diameter (D) by the equation:

$$\dot{Q} = \frac{v_{sa} \cdot \pi \cdot D^2}{4} \tag{13.3}$$

Thus, $\dot{Q}$ can be derived from two independent measurements (v_{sa} and D) determined ultrasonically (Phillips et al., 1980; Loeppky et al., 1981).

Equations (13.2) and (13.3) are deceivingly simple and have led some investigators to apply commercially available ultrasound Doppler systems to blood vessels to arrive at quantitative measurements of v_{sa} and $\dot{Q}$ without appreciation of the complexities involved in making the measurements and processing the data (Strandness, 1978). One must recognize that $\dot{Q}$ is dynamic and cannot be accurately obtained with a single measurement without attention to geometry anatomy and temporal changes. The noninvasive Doppler ultrasound methods of measuring $\dot{Q}$ require the following four distinct steps: (1) location of the vessel, (2) determination of the Doppler incident angle, (3) measurement of the lumen area, and (4) measurement of the spatial average frequency shift, Δf which represents v_{sa}. The first three steps appear to be adequately resolved by the recently developed real-time, 2-dimensional echo-Doppler duplex scanner, which has been described in detail elsewhere (Barber et al., 1974; Baker and Daigle, 1977; Baker, 1980).

The fourth step, determination of the mean value of Δf and hence v_{sa}, can be quite difficult. For the simplest case: if the velocity profile is parabolic with a low Reynolds' number (McDonald, 1974, pp. 101–117) and if there is complete insonation of the entire flow field with an even distribution of acoustic energy, then the calculated blood velocity will be v_{sa} and will represent one-half of the maximum centerline velocity (v_{max}) (Greene et al., 1976). If the velocity profile is flat due to developing boundary layers (Schlichting, 1968), but not turbulent (McDonald, 1974, pp. 71–101), theoretically only one Doppler shift will be present which will represent v_{sa} and v_{max}. In the cardiovascular system, there are several complexities that make the analysis of v_{sa} even more difficult. Due to the pulsatile nature of flow and its reversal in early diastole in many peripheral vessels, flow will be reversed near the vessel walls, although there is still forward flow in the central part of the velocity profile during some phases in the cardiac cycle. Noninvasive measurements taken in our laboratory of the adult common carotid blood velocity waveform and its spatially-distributed velocity profile at given points in the cardiac cycle are shown in Figure 1. Note that the flow velocity at the walls during early diastole, as shown in D, is reversed although the value of v_{sa} at that point is above zero. If turbulence is present, either transient or fully developed, the Doppler spectra becomes quite complex and so the extraction of v_{sa} from the Doppler spectra is unreliable (Lunt, 1975; Baker and Daigle, 1977). Furthermore, even in laminar flow regimens the velocity profile is generally not symmetric, thus making the requirement of uniform insonation of the vessel with acoustic energy for the measurement of the mean Δf even more important.

Even if the hemodynamics of the interrogated blood vessel are well-behaved and understood, it must also be known (Baker and Daigle, 1977), (1) whether there is axial migration of the red blood cells which would weigh the Doppler spectra towards the higher velocities, (2) whether there is a uniform sound beam which is required for uniform insonation of the vessel, and (3) whether there is distortion of the Doppler signal due to band-pass characteristics of the signal processing system which would distort the true measurement of the mean Δf value. Recent technological improvements have provided more control of the blood velocity sensing region, known as the sample volume (SV). Consequently, specific locations of blood velocities can be more uniformly insonated to provide a Doppler spectrum which reflects the true distribution of velocities within the vessel (Greene et al., 1979). From this spectrum, Doppler analysis can yield a more accurate calculation of v_{sa} [Equation (13.2) which can be multiplied by the lumen diameter (assuming a circular geometry) to obtain $\dot{Q}$ [Equation (13.3)].

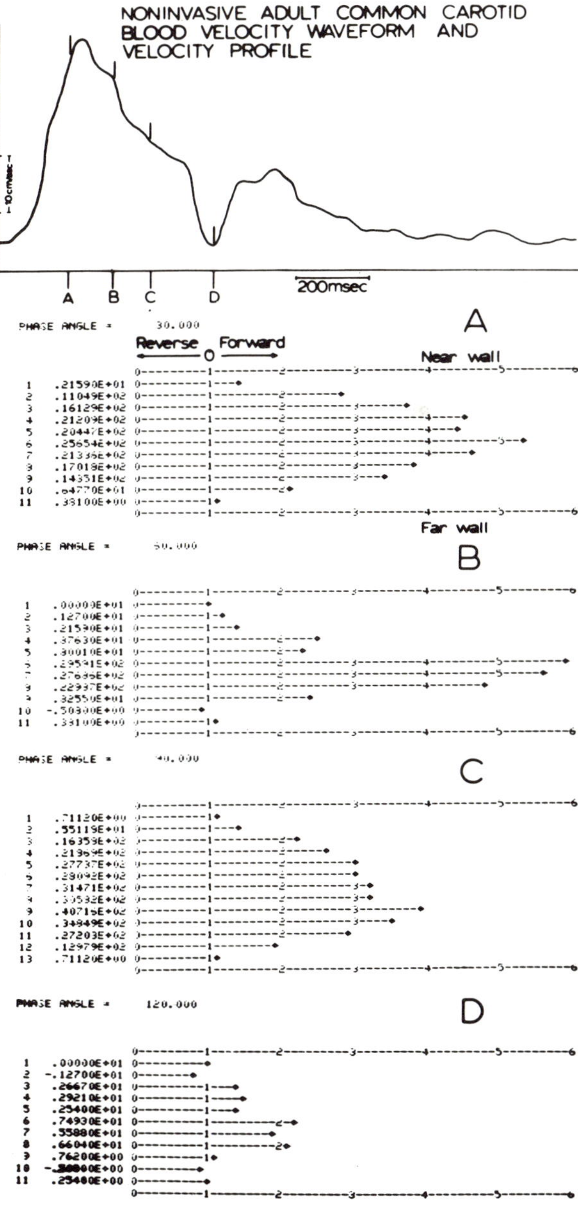

Figure 1. Noninvasive adult common carotid blood spatial averaged velocity waveform (v_{sa}) and corresponding velocity profiles measured at points A, B, C, and D in the cardiac cycle by a 7.0 MHz pulsed Doppler velocimeter. The length of the computer-generated velocity profile arrows are calibrated in cm/sec. Zero velocity is located at the scale of 1.

Although alternative methods of obtaining $\dot{Q}$ from pulsed Doppler flowmetry, with or without vessel imaging, are available (Greene et al., 1976; Blair et al., 1981), the most thorough scheme which considers all the factors one must address in the noninvasive pulsed Doppler determination of $\dot{Q}$ is outlined in Figure 2. With appropriate instrumentation and technique, the influence of these factors on the accuracy and precision of noninvasive measurements of $\dot{Q}$ can be optimized. Systematic and experimental errors can be reduced, and the technique of noninvasive flowmetry can be applied to the human cardiovascular system.

Application of Noninvasive Doppler Flowmetry to the Human Cardiovascular System

With appropriate instrumentation, the pulsed Doppler technique can be applied to a wide range of vessel dimensions ranging in size from 1.0 mm to 4.0 cm in diameter. Both superficial (1.0 mm below skin surface) (Blair et al., 1981) and deep (17 cm below skin surface) vessels (Greene et al., 1981) can be examined. Vessels lying underneath lung or bone tissue are generally unavailable for interrogation due to the inability to pass sufficient acoustic energy through these tissues (Wells, 1977). Generally, a real-time, 2-dimensional image of the examined vessel is required to obtain the vessel diameter and the Doppler incident angle. In particular applications (e.g., ascending aorta), the Doppler angle can be assumed to be near zero and hence the cosine function in the Doppler equation becomes 1.0 (Darsee et al., 1980; Loeppky et al., 1981).

Figure 2. Factors influencing the noninvasive measurment of volume flow rate using pulsed Doppler flowmetry. (*Note*: BW-band width; S/N = signal to noise ratio; PRF = pulse repetition frequency.)

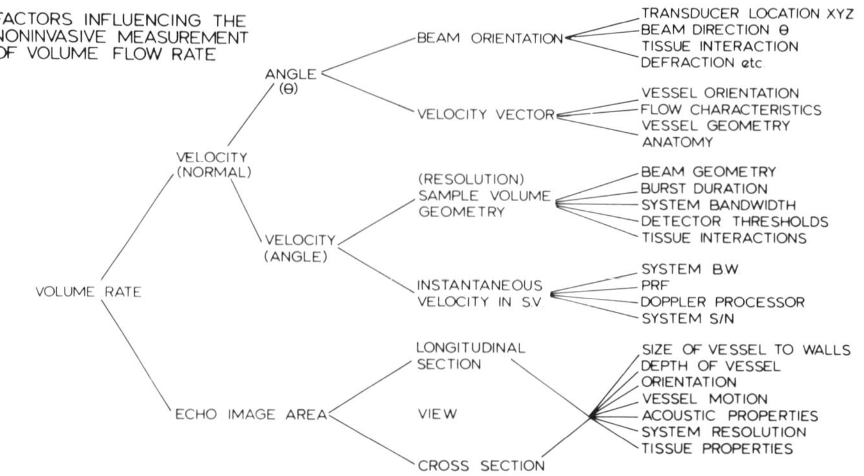

Furthermore, noninvasive flowmetry is not limited to measuring blood velocity and volumetric blood flow. There is also a significant application of Doppler ultrasound in the noninvasive diagnosis of arterial and cardiac disease (Strandness, 1978; Baker, 1980; Greene et al., 1980a). In present clinical applications of identifying vascular disease, flow disturbances created by anatomical lesions are monitored by changes in the recorded Doppler frequency spectra. By this method, hemodynamically and nonhemodynamically significant lesions can be detected noninvasively (Phillips et al., 1980). Until recently, no emphasis was placed on quantitatively measuring $\dot{Q}$ in the presence of atherosclerotic lesions. However, clinical attitudes appear to be changing toward a greater appreciation of the hemodynamic significance of the interaction of distal vascular impedance with changes in $\dot{Q}$ resulting from arterial lesions (Young, 1979).

The following examples of applications of noninvasive pulsed Doppler flowmetry are taken from recent work in our laboratory and represent the capabilities and limitations of this technique applied to the human cardiovascular system.

Left ventricular stroke volume (LVSV) and cardiac output (CO). A noninvasive, dynamic measurement of LVSV and CO has been a goal of cardiovascular researchers for many years (Rushmer, 1976, pp. 36–75). Using a single crystal Doppler transducer placed in the subject's suprasternal notch (Figure 3), mean frequency shift Doppler spectra can be obtained from the ascending aorta. In this application, the value of θ is assumed to be near zero. Since the blood flow profile in the aortic root is blunt (Seed and Wood, 1971), the SV reflects v_{sa} and v_{max}. From the left sternal border, either a multiple crystal real-time

Figure 3. A schematic representation of the pulsed Doppler technique of measuring LVSV and CO. The transducer is angled until the same volume intercepts the blood stream in the ascending aorta 2 to 3 cm from the aortic valve.

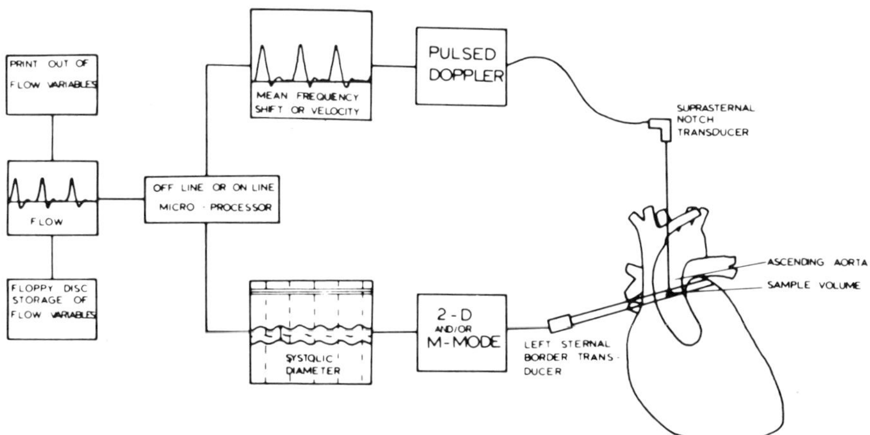

scanhead or a single crystal M-mode echocardiographic transducer can independently obtain the mean systolic diameter (D) of the ascending aorta (Feigenbaum, 1981). By either off-line or on-line computer processing of the Doppler spectra and D, beat-to-beat values of $\dot{Q}$ can be calculated, stored, or displayed. This method of measuring LVSV and CO has been validated *in vitro* (Greene et al., 1980b) and *in vivo* in humans with the direct Fick procedure (Hoekenga et al., 1980) with excellent correlation coefficients and slopes of the regression lines near 1.0 being obtained. Other investigators (Darsee et al., 1980; Steingart et al., 1980) have supported these results. Physiological studies of dynamic changes of LVSV and CO during upright and supine exercise (Loeppky et al., 1981) and lower body negative pressure (Loeppky et al., 1979) have demonstrated that unique, beat-by-beat information can be obtained by this technique. Recently, the method has been applied to patients with various degrees of coronary artery disease during progressive upright ergometric exercise. Results have shown that patients with significant coronary disease in one or more of the main coronary vessels but with good left ventricular function (resting ejection fraction above 55% by invasive ventriculography) show a smaller ($p<0.05$) increase (+11%) in LVSV during submaximal exercise than normal age-matched subjects (+37%). Coronary patients with ejection fractions less than 55% show no increase in LVSV during ergometric exercise at any workload. Changes in global left ventricular function determined serially by noninvasive pulsed Doppler flowmetry during submaximal exercise may provide further insight into the hemodynamic and functional significance of coronary lesions on ventricular function as well as the clinical efficacy of short- and long-term treatment regimens.

Main pulmonary artery blood flow. Since the anatomy of the main pulmonary artery creates a curvilinear conduit which does not allow the assumption of a Doppler incident angle of zero, the pulsed Doppler sample volume can be guided by the real-time, 2-dimensional duplex image developed by three rotating crystals in a hand-held scanhead (Figure 4). The solid white line in the figure is the Doppler beam axis displayed by the duplex scanner (Kalmanson et al., 1979; Phillips et al., 1980), and the white dot represents the location of the SV which can be placed at any location in the sector image. The blood velocity vectors are assumed to be parallel to the imaged vessel walls. At the bottom of the figure, the Doppler shift spectrum representing blood velocities in the PA is displayed and velocity calculated by determining θ from the sector image. This velocity and D of the pulmonary artery determined from the real-time image are then used to calculate $\dot{Q}$. Correlation with invasive thermodilution measurements of CO from the PA in man ($n=15$) has been encouraging with a correlation coefficient of +0.84 (Bommer et al., 1980). Additional information may be available in the analysis of the flow waveform. For example, patients with pulmonary hypertension demonstrate decreased ejection time and an increase in early diastolic flow reversal (Hatle et al., 1981).

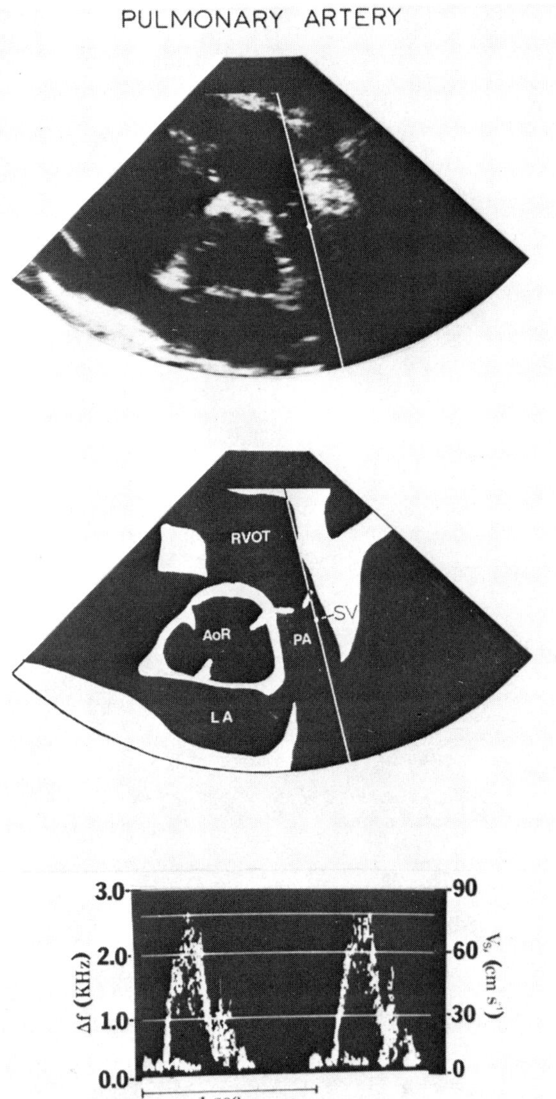

Figure 4. A freeze-frame, 2-dimensional image of the short axis of the base of the heart (top) demonstrating anatomical landmarks as depicted diagrammatically (center). The Doppler spectrum obtained at the point of the SV is shown (bottom) and represents blood velocities in the pulmonary artery (PA). This spectral display is unidirectional so the signals displayed in early diastole are actually reversed. (*Note*: RVOT=right ventricular outflow tract; AoR=aortic root; LA=left atrium; SV=sample volume.)

Extracranial vasculature. From the suprasternal notch, the rotating scanhead transducer of the duplex scanner can be angled (Figure 5) to view the aortic arch and the origin of the innominate artery, left common carotid (LCC) and left subclavian artery (LSA). The SV can be selectively placed in any of these vessels to obtain measurements of Δf, θ, and D to calculate v_{sa} and $\dot{Q}$. Figure 5 illustrates an LCC image and v_{sa} obtained in a healthy adult. Note the continuous forward flow pattern throughout the cardiac cycle (similar to Figure 1) due to the low impedance of the cranial vasculature (McDonald, 1974, pp. 351–388). By simply readjusting the SV into the LSA (Figure 6), the v_{sa} waveform dramatically changes to show significant flow reversal during early diastole due to the relatively high impedance vascular bed of the resting arm (Strandness, 1978). With exercise, the vascular bed dilates and the arterial input impedance of the arm decreases (Murgo et al., 1981). Consequently, the waveform in Figure 6 will lose its reversal stage and appear similar to the LCC waveform in Figure 5. The calculated mean values of $\dot{Q}$ at rest in the LCC in

Figure 5. Freeze-frame images of the branches of the adult extracranial vasculature at their origin with the aortic arch. The sample volume is placed in the left common carotid (LCC) and v_{sa} is displayed. (*Note*: IA=innominate artery; LSA=left subclavian artery; AA=aortic arch.)

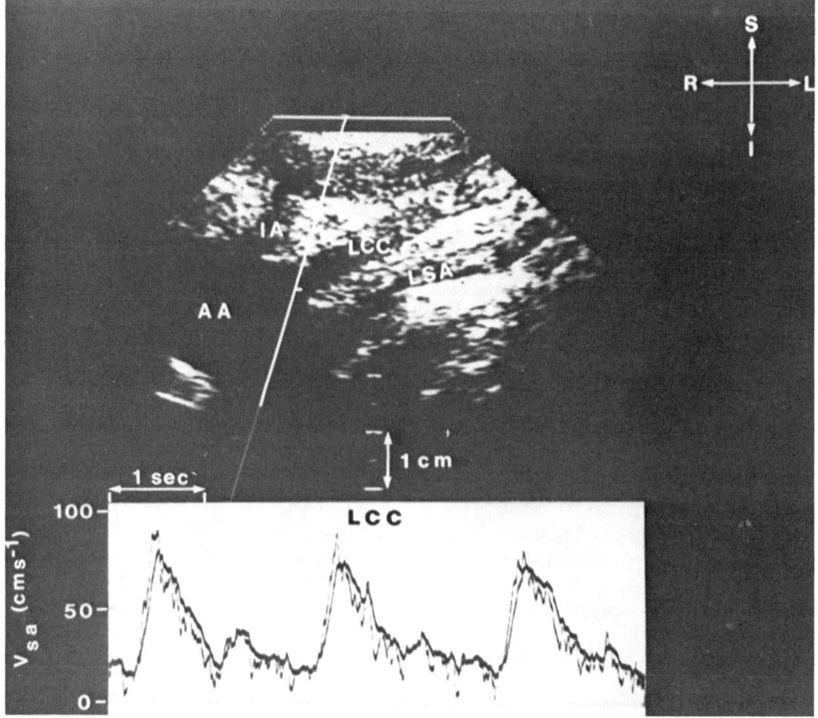

healthy adults are approximately 450 ml/min. During submaximal upright exercise, the value of $\dot{Q}$ in the LCC remains relatively constant but the LCC stroke volume decreases significantly with major alterations in the v_{sa} waveform due to relative changes in cerebral and central vascular impedance.

Renal artery blood flow. The importance of the imaging capability of the duplex scanner coupled with pulsed Doppler flowmetry is again apparent in the determination of blood velocities and $\dot{Q}$ in the vessels of the abdominal cavity. For example, Figure 7 (A) illustrates an anterior-posterior radiological image of the abdominal aorta and its abdominal branches in a 35-yr-old hypertensive adult. In (B), a transverse ultrasonic image depicts the numerous abdominal vessels and illustrates the v_{sa} waveform in the left and right renal arteries. In the normal left renal artery and left kidney, the velocity waveform exhibits a high diastolic component with $\dot{Q}$ being approximately 430 ml/min. In the atrophied right renal vasculature, the diastolic flow pattern is decreased to near zero and the value of $\dot{Q}$ decreased to 180 ml/min, indicating increased

Figure 6. Freeze-frame image of the branches of the adult extracranial vasculature at their origin with the aortic arch. The sample volume is placed in the left subclavian artery (LSA) and v_{sa} is displayed. *Note*: see symbols in Figure 5.)

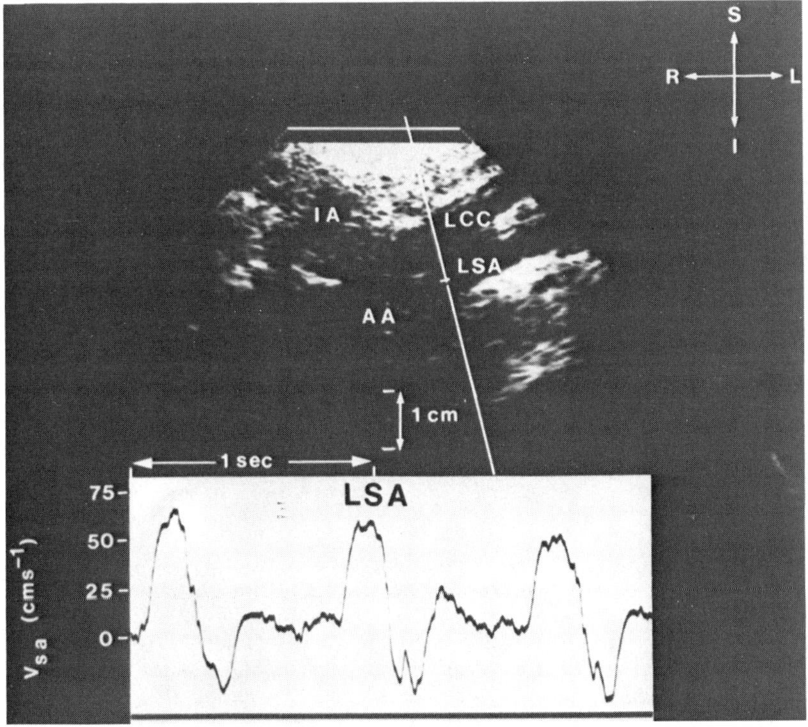

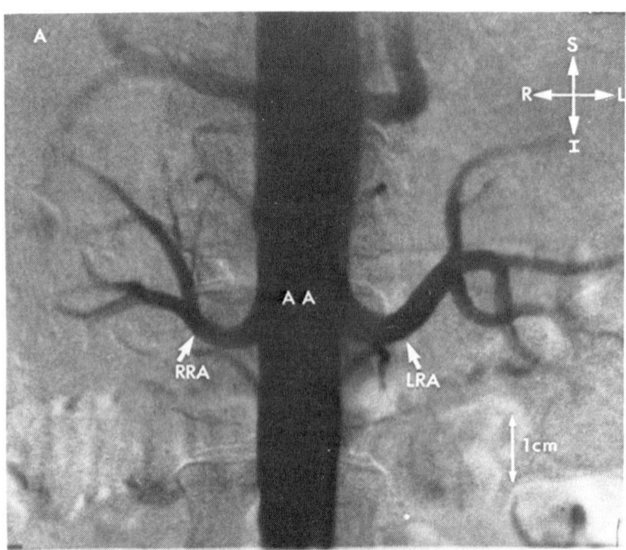

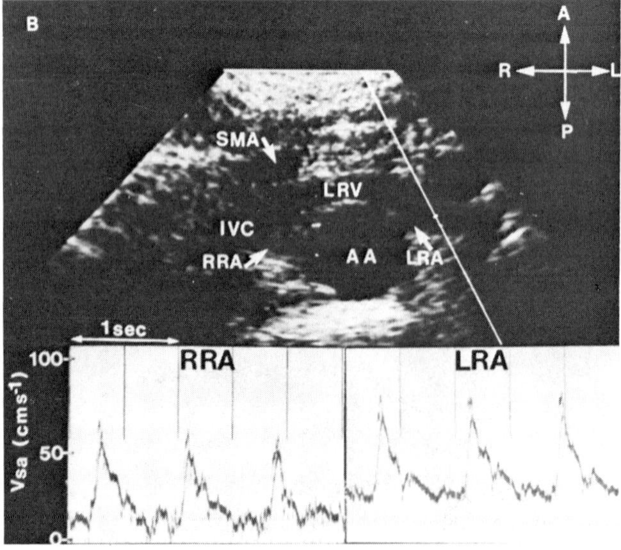

Figure 7. A radiological image of the abdominal vasculature in a 35-yr-old hypertensive adult (A) with reduced lower branches of the right renal artery. A transverse duplex image of the abdominal vessels in the same subject is shown in B. (*Note*: A = anterior; R = right; L = left; P = posterior; S = superior; I = inferior; AA = abdominal aorta; RRA = right renal artery; LRA = left renal artery; SMA = superior mesenteric artery; IVC = inferior vena cava; LRV = left renal vein.)

vascular impedance due to parenchymal kidney disease (Greene et al., 1981). The values of $\dot{Q}$ in normal and diseased renal vasculatures will be affected by orthostatic changes and can be measured by similar techniques (J.A. Loeppky, personal communication).

Femoral blood flow. As a final example of the application of pulsed Doppler flowmetry, Figure 8 illustrates the duplex image associated with a branch of

Figure 8. Freeze-frame duplex image of the bifurcation of the adult common femoral artery into the deep and superficial branches (top). A diagrammatic representation of the image is given below. The sample volume (SV) is placed in the superficial femoral artery and v_{sa} is displayed. (*Note*: M=medial; S=superficial; I=inferior; L=lateral; CFA=common femoral artery; DFA=deep femoral artery; SFA=superficial femoral artery.)

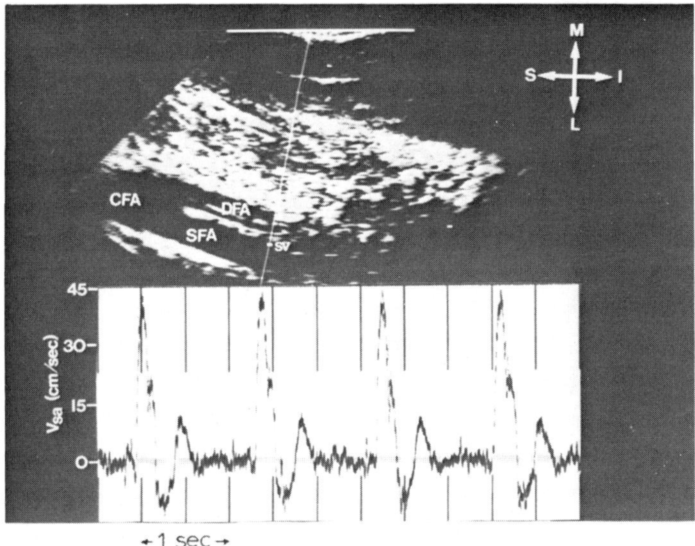

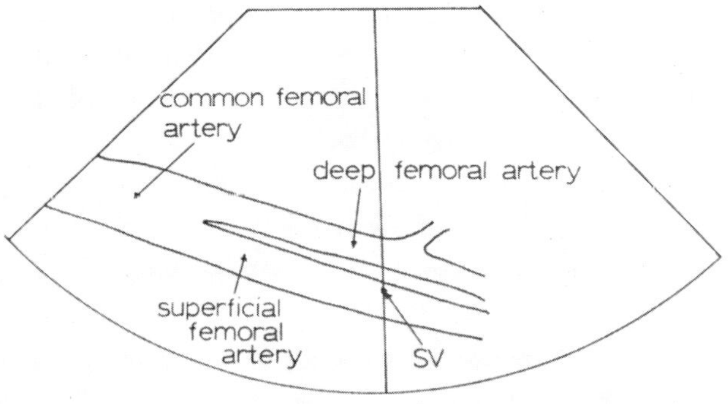

the common femoral artery into the deep and superficial femoral arteries. In this case, the SV is placed in the superficial femoral artery. Note the significant flow reversal in early diastole occurring in the superficial femoral artery due to high input impedance. This pattern of flow is similar to flow patterns in the subclavian artery (Figure 6). In leg exercise by normal subjects, this waveform will lose its reversal stage and show small phasic changes while the value of $\dot{Q}$ can increase up to 10-fold (Rushmer, 1976, pp. 246–280). In patients with arterial lesions, only small increases in $\dot{Q}$ occur with no significant changes in the shape of the v_{sa} waveform (Strandness, 1978). Vessel capacitance (McDonald, 1974, pp. 389–419) can also be evaluated by measurement of the harmonic content of the v_{sa} waveform, allowing a more comprehensive evaluation of the effects of aging and disease on the cardiovascular system.

Summary

It is apparent that pulsed Doppler flowmetry, with or without the imaging capabilities of the duplex scanner, will assume an increasingly important role in the serial evaluation of human cardiovascular physiology and its role in perfusion and oxygen transport. The principle advantages of pulsed Doppler flowmetry are that it: (1) is noninvasive, (2) is nontraumatic, (3) provides anatomical and physiological data, and (4) provides dynamic measurements. Nevertheless, the limitations of the technique are of equal importance: (1) it is difficult to apply in some subjects due to obesity and anatomical variations, (2) it requires operator skill and a thorough knowledge of human anatomy and cardiovascular dynamics, (3) it has a finite spatial resolution which may compromise the measurement of vessel diameter, and (4) it has a finite velocity measuring capability which will affect measurements of blood velocities outside the range of 2 to 200 cm/sec.

With full appreciation of the capabilities and limitations of noninvasive pulsed Doppler flowmetry, a better understanding of the dynamic interplay of anatomy, pressure, flow, and impedance in the normal and diseased human cardiovascular system becomes feasible.

ACKNOWLEDGMENTS

The author would like to thank Jerry Davis, John Adams, Pat Reilly, Treva Miller, Arvind Caprihan, and Isidora Miranda for their technical assistance; Jack Loeppky and Mike Histand for their physiological consultation; Wyatt Voyles and K.L. Richards for their clinical expertise; and Karen Crawford for her excellent secretarial assistance. Their work was supported by Lovelace Medical Foundation Endowment Funds, NIH RIHL26025A, NIH HL2709501, and American Heart Association Grants.

References

Baker, D.W. 1970. Pulsed ultrasonic Doppler blood flow sensing. *IEEE Trans. Sonics and Ultrasonics*. 17:170–185.

Baker, D.W. 1980. Applications of pulsed Doppler techniques. *Radiol. Clin. North Am.* 18:79–103.

Baker, D.W. and Daigle, R.E. 1977. Noninvasive ultrasonic flowmetry. In *Cardiovascular Flow Dynamics and Measurements*. Hwang, N.H. and Norman, N., eds. Baltimore: University Park Press. pp. 151–189.

Barber, F.E., Baker, D.W., and Nation, A.W. 1974. Ultrasonic duplex echo Doppler scanner. *IEEE Trans. Biomed. Eng.* 21:109–113.

Blair, W.F., Greene, E.R., and Omer, G.E., Jr. 1981. A method for the calculation of blood flow in human digital arteries. *J. Hand Surgery*. 6:90–96.

Bommer, W., Miller, L., Keown, M., Mason, D.T., and Demaria, A.N. 1980. Real-time fast Fourier analysis of Doppler spectral information and two-dimensional echocardiography yield a noninvasive estimate of cardiac output. *Circulation* 62 (Part II):III–199.

Darsee, J.R., Walter, P.F., and Nutter, D.O. 1980. Transcutaneous Doppler method of measuring cardiac output II. *Am. J. Cardiol.* 46:613–618.

Davis, J.G., Richards, K.L., and Greene, D. 1979. A sample volume tracking unit for pulsed Doppler echocardiography. *IEEE Trans. Biomed. Eng.* 26:285–288.

Detweiler, D.K. 1973. Circulation. In *Best and Taylor's Physiological Basis of Medical Practice*, Ninth Edition. Brobeck, J.R., ed. Baltimore: William and Wilkins.

Feigenbaum, H. 1981. *Echocardiography*, Third Edition. Philadelphia: Lea and Febiger.

Greene, E.R. and Histand, M.B. 1979. Ultrasonic assessment of simulated atherosclerosis—*in vitro* and *in vivo* comparisons. *ASME J. Biomech. Eng.* 101:73–81.

Greene, E.R., Histand, M.B., and Miller, C.W. 1976. Ultrasonic blood flow measurements: transcutaneous compared with implanted cuff. *ISA Trans.* 15:88–94.

Greene, E.R., Hoekenga, D.E., Richards, K.L., and Davis, J.G. 1980a. Pulsed Doppler echocardiographic audio spectrum analysis: time interval histogram versus multifilter spectrogram and fast Fourier transform. *Biomed. Sci. Instrum.* 16:134–144.

Greene, E.R., Loeppky, J.A., Mathews, E.C., Hoekenga, D.E., Richards, K.L., and Tuttle, W.C. 1980b. Noninvasive Doppler stroke volume during rest and exercise. *Proc. 33rd ACEMB* 22:23.

Greene, E.R., Richards, K.L., and Davis, J.G. 1979. Improved sample volume control per pulsed Doppler echocardiography. *Circulation* 60(II):245.

Greene, E.R., Venters, M.D., Conn, R.L., and Avasthi, P.S. 1981. Noninvasive characterization of renal artery blood flow. *Kidney Int.*, 20:523–529.

Hatle, L., Angelsen, B.A.J., and Tromsdal, A. 1981. Noninvasive estimation of pulmonary artery systolic pressure with Doppler ultrasound. *Br. Heart J.* 45:157–165.

Hoekenga, D.E., Greene, E.R., Loeppky, J.A., Mathews, E.C., Richards, K.L., and Luft, U.C. 1980. A comparison of noninvasive Doppler cardiographic and simultaneous Fick measurements of left ventricular stroke volume in man. *Circulation* 62(Part II):III–199.

Jorgensen, J.E., Campau, D., and Baker, D.W. 1973. Physical characteristics and mathematical modelling of the pulsed ultrasonic flowmeter. *Med. Biol. Eng.* 2:404–421.

Kalmanson, D., Veryrat, C., and Abitbol, G. 1979. Two-dimensional echo-Doppler velocimetry in mitral and tricuspid valve disease. In *Recent Advances in Ultrasound Diagnosis*. Kurjak, A. ed. Amsterdam: Excerpta Medica. pp. 335–348.

Loeppky, J.A., Greene, E.R., Hoekenga, D.E., Caprihan, A., and Luft, U.C. 1981. Beat-by-beat stroke volume assessment by pulsed Doppler in upright and supine exercise. *J. Appl. Physiol.* 50:1173–1182.

Loeppky, J.A., Richards, K.L., Greene, E.R., Eldridge, M.W., Hoekenga, D.E., Venters, M.D., and Luft, U.C. 1979. Instantaneous stroke volume in man during lower body negative pressure (LBNP). *Physiologist* 22(6):s81–s82.

Lunt, M.H. 1975. Accuracy and limitations of ultrasonic Doppler blood velocimeter and zero-crossing detector. *Ultrasound. Med. Biol.* 2:1–10.

McDonald, D.A. 1974. *Blood Flow in Arteries*, Second Edition. Baltimore: William and Wilkins.

Murgo, J.P., Westerhof, N., Giolma, J.P., and Altobelli, S.A. 1980. Aortic input impedance in normal man: relationship to pressure waveforms. *Circulation* 62:105–116.

Murgo, J.P., Westerhof, N., Giolma, J.P., and Altobelli, S.A. 1981. Effects of exercise on aortic input impedance and pressure waveforms in normal humans. *Circ. Res.* 48:334–343.

Phillips, D.J., Powers, J.E., Eyer, M.K., Blacksheas, W.M., Bodily, K.C., Strandness, D.W., and Baker, D.W. 1980. Detection of peripheral vascular disease using the duplex scanner III. *Ultrasound Med. Biol.* 5:205–218.

Rowell, L.B. 1974. Human cardiovascular adjustments to exercise and thermal stress. *Physiol. Rev.* 54:75–159.

Rushmer, R.F. 1976. *Cardiovascular Dynamics*, Fourth Edition. Philadelphia: W.B. Saunders Company.

Schlichting, H. 1968. *Boundary Layer Theory*, Sixth Edition. New York: McGraw-Hill.

Seed, W.A. and Wood, N.B. 1971. Velocity patterns in the aorta. *Cardiovasc. Res.* 5:319–330.

Steingart, R.M., Miller, J., Barovich, J., Patterson, R., Herman, M.V., and Teichholz, L.E. 1980. Pulsed Doppler echocardiographic measurement of beat-to-beat changes in stroke volume in dogs. *Circulation* 62:542–548.

Strandness, D.E., Jr. 1978. The use of ultrasound in the evaluation of peripheral vascular disease. *Prog. Cardiovasc. Dis.* 20:403–422.

Wells, P.N.T. 1977. *Biomedical Ultrasonics*. New York: Academic Press.

Young, D.F. 1979. Fluid mechanics of arterial stenoses. *ASME J. Biomech. Eng.* 101:157–175.

J.A. Loeppky and M.L. Riedesel, editors
OXYGEN TRANSPORT TO HUMAN TISSUES

A Pulmonary CO_2-Sensitive Chemoreceptor

Jerry Franklin Green

The existence of a chemoreceptor in the lung which when stimulated with CO_2 would increase ventilation has been the center of much controversy since it was first proposed by Pi-Suner and Bellido (1919). Riley et al. (1963) rekindled this idea some 20 years ago by demonstrating a high correlation between mixed venous PCO_2 and ventilation during CO_2 breathing and during exercise. The most recent data to support this idea have been those of Kolobow et al. (1977) and Phillipson et al. (1981). Both groups of investigators have demonstrated a tight correlation between alveolar ventilation ($\dot{V}_A$) and CO_2 excretion at the lungs ($\dot{V}CO_2$) under isocapnic conditions in awake animals. Using a venovenous extracorporeal perfusion circuit, Phillipson et al. (1981) were able to load and unload CO_2 from the venous blood of sheep, trained to run on a treadmill. The relationship of $\dot{V}_A$ and $\dot{V}CO_2$ was linear as all points fell on a single line regardless of whether $\dot{V}CO_2$ was altered by exercise, venous CO_2 loading and unloading, or a combination of both. Furthermore, throughout these experiments, $PaCO_2$ remained constant. If we are to accept these experiments, then according to the Fick principle, we must also accept that a change in $\dot{V}CO_2$ and $\dot{V}_A$ can only be correlated with a change in either the CO_2 content of the mixed venous blood or cardiac output, since the arterial CO_2 content would remain constant under isocapnic conditions. Either correlation would suggest the existence of some sort of a pulmonary CO_2-chemoreceptor. To demonstrate unequivocally the absence or existence of such a chemoreceptor, my colleagues and I felt it was mandatory to isolate the systemic and pulmonary circulations in a spontaneously breathing animal. With such a preparation we could not only alter the mixed venous PCO_2 at constant levels of pulmonary blood flow and arterial PCO_2, but we could also alter pulmonary blood flow at constant levels of mixed venous and arterial PCO_2. I would now like to share with you the latest results from such a study currently being conducted by Murray I. Sheldon and myself. Since these experiments are still in progress our conclusions must be considered tentative.

Methods

Mongrel dogs weighing between 18 and 25 kg are anesthetized with ketamine (10 mg/kg), paralyzed with succinylcholine (0.9 mg/kg) for endotracheal intubation and maintained with 0.5 to 1.0% halothane in 100% oxygen. A ventral thoracotomy is performed and sodium heparin (3 mg/kg) administered. The superior and inferior venae cavae are then cannulated through the right atrial wall. The entire systemic venous return is drained by gravity into a reservoir and then passes in succession through an oxygenator, a heat exchanger, and finally an electromagnetic flowmeter, before returning to the ascending aorta via a cannula advanced through the left subclavian artery. Bypass is then begun as blood flow is increased to 0.08 liter/min/kg. Once full flow is achieved in the systemic circuit, the heart is electrically fibrillated. The left atrium is then cannulated by a wide bore Tygon tube which is passed through the left ventricular wall. The entire pulmonary venous return is withdrawn through this cannula and passes in succession through an extracorporeal circuit identical to that of the systemic circuit. Blood in the pulmonary circuit is returned into the pulmonary artery via a cannula placed in the pulmonary artery through the right ventricular outflow tract. The blood flow to this circuit is initially set at 0.08 liter/min/kg. The PCO_2 and PO_2 of both circuits is initially set at 40 mm Hg and greater than 300 mm Hg, respectively, by adjusting the CO_2/O_2 gas mixture delivered to the oxygenators. To maintain anesthesia, 0.5 to 1.0% halothane is delivered to the systemic circulation through the systemic oxygenator. All cannulae are brought out of the chest wall through separate incisions. Two large drainage tubes are placed in the costophrenic angles and connected to a Pleur-evac set at -20 cm H_2O for continuous evacuation of air and blood from the pleural space. All blood from the pleural space is pumped from the Pleur-evac into the systemic reservoir through a bypass blood filter. The chest is closed with pericostal cable ties and the wound closed in two layers with O-silk. Once double bypass is established, the ventilator is stopped and spontaneous ventilation allowed from a reservoir containing 100% oxygen at atmospheric pressure. Expiratory gases are passed through a pneumotach; its signal is then integrated over a 1-min period by an analog integrator giving spontaneous minute ventilation ($\dot{V}_E$).

With this preparation, two series of experiments are being performed. In the first, blood flow through each circuit is maintained at 0.08 liter/min/kg. Systemic arterial CO_2 tension is then held constant at 3 different nonoscillatory levels as pulmonary PCO_2 is randomly varied between 5 and 90 mm Hg. In the second series of experiments, systemic blood flow and both systemic and pulmonary PCO_2 are held constant as pulmonary blood flow is varied between

0.5 and 4.0 liter/min. In both series of experiments, the oxygen tension in each circuit is maintained at values in excess of 300 mm Hg.

Results and Discussion

Series A: Constant Pulmonary Blood Flow

Figure 1 presents a typical CO_2-response curve obtained from one of our animals. Here ventilation is plotted against pulmonary arterial CO_2 tension ($PpCO_2$) at three constant levels of systemic arterial CO_2 tension ($PsCO_2$). When systemic PCO_2 was set low (35 mm Hg), the animal become apneic and remained so at all levels of pulmonary PCO_2, even as high as 100 mm Hg. However, at a normal systemic CO_2 tension of 42 mm Hg, ventilation increased as a function of pulmonary PCO_2. When systemic PCO_2 was raised to a level of 56 mm Hg, ventilation increased as a function of pulmonary PCO_2 with a higher gain in the lower ranges of $PpCO_2$ than at the upper ranges, suggesting some sort of saturation mechanism. Notice also from this figure that in both the normal and hypercapnic ranges of systemic CO_2, ventilation ceased when pulmonary CO_2 tension was lowered to values less than 20 mm Hg. In other words, apnea ensued when either systemic or pulmonary CO_2 was lowered below an apneic threshold which was different for each circuit.

Figure 2 presents a classic type of CO_2-response curve, with ventilation plotted against systemic arterial PCO_2. The three isopleths represent different levels of pulmonary arterial CO_2 tension. Notice that decreasing the level of pulmonary CO_2 served to depress the slope of CO_2-response curve. Once the pulmonary apneic threshold was achieved, ventilation did not increase even in the face of systemic PCO_2 levels as high as 60 mm Hg!

In two animals, we have studied the effects of vagotomy upon the CO_2-response curve. Vagotomy had no effect as long as the respiratory apparatus had been "turned off" by systemic hypocapnea. However, at values of systemic

Figure 1. Pulmonary carbon dioxide-ventilatory response curves. Minute ventilation ($\dot{V}_E$) plotted as a function of pulmonary artery PCO_2 ($PpCO_2$) at constant levels of systemic arterial PCO_2 ($PsCO_2$).

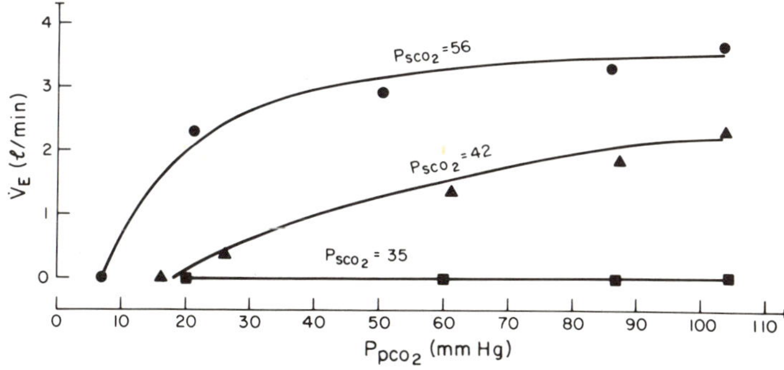

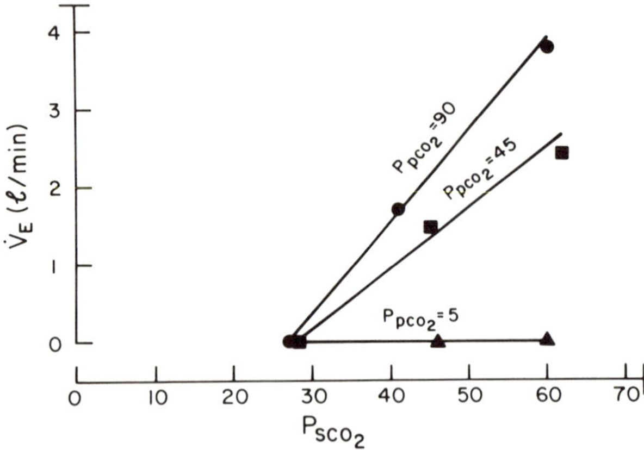

Figure 2. Systemic carbon dioxide-ventilatory response curves. Minute ventilation ($\dot{V}_E$) plotted as a function of systemic arterial PCO_2 ($PsCO_2$) at constant levels of pulmonary arterial PCO_2 ($PpCO_2$).

PCO_2 above the systemic apneic threshold, vagotomy eliminated the effects of changes in pulmonary CO_2 upon ventilation. It is interesting to note that pulmonary hypercapnea, like vagotomy, appears to act such as to remove a vagally mediated inhibition.

With this series of experiments, we believe we are demonstrating the existence, in the canine species, of a vagally mediated CO_2-sensitive pulmonary chemoreceptor. This chemoreceptor is able to reflexly alter ventilation in response to changes in mixed venous CO_2 tension. Furthermore, the pulmonary chemoreceptor appears to interact with the nonpulmonary chemoreceptors such as to respond to the total CO_2 load of the body. Since in our preparation hydrogen ion concentration varies inversely with the CO_2 tension, we are unable to determine whether the stimulus for the ventilatory drive is PCO_2 per se or the hydrogen ion concentration.

Series B: Changes in Pulmonary Blood Flow

With this series of experiments, we are attempting to see if changes in pulmonary blood flow can alter ventilation. Since we have a finite amount of time during which our preparation is responsive, it is impractical to vary pulmonary blood flow at various permutations of systemic and pulmonary PCO_2 levels. We, therefore, hold both systemic and pulmonary PCO_2 constant at two levels. Thus, pulmonary blood flow is randomly varied over a range from 0.5 to 4.0 liter/min, first while both $PsCO_2$ and $PpCO_2$ are held constant at 40 mm Hg and then while CO_2 tensions are held constant at 60 mm Hg. Systemic blood flow is also held constant. Again oxygen tensions in each circuit are maintained at values greater than 300 mm Hg.

Figure 3 shows the effect that changes in pulmonary blood flow have on ventilation. These data, which are typical of the responses we are getting, were obtained from a 20-kg dog. The solid lines were obtained from least square regression. At the 40 mm Hg level of CO_2, ventilation ($\dot{V}_E$) increased as a linear function of pulmonary blood flow ($\dot{Q}_p$). The regression equation for this relationship was: $\dot{V}_E = 3.08 + 1.61\ \dot{Q}_p$, $P < .001$. At the 60 mm Hg level of Co_2, $\dot{V}_E$ also increased as a linear function of $\dot{Q}_p$. The regression equation at this level of CO_2 was: $\dot{V}_E = 11.47 + 1.31\ \dot{Q}_p$, $P < .001$. Raising the level of CO_2 of both the pulmonary and systemic circuits from 40 to 60 mm Hg affected ventilation not by altering the slope of the $\dot{V}_E - \dot{Q}_p$ relationship but by increasing the intercept.

Using the average data presented in Figure 3, we can construct a systemic CO_2-response curve at two different levels of pulmonary blood flow. This was done in Figure 4 for a normal resting level of blood flow of 1.14 liter/min (points A and B) and then again at the highest level of flow obtained which was approximately 3 times normal (points C and D).

The line segment A-B (Figure 4) represents the change in ventilation as a function of systemic PCO_2 at the low level of pulmonary blood flow. The line segment C-D shows how this relationship changed when pulmonary blood flow was increased threefold and all other variables remained constant. Increasing pulmonary blood flow serves to shift the CO_2-response curve in a parallel fashion to the left. The shaded areas show the regions through which the systemic CO_2-response curve would be expected to rotate at different levels of pulmonary CO_2 from 40 to 60 mm Hg. This information can be estimated from our first series of experiments (Figure 2) which demonstrates that decreasing the pulmonary CO_2 at constant blood flow depresses the slope of the CO_2-response curve.

Figure 3. Minute ventilation ($\dot{V}_E$) versus pulmonary blood flow ($\dot{Q}_p$) at two levels of CO_2.

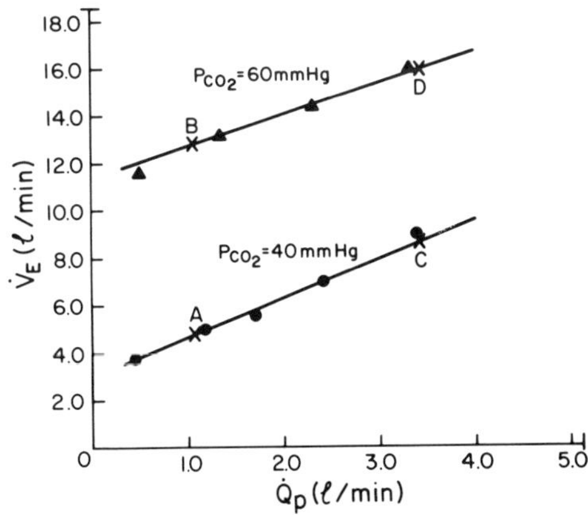

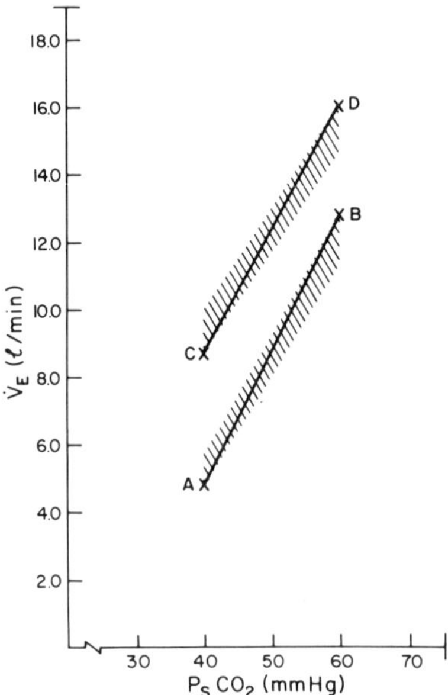

Figure 4. Systemic CO_2-response curves to two different levels of pulmonary blood flow ($\dot{Q}_p$). For line A-B, $\dot{Q}_p$ is normal, for line C-D it is 3 times normal.

With this second series of experiments, we are demonstrating that increases in pulmonary blood flow, independent of changes in mixed venous PCO_2, significantly augment ventilation and that changes in pulmonary blood flow alter the position of the systemic CO_2-response curve and not its slope. Incidentally, once again vagotomy abolishes the response. That is, following vagotomy changes in pulmonary blood flow have no effect upon ventilation.

The next question which concerns us is one of mechanism. That is, does our pulmonary receptor sense the change in blood flow per se or is it some sort of mechanoreceptor which senses the increase in transmural vascular pressure which accompanies an augmentation of blood flow? Our preparation allows us to answer this question. We reason that if the pulmonary receptor responds to stretch, it should make no difference whether the transmural vascular pressures are increased by augmenting the blood flow at constant left atrial pressure or increased by elevating the left atrial pressure at constant blood flow. To date, we have completed one experiment in which this idea was tested. Elevating transmural vascular pressures by increasing pulmonary blood flow at constant left atrial pressure increased ventilation as expected. However, when transmural vascular pressures were elevated by raising left atrial pressure at constant pulmonary blood flow, there was no change in ventilation. On the basis of this one experiment, we draw the preliminary conclusion that the pulmonary receptor that senses blood flow is not a mechanoreceptor. If flow is not sensed by stretch receptors, perhaps flow, like mixed venous CO_2, is sensed in some way by CO_2 exchange in the lungs, even when mixed venous CO_2 is constant (Filley et al., 1978).

I would now like to address the inevitable question, "Can our findings account for the mechanism of exercise hyperpnea?" It is still too early to answer this question definitively, but we feel that the CO_2-sensitive pulmonary chemoreceptor can at least in large part account for the phenomenon of exercise hyperpnea. The sine quo non of exercise hyperpnea is a parallel shift in the systemic CO_2-response curve to the left of the resting curve (Asmussen and Nielsen, 1958; Lambertsen et al., 1959). In our experiments (Figure 4), we are able to simulate this exact response by increasing the pulmonary blood flow at constant $PsCO_2$, $PpCO_2$, and systemic blood flow.

Summary

By isolating the pulmonary and systemic circulations in the canine model, we are controlling the blood flow, blood gases, and atrial pressures of each circuit independently as we measure minute ventilation. Using this technique, we are demonstrating that as long as the CO_2 partial pressure of each circuit is above its apneic threshold, increasing either mixed venous PCO_2 or pulmonary blood flow significantly augments ventilation. When these stimuli are increased together, their effects are additive. We believe that both stimuli act by exciting a CO_2-sensitive, vagally mediated, pulmonary chemoreceptor.

ACKNOWLEDGMENTS

This work was supported by NHLBI Grant No. 20371. I would like to thank Eric Q. Parsons who provided expert technical assistance and Phoebe Ling who cheerfully and skillfully prepared the manuscript.

References

Asmussen, E. and Nielsen, M. 1958. Pulmonary ventilation and effect of oxygen breathing in heavy exercise. *Acta Physiol. Scand.* 43:365–378.

Filley, G.F., Hale, R.C., Kratochvil, J., and Olson, D.E. 1978. The hyperpnea of exercise and chemical disequilibria. *Chest.* 73 (Suppl. February):267–269.

Kolobow, T., Gattinoni, L., Tomlinson, T.A., and Pierce, J.E. 1977. Control of breathing using an extracorporeal membrane lung. *Anesthesiology* 46:138–141.

Lambertsen, C.J., Owen, S.G., Wendel, H., Stroud, M.W., Lurie, A.A., Lochner, W., and Clack, G.F. 1959. Respiratory and cerebral circulatory control during exercise at .21 and 2.0 atmospheres inspired PO_2. *J. Appl. Physiol.* 14:966–981.

Phillipson, E.A., Bowes, G., Townsend, E.R., Duffin, J., and Cooper, J.D. 1981. Critical dependence of exercise ventilation on metabolic CO_2 production. *Fed. Proc.* 40:567.

Pi-Suner, A. and Bellido, J.M. 1919. Segona notá sobre la sensibilitat quimica del neumogastric pulmonar. *Treb. Soc. Biol. Barcelona.* 4:311–314.

Riley, R.L., Dutton, Jr., R.E., Fulcihan, F.J., Nath, S., Hurt, Jr., H.H., Yashimoto, C., Sipple, J.H., Permitt, S., and Bromberger-Barnea, B. 1963. Regulation of respiration and blood gases. *Ann N.Y. Acad. Sci.* 109:829–851.

J.A. Loeppky and M.L. Riedesel, editors
OXYGEN TRANSPORT TO HUMAN TISSUES

The Effect of Sudden Inhalation of CO_2 in N_2O on the Early Breaths of Exercise

Giles F. Filley

The abruptness of the onset of exercise hyperpnea which gave rise to the neurogenic theory (Krogh and Lindhard, 1913; and many others) has recently been explained by stimuli related to venous return. Although an increase in pulmonary blood flow increases "cardiodynamic" gas exchange and might act as a stimulus by some function of the CO_2 load to the lungs (Wasserman et al., 1981) or by traditional carotid body mechanisms (Fordyce and Grodins, 1980), the flow component may be separate from the chemical component (Ponte and Purves, 1978) and perhaps drive the first breaths before the metabolic CO_2 load arrives from the tissues. The work of Loeppky and Luft (1980) shows the importance of exact timing in analyzing blood flow and chemical stimuli on early breaths.

We have introduced CO_2, carried by N_2O, into alveoli rapidly enough to reveal inhibitory effects (by the initial reduction in mixed venous to alveolar CO_2 gradient) which suggest that CO_2-related stimuli acting in the lungs at least partly initiate exercise hyperpnea and largely maintain it as exercise proceeds.

Methods

Data were gathered in the classical manner used by Luft and his colleagues; that is, experiments were carried out with conscious subjects and experimenter and the untouched records were first examined by the experimenter. Twenty-seven nonsmokers, ages 24 to 64 yr, all of whom except the experimenter were ignorant of the study's aim, stood quietly breathing through the respiratory apparatus and then suddenly began walking for a few seconds to minutes on a treadmill at 3.5 mph and 4% grade. Exercise was begun by abruptly starting the treadmill without warning. After one practice start, all subjects made well-coordinated transitions from rest to exercise. Most subjects were exposed only once to CO_2 and/or N_2O to minimize phychological effects of the taste of the gases.

A special CO_2 delivery system was designed to achieve as sudden a step increase in alveolar PCO_2 as possible. The mouthpiece, punctured by a needle leading to a CO_2 analyzer (Beckman LB-2) was connected to a bellows-operated 4-way valve which permitted a silent and imperceptible switch from inspiring air to inspiring a test gas from a bag for a single breath. The total dead space from lips to bag entrance was 98 ml. Figure 1 shows that CO_2 entered the mouthpiece so rapidly that its PCO_2 fell only a few mm Hg or not at all at the start of inspiration.

The carrier gas for CO_2 was N_2O which was used both to disguise the taste of CO_2 and to increase, by its concentrating effect, the speed with which alveolar PCO_2 could be raised. Pneumotachygraph (PNT) and PCO_2 records were traced on 12-in. wide ruled paper so that accurate monitoring and timing of the switching to test gases could be done by one observer and reproduction of records achieved without retouching. The differing viscosities of the gases had no measurable effect on the PNT flow signals.

The indices of chemical ventilatory drive chosen were the inspiratory volume (V_I) and mean inspiratory flow rate (V_I/T_I) where T_I is the duration of inspiration. The relative magnitude of this drive during an exercise breath was measured as the change from the average value of previous breaths.

Figure 1. Records of a naive subject switched to the test mixture toward the end of expiration at the instant the treadmill was started (left vertical arrow). The first breath seems to be little affected. Compare with the first breaths of Figure 3. In a second exercise start, right, the first breath shows a slowing during the last half of inspiration. The PCO_2 recorded from the mouthpiece drops slightly or not at all at the beginning of the inspiration of the test breath.

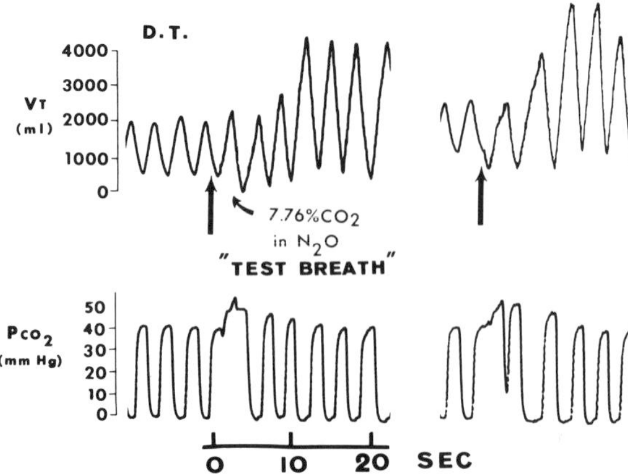

The effect of 7.76% CO_2 in N_2O on the first breath of exercise was studied in 9 subjects. One or two control runs were carried out with air to determine the spontaneous change of the first breath from the average of the 10 previous breaths. A few minutes later, after another recorded rest period, the subject was switched to the gas mixture during a resting expiration at the moment the treadmill was started (Table 1).

In separate exercise starts in 12 subjects, this test mixture was administered during the expirations preceding the 3rd, 4th, 5th, and 10th breaths (8 exercise starts, each of the 4 test breaths being studied twice). For each start, the average of the previous 2, 3, 4, or 9 breaths, respectively, was subtracted from the test measurement. The same 12 subjects participated in 2 additional control starts. Because normal people often transiently lower their ventilation after exercise has started (Krogh and Lindhard, 1913), usually after 4 to 6 breaths, we chose the change in the 6th breath from the average of the 5 previous breaths as a control change. The 10 changes per subject (8 test and 2 control) were analyzed in Table 2 using a 2-way analysis of variance (12 subjects by 5 conditions with 2 replications (Snedecor and Cochran, 1971).

Single breaths of pure N_2O were administered for one breath in 8 subjects during steady state exercise. For the N_2O breaths, the inspired volumes, flow rates, and end-tidal PCO_2's were compared with the means of the 10 previous breaths as shown in Table 3. In a few subjects, other early and late breaths were tested with the test mixture in the same exercise start.

Results

The first inspiration of exercise was not affected in some and variably depressed in other subjects by the test mixture. Even in the same subject the effect was variable (Figure 1). The mean absolute reduction of the first breath by the mixture was not statistically significant, but the difference between the changes from the rest was significant both for V_I and V_I/T_I (Table 1).

Table 1. Effect of Test Mixture on the First Breath of Exercise.[a]

		Resting[b] breaths	**1st exercise breath**	**Change from rest**
V_I (liter)	Control	.91 ± .178	1.13 ± .240	.22 ± .218
	Test	.99 ± .150	1.01 ± .297	.02 ± .288
	p[c]	NS	NS	<.02
V_I/T_I (liter/sec)	Control	.58 ± .125	.87 ± .225	.29 ± .204
	Test	.63 ± .126	.74 ± .181	.11 ± .174
	p[c]	NS	NS	<.03

[a] Mean values (± S.D.) found in 9 subjects.

[b] For each subject the 10 resting breaths before exercise began were averaged.

[c] The two-tailed paired t-test was used to calculate P.

Table 2. Effect of Test Mixture on 4 Later Exercise Breaths.[a]

	Control breath change[b]	Test breath changes[c]				
		3rd	4th	5th	10th	L.S.D.[d]
Δ_I(ml)	−22 ± 259	−105 ± 193	−196 ± 179	$-276^e \pm 223$	$-269^e \pm 253$	183
Δ%	+2.1 ± 14.2	$-10.2^e \pm 17.2$	−17.6 ± 13.4	$-20.7^e \pm 14.7$	$-22.1^e \pm 14.3$	12.1
ΔT_I(sec)	+.186 ± .263	+.351 ± .370	+.304 ± .270	+.285 ± .274	+.268 ± .240	.235
Δ%	+16.8 ± 19.9	+27.9 ± 26.0	+22.1 ± 23.4	+19.0 ± 19.5	+20.3 ± 20.2	18
$\Delta V_I T_I$ (ml/sec)	−120 ± 124	$-241^e \pm 112$	$-244^e \pm 134$	$-300^e \pm 178$	$-312^e \pm 174$	120
Δ%	−11.3 ± 11.2	$-28.2^e \pm 7.9$	$-30.5^e \pm 14.6$	$-32.2^e \pm 12.7$	$-34.1^e \pm 12.5$	9.8

[a] Mean values (± S.D.) of changes from previous exercise breaths in 12 subjects.

[b] For each subject, the control breath change is the spontaneous (or random) change (6th breath on air-average of 5 previous breaths of air).

[c] For each subject, the 3rd (4th, 5th, 10th) test breath change is the test breath minus the average of the 2 (3, 4, 9) previous breaths on air.

[d] Least significant difference from a 2-way analysis of variance for two-tailed comparisons with $P = 0.05$.

[e] Difference from control exceeds the least significant difference.

Table 3. Effect of N_2O in Steady State Exercise.[a]

	Previous[b] breaths	Test breath	Change	Percent change	p[c]
V_I (liter)	2.41 ± .80	2.24 ± .86	− .17		.10
				− 7.8	.07
V_IT_I (liter/sec)	1.03 ± .23	.83 ± .30	− .20		.005
				−20.0	.003
PCO_2 (mm Hg)	34.26 ± 2.50	35.70 ± 2.18	+1.44		.01

[a] Mean (± S.D.) for inspired volume, flow rate, and end-tidal PCO_2 in 8 subjects 100% N_2O for *breath.*

[b] For each subject, the 10 breaths previous to the test were averaged.

[c] The two-tailed paired t-test was used to calculate P.

In irregular breathers, the test mixture's effect was only clearly evident in later breaths (Figure 2), but in some subjects a depression was consistent and obvious (Figure 3). In 12 subjects systemically studied, the CO_2 mixture progressively lowered breaths 3, 4, 5, and 10 (Table 2). The inspiratory volume of these breaths was reduced by 10.2 to 22.1% and the inspiratory rate by 28.2 to 34.1%. All of these changes significantly exceeded the control change. None of the differences between the T_I changes from control were significant.

Nitrous oxide for one breath during exercise slightly lowered V_I and V_I/T_I of that breath, the latter significantly (Figure 4 and Table 3). The end-tidal PCO_2 of the N_2O breath rose in all subjects (range 0.6 to 3.4 mm Hg).

Discussion

Statistical Significance of Observations

The inherent variability of the first few breaths of exercise (Krogh and Lindhard, 1913; Paulev, 1971) largely accounts for the variations in Table 1. This variability is dependent on the "degree of naivete" of the subjects (Wasserman et al., 1981) and is less within than between subjects, but the similarly insignificant depressive effect of CO_2 on the absolute value of the first breath ($\dot{V}_E$) found by Ward (1979) in 3 subjects studied repeatedly is also probably ascribable to this variability. Since she found, as we did, that the resting baseline minute ventilation was higher in the CO_2 than in the control runs, it is possible that the relative value of $\dot{V}_E$ (i.e., the difference between the change from the rest with and without CO_2) was statistically significant.

Breathing irregularity becomes less pronounced as exercise proceeds, but random reductions in individual inspirations during the first 10 breaths are frequent enough that an analysis of variance is appropriate. Table 2 shows that the control breath volume was only 22 ml less than the previous average V_I but (barely) significantly less with respect to V_I/T_I (−120 ml/sec). However, the reductions by the test mixture were large enough so that the change in V_I was

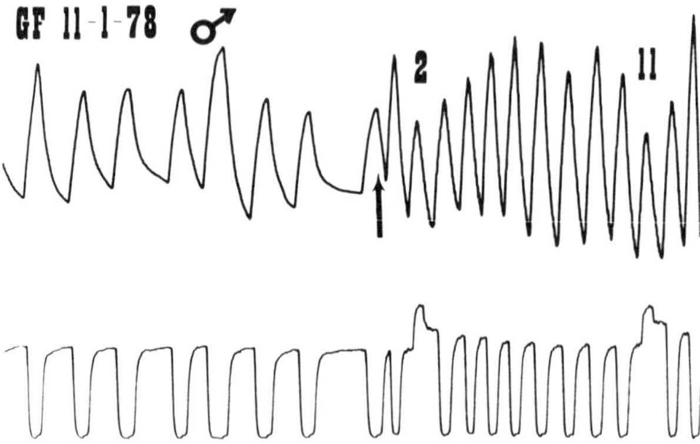

Figure 2. Records of an irregular breather standing on the treadmill (left of arrow) and switched to CO_2 in N_2O during the expirations preceding the 2nd and 11th breaths of exercise (which was started at arrow). Scales as in Figure 1.

significantly greater than the control change in the 5th and 10th breaths, and the V_I/T_I changes were significantly greater than control in all breaths studied.

Physiological Validity

This depends on avoidance of experimental artifact and minimization of psychological influences. The effect of inhaled N_2O in concentrating other lung gases (because of its rapid extraction from alveoli by blood) also increases inspiratory flow at the mouth (Rackow and Salanitre, 1976). The ventilatory depression we find would be even greater if the same step jump in alveolar PCO_2 were achieved with high CO_2 concentrations without N_2O. The artifact of differing gas viscosities affecting PNT performance was ruled out, and in any event CO_2 given in other mixtures via a spirometer system (Filley, 1976), has produced a similar respiratory depression. Esophageal balloon studies have shown lower, not higher, pressure swings in the CO_2 breaths, tending to eliminate changes in pulmonary mechanics as being responsible for inspiratory slowing (Filley et al., 1978).

Conscious men can taste CO_2 if it is introduced suddenly enough into the mouth. Because of this, we have compared the response of subjects exposed to test gases only once with that of other subjects repeatedly tested. The single-breath depression was of the same type and magnitude in the two groups and seemed independent of a subject's "knowing what to expect." In traditional CO_2 inhalation experiments, the gas does not enter as a bolus. As Berger (1981) observed, "When the immediacy of the response can be gauged from earlier work, inspiration of CO_2 has generally been found not to affect $\dot{V}_I$ until the second breath of exposure or later [in birds]... the gas mixing systems used might have delivered CO_2 to the trachea well after the start of the first

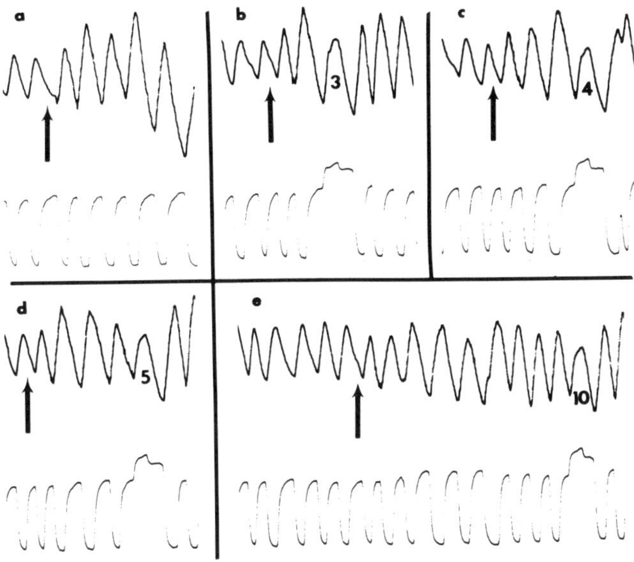

Figure 3. Records of 5 separate runs in a regular breather studied by the protocol used for the data of Table 2. The arrows indicate the moment the treadmill was started.

Figure 4. Records of a subject showing the effect of N_2O on end-tidal PCO_2 and on the respiratory pattern.

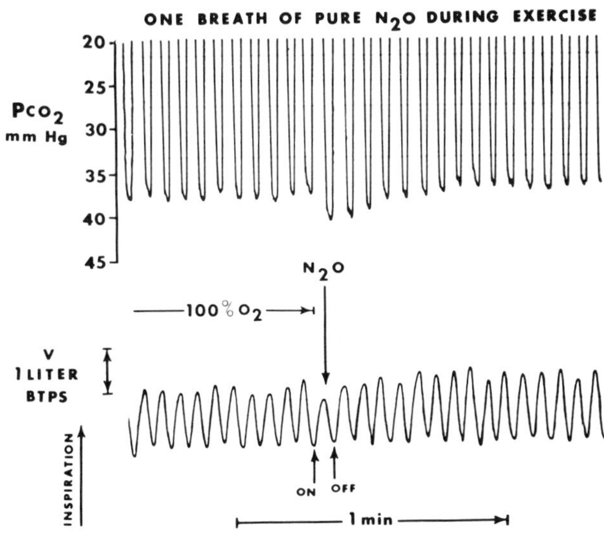

inspiration." In the single study comparable to this one (Ward, 1979), the volume of the inspired line delayed the arrival of CO_2 by one breath; such a delivery system may explain why the 3 subjects were unaware of the CO_2. By imposing sudden moderate exercise, by avoiding perceptible switching of valves, and by studying many naive subjects, we believe we have minimized psychological factors.

Regulatory Implications

Since exercise hyperpnea is proportional to CO_2 flux (Wasserman et al., 1981), it is proportional to the PCO_2 gradient across alveolar walls. Lowering this gradient by raising alveolar PCO_2 fast enough to avoid stimulation via the carotid body should depress ventilation, as herein reported, if breathing is driven by intrapulmonary chemoreception.

Can the respiratory depression we find be mediated by the CO_2-sensitive laryngeal receptor of Boushey and Richardson (1973)? Their reflex takes at least several breaths to be manifest, and unless N_2O acts like CO_2 on upper airways, a laryngeal response seems not to explain our findings.

Part of the current confusion as to why CO_2 seems to affect breathing differently when air-borne rather than blood-borne may stem from neglect of the warnings of Dejours (1959) regarding the need to study CO_2 reactions "in natural conditions" and of Comroe (1974) that when CO_2 is inspired, "it clogs the mechanism for CO_2 elimination." In reviewing unretouched records and variously presented measurements in the CO_2 inhalation literature, we have examined the immediate response (Filley et al., 1980) and have found many instances in which, before carotid body effects are evident, ventilation is reduced rather than increased. Loeppky and Luft (1980) have paid attention to the difference between early effects of CO_2 given by the 2 routes, but have only partly confirmed the present findings. Their cardiodynamic stimulus from venous CO_2 loading either overwhelmed any clogging effect of inhaled CO_2 or was augmented by it, probably depending on the exact timing of the stimuli.

In conclusion, the reductions we find in inspiratory volume and flow rate by sudden increases in alveolar PCO_2 are consistent with a pulmonary receptor vectorially sensitive to ΔPCO_2 between gas and blood, i.e., a differential chemical pressure transducer. Because the first breath of exercise is so variably reduced by CO_2, neural or "cardiodynamic" stimuli probably contribute to early breaths. Whether or not acid-base disequilibria, as we have originally postulated, underlie the observations and how afferent information needed to explain them is carried from lungs to brain during inspiration still remain speculative questions.

ACKNOWLEDGMENTS

The author is grateful for the advice of Drs. Gary Zerbe and Strother Walker and for the assistance of Clark Hale and Marjorie James. This work was supported by Grant No. 16-P-56815/8-13 from the National Institute of Handicapped Research, Department of Education, Washington, D.C.

References

Berger, P.J. 1981. Changes in ventilatory flow rate in ducks in response to a single inspiration of air containing 5% CO_2. *Respir. Physiol.* 43:241–248.

Boushey, H.A. and Richardson, P.S. 1973. The reflex effects of intralaryngeal carbon dioxide on the pattern of breathing. *J. Physiol (London).* 288:181–191.

Comroe, J.G., Jr. 1974. *Physiology of Respiration.* Chicago: Year Book Medical Publishers.

Dejours, P. 1959. La régulation de la ventilation au cours de l'exercice musculaire chez l'homme. *J. Physiol. (Paris)* 51:163–261.

Filley, G.F. 1976. Blood gas disequilibria and exercise hyperpnea. *Trans. Am. Clin. Climatol. Assoc.* 87:48–59.

Filley, G.F., Hale, R.C., Kratochvil, J., and Olson, D.E. 1978. The hyperpnea of exercise and chemical disequilibria. *Chest* 73 (Suppl.):267–270.

Filley, G.F., Swanson, G.D., and Kindig, N.B. 1980. Chemical breathing controls: slow, intermediate, and fast. *Clin. Chest Med.* 1:13–32.

Fordyce, W.E. and Grodins, F.S. 1980. Ventilatory responses to intravenous and airway CO_2 administration in anesthetized dogs. *J. Appl. Physiol.* 48:337–346.

Krogh, A. and Lindhard, J. 1913. The regulation of respiration and circulation during the initial stages of muscular work. *J. Physiol. (London)* 47:112–136.

Loeppky, J.A. and Luft, U.C. 1980. Effect of lower body negative pressure release on hyperpnea induced by inhaled gas. *Respir. Physiol.* 41:349–365.

Paulev, P.E. 1971. Respiratory and cardiac responses to exercise in man. *J. Appl. Physiol.* 30:165–172.

Ponte, J. and Purves, M.J. 1978. Carbon dioxide and venous return and their interaction as stimuli to ventilation in the cat. *J. Physiol. (London)*274:455–475.

Rackow, H. and Salanitre, E. 1976. The pulmonary absorption excretion volume effect. *Anesth. Analg.* 55:51–56.

Snedecor, G.A. and Cochran, W.G. 1971. *Statistical Methods.* Sixth edition. Ames, Iowa: Iowa State University Free Press.

Ward, S.A. 1979. The effects of sudden airway hypercapnia on the initiation of exercise hyperpnea in man. *J. Physiol. (London).* 296:203–214.

Wasserman, K., Whipp, B.J., and Davis, J.A. 1981. Respiratory physiology of exercise: metabolism, gas exchange, and ventilatory control. In *International Review of Physiology, Respiratory Physiology III, Vol. 23.* Widdicome, J.G., ed. Baltimore: University Park Press.

Copyright 1982 by Elsevier North Holland, Inc.
J.A. Loeppky and M.L. Riedesel, editors
OXYGEN TRANSPORT TO HUMAN TISSUES

Regulation of Cerebral Perfusion and PO_2 in Normal and Edematous Brain Tissue

Jürgen Grote and Roland Schubert

Introduction

A decrease of arterial oxygen content due to hypoxia or anemia produces cerebral vasodilation and at normal perfusion pressure a subsequent increase of cerebral blood flow (Kety and Schmidt, 1948; Opitz and Schneider, 1950; Betz, 1972; Grote, 1978; Kuschinsky and Wahl, 1978). Significant brain blood flow reactions occur during hypoxemia when mean cerebral venous oxygen tension falls below 28 to 25 mm Hg, which is the reaction threshold according to Noell and Schneider (Noell and Schneider, 1942; Noell, 1944; Opitz and Schneider, 1950). In the case of arterial hypoxia, an additional PaO_2 threshold for the response of cerebral blood flow was determined to be between 60 and 50 mm Hg (Kety and Schmidt, 1948; Opitz and Schneider, 1950; Kogure et al., 1970; Betz, 1972; Grote, 1978; Kuschinsky and Wahl, 1978).

The lowering of cerebral vascular tone during hypoxemia is assumed to be mainly mediated by local mechanisms, among which the increase in the concentrations of hydrogen and potassium ions in the perivascular space as well as the elevation of the brain tissue adenosine content seem to be of great importance. The experimental results of different investigations have been summarized in a metabolic hypothesis of cerebral blood flow regulation according to which an imbalance of brain tissue oxygen supply and brain tissue oxygen consumption causes the release of the vasodilator products (Schmidt et al., 1945; Lassen, 1968; Betz, 1972; Rubio et al., 1975; Grote, 1978; Kuschinsky and Wahl, 1978). The general validity of the above hypothesis has been recently questioned, since new findings are partially in disagreement with the assumptions on which it is based. Measurements of brain extracellular H^+ and K^+ activity performed during arterial hypoxia or during and after direct electrical stimulation of the brain cortex showed an initial alkalotic change of extracellular pH while the K^+ activity and the blood flow simultaneously increased (Astrup et al., 1976; Silver, 1976; Urbanics et al., 1977; Urbanics et al., 1978). According to brain metabolite assays of Nilsson and coworkers (Nilsson et al., 1977; Seisjö et al., 1979), neither extracellular acidosis nor adenosine accumulation seem to be responsible for the increase of brain vascular conductance in the first phase of hypoxia and in epileptic seizures. However, these findings are partly in contrast to results of Schrader et al. (1980), who observed a significant increase of cortical adenosine level only 15 sec after beginning of seizure activity induced by bicuculline. Today, we are far from having conclusive evidence showing which coupling mechanisms are responsible for the cerebral vascular adjustment observed during hypoxemia. Besides the discussed intrinsic regulatory mechanisms, neurogenic and humoral factors may be involved (Klatzo et al., 1967; Edvinsson and MacKenzie, 1976).

During our current experiments, the effect of decreasing arterial O_2 tension on regional blood flow and tissue PO_2 of the brain cortex was investigated under conditions of normal and increased tissue water content. Since during arterial hypoxemia, the imbalance between cerebral O_2 supply and consumption (as described by the metabolic hypothesis of cerebral blood flow regulation) should result in brain tissue hypoxia, we tried to answer the question of whether pronounced hypoxia or anoxia is detectable in parts of the brain cortex at arterial O_2 tensions at which flow rates begin to increase.

Methods

The investigations were performed on 32 cats with normal brain tissue water content (group 1) and on 24 cats (group 2) in which local brain edema was induced by a cryolesion according to Klatzo 24 hr before (Kety and Schmidt, 1948; Elliot and Jasper, 1949; Klatzo et al., 1967). All animals were lightly anesthetized with sodium pentobarbital (Nembutal, 25 to 30 mg/kg body wt i.v.) and tracheotomized and artificially ventilated after complete relaxation with hexcarbacholinbromide (Imbretil, 1.6 to 2.0 mg initially, 0.2–0.3 mg every 30 min during the experiments). In the course of the experiments, normocapnic normoxia as well as normocapnic hypoxia conditions were established by adjusting the O_2 fraction of the respiratory gas mixture. End-tidal CO_2 was monitored continuously by an infrared CO_2 analyzer. In order to directly measure blood pressure, catheters were inserted into the left femoral artery and into the superior sagittal sinus. The same catheters allowed intermittent blood sampling for PO_2, PCO_2, and pH determinations.

Following bilateral craniotomy and catheterization of both lingual arteries for tracer injection, regional cerebral blood flow (rCBF) was simultaneously measured in two corresponding areas of the left and right suprasylvian gyri in group 1. In group 2, the rCBF measurements were performed in perifocal edematous brain tissue of the right gyrus suprasylvius and in the corresponding zone of the unaffected left hemisphere. In 15 cats from group 1 and 13 cats from group 2, the dura was kept intact, while being opened in the remaining 17 and 11 animals, respectively, to permit additional tissue PO_2 measurements. Regional cortical blood flow was determined using the Kr^{85}-clearance method with bolus injection of the indicator (Lassen and Ingvar, 1961; Zierler, 1965; Hutten and Brock, 1969).

In order to measure the tissue O_2 tension in the upper cortical layers, multiwire surface microelectrodes were used (Kessler and Grunewald, 1969; Lübbers et al., 1969; Lübbers, 1973). The electrodes consisted of 8 individual platinum cathodes of 15 μm tip diameter with a spacing ranging between 350 and 700 μm. The electrode system was calibrated at brain surface temperature with saline solutions of 3 different O_2 tensions. Since the electrodes were mounted on a counterbalanced system, no blood flow restriction occurred in the measuring field. At all PaO_2 levels, 60 to 80 tissue PO_2 measurements were conducted in each brain area under investigation. Body temperature and the temperature of the brain surface, both continuously monitored with thermistor probes, were kept within the normal range.

After completion of the initial rCBF and tissue PO_2 measurements during arterial normoxia and normocapnia, the arterial O_2 tension was decreased stepwise to approximately 50 mm Hg and 30 mm Hg at normal CO_2 tension. Both hypoxic levels were maintained for about 30 to 45 min and the measurements repeated. At the end of the experiments, frozen tissue samples were taken from the gray and the subcortical white matter for determination of tissue water content (Frei et al., 1973; Grote et al., 1981). In the first group of cats, the occurrence of edema could be ruled out in all cases. In the second group, the measured values of dry and wet weight permitted the calculation of the amount of brain swelling present in the edematous tissue (Elliot and Jasper, 1949).

Additionally, in 18 cats of group 1 the frozen tissue samples were utilized to enzymatically assay metabolite concentrations in the cortical gray matter (Grote et al., 1981). Five of these animals were sacrificed at moderate arterial hypoxia ($PaO_2 = 50$ mm Hg) and 13 at pronounced hypoxia ($PaO_2 = 30$ mm Hg). Normal values for brain cortex metabolite concentrations were derived from earlier experiments, conducted in 10 cats under comparable conditions (Grote et al., 1981).

Results and Discussion

Influence of Steady State Arterial Hypoxia on rCBF, Tissue PO_2, and Tissue Metabolites in Normal Cortical Tissue

The stepwise decrease of arterial oxygen tension from normal levels to approximately 50 mm Hg and 30 mm Hg induced in all cases the typical hypoxic blood flow reactions in animals with intact as well as opened dura. Figure 1 summarizes the mean values for rCBF determined during arterial normocapnic normoxia and normocapnic hypoxia at normal arterial blood pressure. In experiments with opened dura, the blood flow rates of the brain cortex were greater than those determined in cats with intact dura, which may in part be attributable to the concomitant tissue pressure decrease. In both experimental series, elevated rCBF values were found when the arterial oxygen tension reached approximately 50 mm Hg.

The results of tissue PO_2 measurements performed parallel to the regional blood flow determinations are shown in the frequency histograms of Figure 2. During arterial normoxia and normocapnia, the oxygen tension measurements on the brain surface resulted without exception in typical PO_2 histograms. Cortical oxygen tensions ranged from very low values between 0 and 2.5 mm Hg to values near the arterial PO_2. The frequency maximum of the histogram was found to be between 25 and 30 mm Hg, while the mean tissue PO_2 was 27.7 mm Hg. The PO_2 distribution agrees with the results of needle electrode and surface electrode measurements by other authors performed in the brain cortex under similar conditions (Lübbers, 1968; Lübbers, 1973; Leniger-Follert et al., 1975; Silver, 1976) as well as with theoretical calculations (Thews, 1960; Grote, 1967). Under moderate arterial hypoxia, along with the increase in regional blood flow, a pronounced left shift of the tissue PO_2 histograms was observed with a significant increase of oxygen tensions between 0 and 2.5 mm Hg. The fact that the shift of the PO_2 distribution to low values was found

Figure 1. Effect of arterial hypoxia on rCBF in the brain cortex of cats with opened (—) and intact dura (---).

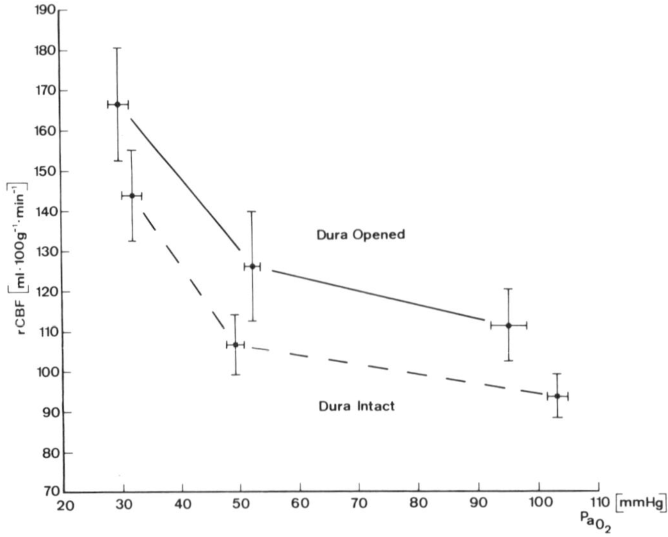

under steady state conditions in which blood flow rates were already elevated suggests a more pronounced tissue hypoxia was present before blood flow regulation was initiated. Moreover, these very low tissue oxygen tensions may act as the stimulus to maintain the hyperemia. At arterial oxygen tensions of approximately 30 mm Hg, the frequency maximum of the tissue PO_2 values was between 0 and 5 mm Hg, indicating severe tissue hypoxia.

The results of tissue metabolite assays are consistent with the above findings. In comparison to the control data, which were in agreement with values measured by different authors (Schmahl et al., 1966; Duffy et al., 1972; Schmiedek et al., 1974; Siesjö, 1978), PaO_2 reduction to 50 mm Hg resulted in significant increases in lactate and pyruvate tissue concentrations and in the lactate/pyruvate ratio as well as in a significant decrease of the phosphocreatine level (Table 1). Slightly elevated ADP and AMP concentrations were also found. Since phosphofructokinase, the major regulatory enzyme of the glycolytic pathway, is activated by a very small decrease in phosphocreatine and a very small increase in ADP (Norberg and Siesjö, 1975; Norberg et al., 1975;

Figure 2. Tissue PO_2 frequency histograms in the brain cortex of cats determined at mean PaO_2 levels of 95.6 mm Hg (A); 52.3 mm Hg (B); and 31.3 mm Hg (C).

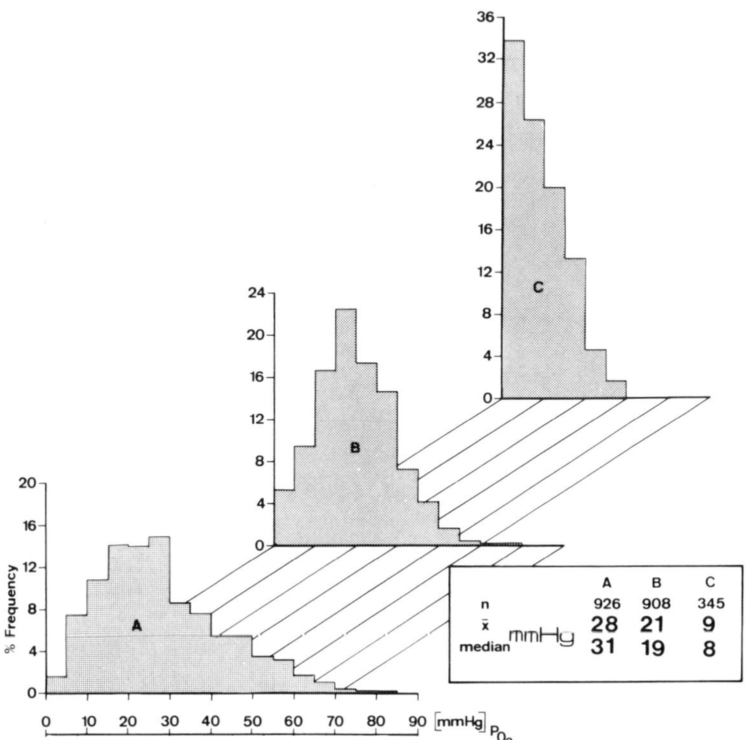

Table 1. Effect of Moderate and Pronounced Arterial Hypoxia on Metabolite Concentrations in the Brain Cortex of Cats.

n	**10**	**5**	**13**
PaO_2 (mm Hg)	**(85 - 125)**	**(45 - 60)**	**(25 - 35)**
Glu	4.88 ± 0.49	4.02 ± 1.05	2.71 ± 0.60
La	1.244 ± 0.141	10.166 ± 2.727	23.737 ± 3.674
Py	0.096 ± 0.020	0.247 ± 0.044	0.264 ± 0.019
PCr	4.59 ± 0.20	2.24 ± 0.52	1.07 ± 0.25
ATP	2.53 ± 0.15	2.26 ± 0.08	1.96 ± 0.22
ADP	0.33 ± 0.03	0.53 ± 0.06	0.75 ± 0.11
AMP	0.04 ± 0.01	0.18 ± 0.03	0.15 ± 0.03
La/Py	15.6 ± 2.9	41.2 ± 10.1	61.1 ± 8.4

NOTE: Mean values ± S.E. are given. Concentrations are in μmol/g wet. wt.

Siesjö, 1978), the observed concentration changes of both phosphate compounds indicate the acceleration of glycolysis. Under conditions of pronounced arterial hypoxia, all metabolic alterations were enhanced (Schmahl et al., 1966; Duffy et al., 1972; Norberg and Siesjö, 1975; Norberg et al., 1975; Siesjö, 1978). In addition, a significant decrease in the glucose concentration was found.

Influence of Steady State Arterial Hypoxia on rCBF and Tissue PO_2 in Edematous Brain Cortex

During arterial normocapnic normoxia and normal arterial blood pressure in the animals with intact as well as in those with opened dura, rCBF was significantly reduced in the edematous brain cortex in comparison to the control values of the unaffected hemisphere (Figure 3). In both experimental groups, tissue water content was normal in the uninjured cortical regions and increased to 80 ml/100g wet wt. in the perifocal areas. Considering the calculated regional swelling of the edematous cortical tissue of 7 to 10%, one would expect a similar difference between the rCBF values of the compared brain regions. The determined mean reduction of regional blood flow, however, was approximately 35% which demonstrates that a depression of regional blood flow does indeed take place in cortical areas with increased water content. As can be seen in Figure 3, the reduction of arterial oxygen tension had little or no effect on regional blood flow of the perifocal cortical regions. However, the hypoxia-induced blood flow response of the control region was normal, indicating impaired or eliminated blood flow regulation in the edematous brain tissue.

Under normoxic conditions, the tissue oxygen tension measurements in the brain cortex resulted in normal PO_2 histograms for the control areas while those of the edematous tissue were slightly shifted to lower PO_2 values (Figure 4). Arterial hypoxia induced progressive tissue hypoxia in both compared brain

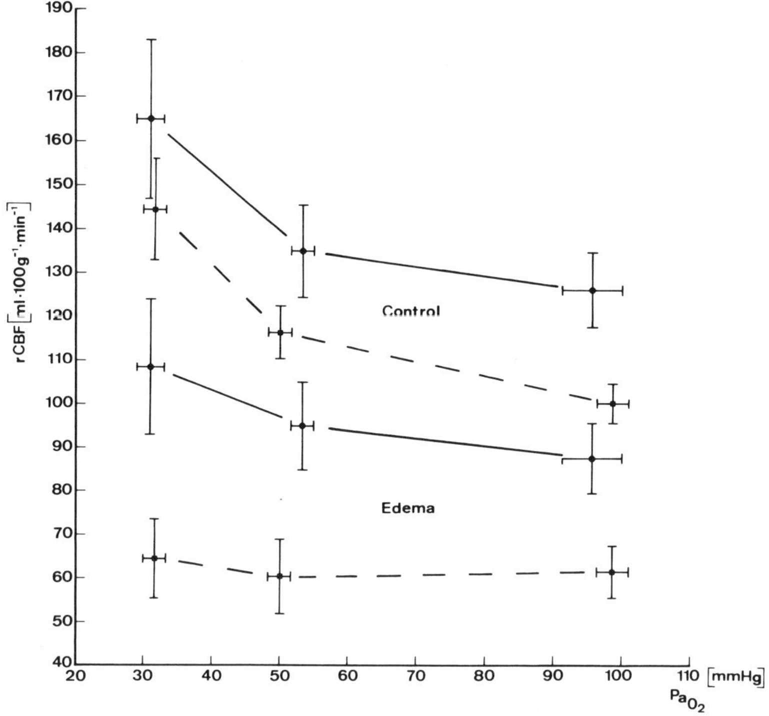

Figure 3. Effect of arterial hypoxia on rCBF of perifocal edematous tissue of brain cortex and of the corresponding area of the undamaged hemisphere of cats with opened (—) and intact dura (---).

regions. However, the injured hemisphere showed a less pronounced increase in the frequency of tissue oxygen tensions between 0 and 2.5 mm Hg. These findings can be interpreted to be a consequence of a decrease in oxygen consumption in the edematous brain tissue due to an alteration in metabolism. The metabolic changes are characterized by significantly greater tissue levels of lactate and pyruvate and a decrease in the concentrations of phosphocreatine and ATP (Frei et al., 1973; Schmiedek et al., 1974; Grote et al., 1978).

In conclusion, the above results of tissue PO_2 measurements as well as tissue metabolite assays demonstrate the presence of brain cortex hypoxia with anoxia in single cells when the decrease in arterial O_2 tension induced a significant elevation of rCBF. Since under these conditions (PaO_2 45 to 60 mm Hg), O_2 deficiency and diminished oxidative metabolism were observed in cortical tissue, the findings support the metabolic hypothesis of cerebral blood flow regulation during arterial hypoxia. The normal behavior of cerebral vascular resistance under hypoxic conditions is impaired in edematous brain areas. The decrease of arterial O_2 tension to values below 50 mm Hg resulted in

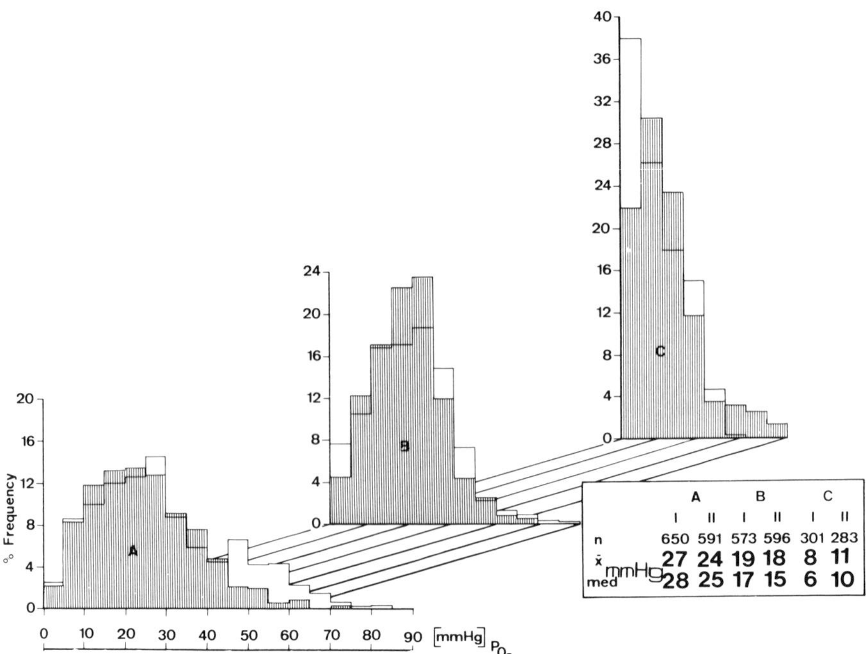

Figure 4. Tissue frequency histograms in perifocal edematous tissue of brain cortex (shaded, II) and in the corresponding area of the undamaged hemisphere (I) of cats determined at mean PaO_2 levels of 95.9 mm Hg (A); 52.7 mm Hg (B); and 33.6 mm Hg (C).

tissue hypoxia in brain areas with both increased and normal water content. However, less pronounced or no blood flow reactions could be observed in the edematous tissue whereas in the control region the blood flow regulation was normal.

References

Astrup, J., Heuser, D., Lassen, N.A., Nilsson, B., Norberg, K., and Siesjö, B.K. 1976. Evidence against H^+ and K^+ as the main factors in the regulation of cerebral blood flow during epileptic discharges, acute hypoxemia, amphetamine intoxication, and hypoglycemia. A micro-electrode study. In *Ionic Actions on Vascular Smooth Muscle*. Betz, E., ed. New York: Springer. pp. 110–116.

Betz, E. 1972. Cerebral blood flow: its measurement and regulation. *Physiol. Rev.* 52:595–630.

Duffy, T.E., Nelson, S.R., and Lowry, O.H. 1972. Cerebral carbohydrate metabolism during acute hypoxia and recovery. *J. Neurochem.* 19:959–977.

Edvinsson, L. and MacKenzie, E.T. 1976. Amine mechanisms in the cerebral circulation. *Pharmacol. Rev.* 28:275–348.

Elliot, K.A. and Jasper, H. 1949. Measurement of experimentally induced brain swelling and shrinkage. *Am. J. Physiol.* 157:122–129.

Frei, H.J., Wallenfang, T., Pöll, W., Reulen, H.J., Schubert, R., and Brock, M. 1973. Regional cerebral blood flow and regional metabolism in cold-induced edema. *Acta Neurochir (Wien)* 29:15–28.

Grote, J. 1967. Die Sauerstoffspannung im Gehirngewebe. In *Hydrodynamik, Elektrolyt- und Säure-Basen-Haushalt im Liquor und Nervensystem*. Kienle, G., ed. Stuttgart: Thieme. pp. 41–50.

Grote, J. 1978. Cerebral blood flow regulation under the conditions of arterial hypoxia. In *The Arterial System*. Bauer, R.D. and Busse, R., eds. New York: Springer. pp. 209–215.

Grote, J., Reulen, J.H., and Schubert, R. 1978. Increased tissue water in the brain: influence on regional cerebral blood flow and oxygen supply. *Advances in Neurology, Vol.* 20. Cervós-Navarro, J., Betz, E., Ebhardt, G., Ferszt, R., and Wüllenweber, R., eds. New York: Raven Press. pp. 333–339.

Grote, J., Zimmer, K., and Schubert, R. 1981. Effects of severe arterial hypocapnia on regional blood flow regulation, tissue PO_2, and metabolism in the brain cortex of cats. *Pflügers Arch.*, in press.

Hutten, H. and Brock, M. 1969. The two-minutes-flow index (TMFI). In *Cerebral Blood Flow, Clinical and Experimental Results*. Brock, M., Fieschi, C., Ingvar, D.H., Lassen, N.A., and Schürmann, K., eds. New York: Springer. pp. 19–23.

Kessler, M. and Grunewald, W. 1969. Possibilities of measuring oxygen pressure fields in tissue by multiwire platinum electrodes. *Progr. Respir. Res.* 3:147–152.

Kety, S.S. and Schmidt, C.F. 1948. The effects of altered arterial tensions of carbon dioxide and oxygen on cerebral oxygen consumption of normal young men. *J. Clin. Invest.* 27:484–492.

Klatzo, I., Wiśniewski, H., Steinwall, O., and Streicher, E., 1967. Dynamics of cold injury edema. In *Brain Edema*. Klatzo, I. and Seitelberger, F., eds. New York: Springer. pp. 554–563.

Kogure, K., Scheinberg, P., Reinmutz, O.M., Fujishima, M., and Busto, R. 1970. Mechanism of cerebral vasodilation in hypoxia. *J. Appl. Physiol.* 29:223–229.

Kuschinsky, W. and Wahl, M. 1978. Local chemical and neurogenic regulation of cerebral vascular resistance. *Physiol. Rev.* 58:656–689.

Lassen, N.A. 1968. Brain extracellular pH: the main factor controlling cerebral blood flow. *Scand. J. Clin. Lab. Invest.* 22:247–251.

Lassen, N.A. and Ingvar, D.H. 1961. The blood flow of the cerebral cortex determined by radioactive Krypton^{85}. *Experientia* 17:42–43.

Leniger-Follert, E., Lübbers, D.W., and Wrabetz, W. 1975. Regulation of local tissue PO_2 of brain cortex at different arterial O_2 pressures. *Pflügers Arch.* 359:81–95.

Lübbers, D.W. 1968. The oxygen pressure field of the brain and its significance for the normal and critical oxygen supply of the brain. In *Oxygen Transport in Blood and Tissue*. Lübbers, D.W., Luft, U.C., Thews, G., and Witzleb, E., eds. Stuttgart: Thieme. pp. 124–139.

Lübbers, D.W. 1973. Local tissue PO_2: its measurement and meaning. In *Oxygen Supply, Theoretical and Practical Aspects of Oxygen Supply and Microcirculation of Tissue*. Kessler, M., Bruley, D.F., Clark, L.C., Lübbers, D.W., Silver, I.A., and Strauss, J., eds. Munich: Urban u. Schwarzenberg. pp. 151–155.

Lübbers, D.W., Baumgärtl, H., Fabel, H., Huch, A., Kessler, M., Kunze, K., Riemann, H., Sieler, D., and Schuchardt, S. 1969. Principle and construction of various platinum electrodes. *Progr. Resp. Res.* 3:136–146.

Nilsson, B., Rehncrona, S., and Siesjö, B.K. 1977. Coupling of cerebral metabolism and blood flow in epileptic seizures, hypoxia, and hypoglycemia. In *The Control of Cerebral Vascular Smooth Muscle*. Purves, M., ed. CIBA Foundation Symposium, No. 56. New York: Exerpta Medica. pp. 199–218.

Noell, W. 1944. Über die Durchblutung und die Sauerstoffversorgung des Gehirns; Einfluss der Hypoxämie und Anämie. *Pflügers Arch. Ges. Physiol.* 247:55–575.

Noell, W. and Schneider, M. 1942. Über die Durchblutung und die Sauerstoffversorgung des Gehirns im akuten Sauerstoffmangel. III. Die arteriovenöse Sauerstoff- und Kohlensäuredifferenz. *Pflügers Arch. Ges. Physiol.* 246:207–249.

Norberg, K., and Siesjö, B.K. 1975. Cerebral metabolism in hypoxic hypoxia. I. Pattern of activation of glycolysis: a reevaluation. *Brain Res.* 86:31–44.

Norberg, K., Quistorff, B. and Siesjö, B.K. 1975. Effects of hypoxia of 10–45 seconds duration on energy metabolism in the cerebral cortex of unanesthetized and anesthetized rats. *Acta Physiol. Scand.* 95:301–310.

Opitz, E. and Schneider, M. 1950. Über die Sauerstoffversorgung des Gehirns und den Mechanismus von Mangelwirkungen. *Erg. Physiol.* 46:126–260.

Rubio, R., Berne, R.M., Bockman, E.L., and Curnish, R.R. 1975. Relationship between adenosine concentration and oxygen supply in rat brain. *Am. J. Physiol.* 228:1896–1902.

Schmahl, F.W., Betz, E., Dettinger, E., and Hohorst, H.J. 1966. Energiestoffweschsel der Grosshirnrinde und Elektroencephalogramm bei Sauerstoffmangel. *Pflügers Arch. Ges. Physiol.* 292:46–59.

Schmiedek, P., Baethmann, A., Sippel, G., Oettinger, W., Enzenbach, R., Marguth, F., and Brendel, W. 1974. Energy state and glycolysis in human cerebral edema. The application of a new freeze-stop technique. *J. Neurosurg.* 40:251–264.

Schmidt, C.F., Kety, S.S., and Pennes, H.H. 1945. The gaseous metabolism of the brain of the monkey. *Am. J. Physiol.* 143:33–52.

Schrader, J., Wahl, M., Kuschinsky, W., and Kreutzberg, G.W. 1980. Increase of adenosine content in the cerebral cortex of the cat during bicuculline-induced seizure. *Pflügers Arch.* 387:245–251.

Siesjö, B.K. 1978. *Brain Energy Metabolism.* New York: Wiley.

Seisjö, B.K., Berntman, L., and Rehncrona, S. 1979. Effect of hypoxia on blood flow and metabolic flux in the brain. *Advances in Neurology, Vol.* 26. Fahn, S., Davis, J.N., and Rowland, L.P., eds. New York: Raven press. pp. 267–283.

Silver, I.A. 1976. Tissue responses to hypoxia, shock, and stroke. In Oxygen Transport to Tissue-II. Grote, J., Reneau, D., and Thews, G., eds. *Adv. Exp. Med. Biol.* 75:325–333.

Thews, G. 1960. Die Sauerstoffdiffusion im Gehirn. Ein Beitrag zur Frage der Sauerstoffversorgung der Organe. *Pflügers Arch. Ges. Physiol.* 271:197–266.

Urbanics, R., Leniger-Follert, E., and Lübbers, D.W. 1977. Extracellular K^+ and H^+-activities of the brain cortex during and after a short period of ischemia and arterial hypoxia. In Oxygen Transport to Tissue-III. Silver, I.A., Erecinska, M., and Bicher, H.I., eds. *Adv. Exp. Med. Biol.* 94:611–616.

Urbanics, R., Leniger-Follert, E., and Lübbers, D.W. 1978. Time-course of changes of extracellular H^+ and K^+-activities during and after direct electrical stimulation of the brain cortex. *Pflügers Arch.* 378:47–53.

Zierler, K.L. 1965. Equations for measuring blood flow by external monitoring of radioisotopes. *Circ. Res.* 16:309–321.

J.A. Loeppky and M.L. Riedesel, editors
OXYGEN TRANSPORT TO HUMAN TISSUES

Tissue O_2 Utilization

Eugene D. Robin

Oxygen depletion is extraordinarily common in biological systems (Hochachka, 1980). High altitude exposure represents one special case of O_2 depletion. In this presentation, the following aspects of O_2 depletion will be discussed: (1) What is the ultimate cause of the physiologic manifestations associated with O_2 depletion? (2) What are the general characteristics of cellular O_2 consumption? (3) What kind of processes lead to limitation of cellular O_2 supply? (4) Is diffusion a limiting factor for O_2 uptake in the tissues? (5) What are the interrelations among the various processes involved in O_2 transport by the blood? (6) What kind of processes underlie adaptive changes in response to O_2 depletion?

Ultimate Cause of Physiologic Abnormalities

Oxygen depletion ultimately produces abnormalities of cell, organ, and whole body function by producing abnormalities of cell O_2 metabolism. The term dysoxia has been proposed to characterize abnormalities of cell O_2 metabolism and the group of dysoxic disorders which are related to limitations of O_2 supply are collectively considered as forms of hypoxic dysoxia (Robin, 1977).

Hypoxic dysoxia results from sufficient limitation of O_2 supply so that the rate of O_2-requiring biochemical reactions is reduced, ultimately leading to abnormal cell function. In a fundamental sense, O_2 depletion produces a series of biochemical abnormalities and should be regarded as a biochemical disorder. It should be emphasized that the primary biochemical abnormalities evoked by O_2 depletion usually evoke a series of secondary biochemical changes which reflect the effects of metabolic control mechanisms, adaptive changes, alterations in the composition of the cell, and alterations in the rates of various reactions that do not require O_2. As a result, the biochemical consequences of hypoxia tend to be complex. The concept of dysoxia is probably of value because it suggests that the biochemical processes involved in O_2 uptake are of primary importance in O_2 depletion and that it is desirable that we do not deal with these biochemical processes as a "black box."

General Characteristics of Cell O_2 Consumption

The major site of utilization of molecular O_2 within the cell is the mitochondrion. For an "average" cell, perhaps 80% of total O_2 consumption is by the mitochondria. The O_2 combines with electrons derived from various substrates to release free energy. The free energy made available is then used to pump H^+ from the inside to the outside of the mitochondrion against an electrochemical gradient. As H^+ diffuses back along a favorable gradient, the free energy is made available to phosphorylate ADP and ATP is generated (Mitchell, 1961). The ATP so generated is ultimately used to provide energy for most energy requiring biological processes.

An important property of the mitochondrial enzyme which catalyzes the reaction between molecular O_2 and electrons (cytochrome aa_3) is that the enzyme appears to possess a high affinity for O_2. Half maximal velocity of the reaction occurs at less than 1.0 Torr (Chance, 1965). The implication is that for this reaction there should be no decrease in O_2 consumption until the depression of O_2 supply is extraordinarily severe. That appears to be the case, at least in isolated cell systems (Wilson et al., 1979). Direct impairment of bioenergetics because of a simple decrease in PO_2 is presumably uncommon. However, even with the rate of mitochondrial O_2 consumption maintained constant, moderate to severe O_2 depletion evokes a series of secondary reactions with important consequences for cell energy supply. The rate of glycolysis accelerates, thereby increasing ATP generation (Racker, 1980), and cell pH falls as lactic and pyruvic acid accumulate. The metabolic regulation which results in accelerated glycolysis does not appear to depend on molecular O_2 directly, but rather is evoked by antimycin A and cyanide in the face of a normal O_2 supply (Racker, 1980). In addition to glycolysis, there is another potential source of ATP. The Krebs cycle may become split into 2 linear reaction sequences with the generation of succinic acid possibly increasing anaerobic ATP generation further (Wilson and Cascarano, 1969; Hochachka and Storey, 1975; Sanborn et al., 1979). During severe depletion, phosphocreatine and inorganic phosphate concentrations increase progressively. The link between a reduced O_2 supply, maintained mitochondrial O_2 utilization and an extensive series of secondary energy supplying reactions is not clear (to me).

In addition to the utilization of O_2 in the mitochondria, cellular O_2 consumption takes place in a variety of other subcellular organs (microsomes, nucleus, plasma membrane, lysosomes, etc.). In an "average" cell, these reactions may account for some 20%of cell O_2 consumption. The biochemical reactions in these locations subserve a variety of biosynthetic, biodegradative, and detoxification oxidations (Bloch, 1962). Some of the enzymes involved in these reactions resemble cytochrome aa_3 and have high affinities for O_2. Others have low affinities and presumably the reactions subserved by these enzymes are sensitive to even moderate O_2 depletion. This, for example, is true of the metabolic sequences by which the neurotransmitters (DOPA, the cathecholamines, and serotonin) are synthesized.

It is reasonable to consider that the basis of a number of the manifestations of high altitude exposure are related to the decreased rates of biochemical reactions included in this group of reactions. It has been suggested that some of the manifestations of O_2 depletion are related to so-called "transmitter" failure (decreased availability of neurotransmitters) rather than bioenergetic failure (Siesjö, 1978).

Processes Leading to Decreased O_2 Supply

The etiologic background of impaired O_2 supply may be classified as follows: (1) abnormal pulmonary O_2 exchange, (2) abnormal blood O_2 exchange, (3) abnormal systemic capillary O_2 exchange, (4) abnormal interstitial O_2 exchange, (5) abnormal transmembrane O_2 exchange, and (6) abnormal intracellular O_2 exchange. In turn, each of these can develop as a result of a wide variety of individual disorders. Some of these disorders are listed in Table 1.

An adequate O_2 supply depends on a combination of bulk flow of fluids and direct diffusional flow of O_2 molecules. Bulk flow, whether in gases or liquids, tends to be a highly regulated process with regulation usually occurring at the level of individual organs. Diffusional flow is obviously a largely passive process.

Diffusion Limitation

An interesting issue concerning tissue gas exchange is to what extent diffusion may operate as a rate limiting process for tissue O_2 uptake. One may contrast diffusion across pulmonary capillaries with that across systemic capillaries.

In the lung, it is considered that, at least under normal conditions, diffusion is not rate limiting (Figure 1). This conclusion follows from two facts. One is the evidence that the PO_2 of alveolar air and end-pulmonary capillary plasma are in equilibrium. The second is that prolonging the length of time blood spends in the pulmonary capillary does not increase the O_2 tension of end-capillary plasma (Forster, 1957).

In the case of systemic capillary O_2 transport, an indirect analysis is required, as no accurate measurements of mean cell PO_2 are available. However, most estimates suggest values of 20 Torr or less. That is, cell PO_2 is substantially lower than the PO_2 of blood leaving the venous end of the

Table 1. Etiological Basis of Hypoxic Dysoxia.

Process	Disorders
Pulmonary O_2 uptake	Reduced ambient O_2 Global alveolar hypoventilation Reduced V/Q, regional Absent V/Q, parenchymal shunt Pulmonary vascular shunt Intracardiac right to left shunt Diffusion limitation (?) Reduced cardiac output with right to left shunt Decreased affinity of Hb for O_2 Decreased pH, acute Increased PCO_2 Increased temperature Increased 2,3-DPG Increased pH (chronic), hypoxemia, anemia phosphate retention, red cell pyruvate kinase deficiency Abnormal Hbs Kansas, Seattle, S
Carriage of O_2 combined with Hb	Reduced hematocrit Reduced red cell mass Reduced effective Hb concentration CarboxyHb MetHb
Cardiac output	Global reduction of cardiac output
Regional blood flow	Maldistribution of cardiac output Organic reduction of systemic vascular cross sectional area Functional reduction of systemic vascular cross sectional area Systemic arteriovenous shunts
Altered rheologic properties of blood	Individual red cell disorders Reduced surface/volume Abnormal red cell content Stiff cell membranes Bulk red cell increase Polycythemia White cell abnormalities White cell aggregates Bulk white cell increase
Increased affinity of Hb for O_2	Increased pH, acute Decreased PCO_2 Decreased temperature Decreased red cell organic phosphates (2,3-DPG) Decreased pH (chronic), stored blood, increased ADP, phosphate depletion, red cell pyruvate kinase excess, red cell hexokinase deficiency, heritable absence of 2,3-DPG, decreased 2,3-DPG binding to Hb (fetal Hb) Abnormal Hbs Ranier, Barts, H, Yakima, Capetown, Chesapeake, Hiroshima, Little Rock, McKees Rock

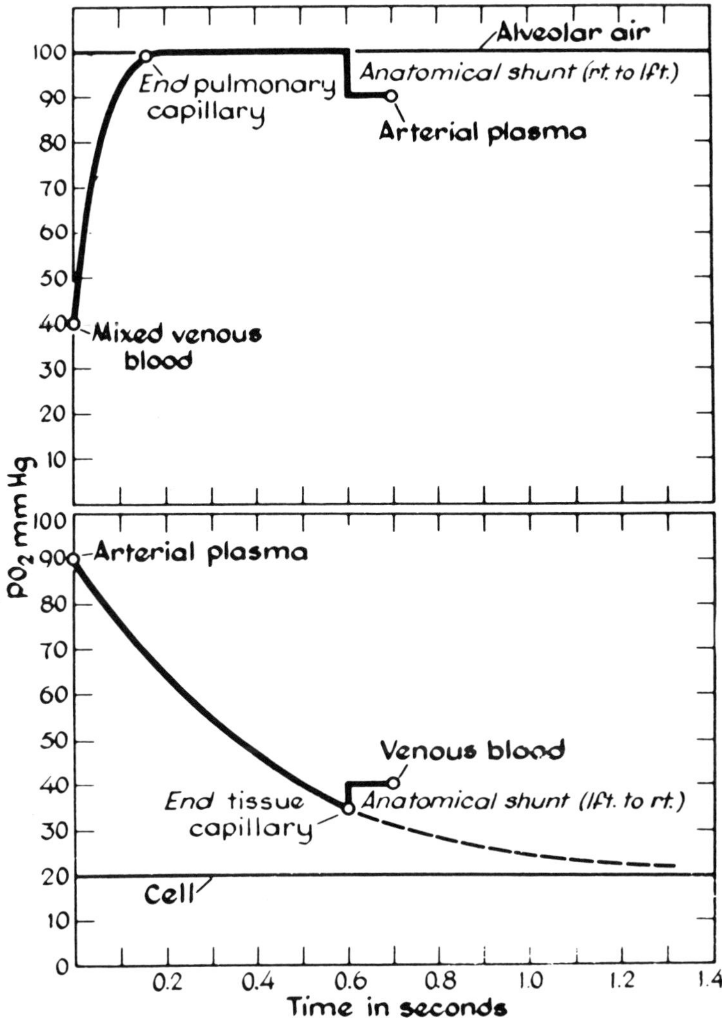

Figure 1. Diffusion is not limiting for O_2 exchange between alveolar air and pulmonary capillary plasma (top). Equilibrium of PO_2 is attained within the time available in the pulmonary capillary. This may not be true in systemic capillaries (bottom). There is a substantial PO_2 gradient between end capillary PO_2 and "mean" intracellular PO_2. (*Note*: rt. = right; lft. = left).

capillary in most organs. The failure to demonstrate equilibrium between cell and capillary of course suggests that the time available for diffusion in such capillaries is inadequate for equilibrium and that the process of diffusion is rate limiting. The second feature of tissue O_2 exchange is that prolonging the time which blood spends in tissue capillaries may result in increased O_2 extraction. For example, most maneuvers which decrease cardiac output are associated with reductions in venous O_2 tensions. This of course is a necessary but not sufficient characteristic of systems in which diffusion is rate limiting. On the other hand, there is increased O_2 extraction during severe exercise (Vatner and Murray, 1980). This might be related either to an increased surface area of capillaries or conceivably a "mitochondrial reserve" which is only mobilized during maximal exercise (Robin and Hance, 1980). This reserve might be mobilized during maximal exercise leading to a steeper gradient for diffusion. If diffusion is indeed rate limiting for tissue O_2 exchange, then of course the maintenance of adequate bulk flow becomes a critical determinant of tissue O_2 supply.

Interrelations Among the Various Processes Involved in Blood O_2 Transport

A list of individual disorders which can be associated with abnormalities of the transport of O_2 in the blood are shown in Table 1. Several general points need to be made. We know little about the quantitative impact of alterations of any of these processes on tissue O_2 utilization. For example, consider one of the most simple and most intensively studied factors, the hematocrit. Can we define a hematocrit value which optimizes tissue O_2 metabolism? The best answer that we have is that there is no single value for an optimal hematocrit. Its value depends on a variety of factors including the organ involved, the values of other variables involved in blood O_2 transport as well as other undefined processes (Gaehtgens and Kreuzer, 1981). Thus our information is quite primitive and largely based on indirect inferences. Or consider the impact of a shift in the affinity of hemoglobin for O_2. Increased affinity may improve and not impair tissue O_2 delivery when arterial PO_2 is low, when the cardiac output is low or when mixed venous PO_2 is low (Duhm, 1981). For most alterations in blood transport, a similar interplay exists and analyses which ignore these interrelationships tend to be simplistic and misleading. The second point is that there is a close interrelationship among the various processes which are involved in blood O_2 transport and as a result the impact on O_2 supply is rarely simple. It should be emphasized that an understanding of the processes involved in blood O_2 transport will require methods which permit us to evaluate tissue O_2 utilization precisely. Such methods are not currently available.

Adaptive Processes

One of the most interesting aspects of high altitude exposure is that it provides a model to examine the nature of adaptive processes which are evoked by O_2 depletion in otherwise normal subjects. A study of biologic adaptive processes is a study of the impact of the dimension of time on the effect of various biologic pertubations. As previously pointed out (Robin, 1980), adaptations to O_2 depletion can be analyzed in 3 categories (Table 2).

Table 2. Classification of Adaptive Responses to Chronic Oxygen Depletion.

I. Improved O_2 Transport/Supply
   1. Increased alveolar ventilation
   2. Increased cardiac output
   3. Increased erythrocyte mass
   4. Altered hemoglobin affinity
   5. Increased myoglobin
   6. O_2 conservation by arterial constriction

II. Improved Substrate Supply
   1. Increased substrate delivery
   2. Glucose conservation by arterial constriction
   3. Substrate conservation by endocrine or paracrine regulation

III. Direct adaptations of cell metabolism to hypoxic dysoxia.

There are adaptations which usually operate at a physiological level and serve to maximize O_2 supply. These adaptations have been extensively studied and are conventionally the focus of attention at meetings like this. A second group of adaptations serves to maximize substrate supply. Oxygen depletion is frequently associated with increased requirements for a variety of substrates (glucose, amino acids, fatty acids). It has only recently been appreciated that a variety of hormonal, neural, and humoral mechanisms operate in various forms of O_2 depletion to improve substrate provision. This area is in its infancy and will presumably be found to be important during adaptation to high altitude exposure. Finally, as anticipated by Paul Bert a hundred years ago, it is becoming clear that there is a series of adaptations which operate at a cellular level which modulate the deleterious effects of O_2 depletion. It may be anticipated that unravelling these will provide a major contribution to understanding the alterations in biologic function related to high altitude exposure.

References

Bloch, K. 1962. Oxygen and biosynthetic patterns. *Fed. Proc.* 21:1058–1063.

Chance, B. 1965. Reaction of oxygen with the respiratory chain in cells and tissue. *J. Gen. Physiol.* 49(Suppl.):163–188.

Duhm, J. 1981. Effects of high altitude (arterial PO_2) and of displacements of the O_2 dissociation curve of blood on peripheral O_2 extraction and PO_2. In *High Altitude Physiology and Medicine. Topics in Environmental Physiology and Medicine.* Brendel, W. and Zink, R.A., eds. Heidelberg: Springer, in press.

Forster, R.W. 1957. Exchange of gases between alveolar air and pulmonary capillary blood: pulmonary diffusing capacity. *Physiol. Rev.* 37:391–452.

Gaehtgens, P. and Kreuzer, F. 1981. Skeletal muscle perfusion, exercise capacity, and the optimal hematocrit. *Eur. J. Appl. Physiol.*, in press.

Hochachka, P.W. 1980. *Living Without Oxygen; Closed and Open Systems in Hypoxia Tolerance.* Cambridge: Harvard University Press. pp. 27–41.

Hochachka, P.W. and Storey, K.B. 1975. Metabolic consequences of diving in animals and man. *Science* 187:613–621.

Mitchell, P. 1961. Coupling of phosphorylation to electron and hydrogen transfer by a chemiosmotic type of mechanism. *Nature* 191:144–148.

Racker, E. 1980. From Pasteur to Mitchell: a hundred years of bioenergetics. *Fed. Proc.* 39:210–215.

Robin, E.D. 1977. Dysoxia: abnormal tissue O_2 utilization. *Arch. Intern. Med.* 137:905–910.

Robin, E.D. 1980. Of men and mitochondria: coping with hypoxic dysoxia. *Amer. Rev. Respir. Dis.* 122:517–531.

Robin, E.D. and Hance, A.J. 1980. Skeletal muscle as a facultative anaerobic system. In *Exercise Bioenergetics and Gas Exchange*. Cerretilli, P. and Whipp, B.J., eds. Amsterdam: Elsevier North Holland. pp. 101–119.

Sanborn, T., Gavin, W., Berkowitz, S., Perille, T., and Lesch, M. 1979. Augmented conversion of aspartate and glutamate to succinate during anoxia in rabbit heart. *Am. J. Physiol.* 237:H535–H541.

Siesjö, B.K. 1978. *Brain Energy Metabolism.* New York: John Wiley and Sons. pp. 398–526.

Vatner, S.F. and Murray, P.A. 1980. Cardiocirculatory adaptations to severe exercise in the conscious dog. In *Exercise Bioenergetics and Gas Exchange*. Cerretilli, P. and Whipp, B.J., eds. New York: Elsevier North Holland. pp. 253–265.

Wilson, M.A. and Cascarano, J. 1970. Energy-yielding oxidation of NADH by fumerate in submitochondrial particles of rat tissues. *Biochem. Biophys. Acta* 216:54–56.

Wilson, D.F., Erecińska, M., Drown, C., and Silver, I.A. 1979. The oxygen dependence of cellular energy metabolism. *Arch. Biochem. Biophys.* 195:485–493.

J.A. Loeppky and M.L. Riedesel, editors
OXYGEN TRANSPORT TO HUMAN TISSUES

Muscle Oxygen Supply in Exercise

Per-Olof Åstrand

At rest, the skeletal muscles consume 15 to 20% of the body's total oxygen uptake. The muscles are, however, the only tissue which can markedly increase its metabolic rate. From a resting aerobic power of 15 W, they can be activated to reach an aerobic power of 1000 W or higher. The highest oxygen uptake which has been reported is 7.4 liter/min and the corresponding aerobic power output of 2400 W is mainly produced by the skeletal muscles. During strenuous exercise of short duration, the oxygen transport from environmental air to the mitochondria becomes the primary task of the respiratory and circulatory systems. The muscles have enough substrates stored for the energy required to regenerate ATP; the problem is to supply the oxygen in an adequate quantity and at an adequate tension. The blood flow delivering the oxygen to the activated muscles is enough to take care of the CO_2 and heat produced. In prolonged exercise, the transport of fuel, mainly free fatty acids, to the muscles becomes more and more important. But again, the local blood flow is basically regulated to secure the oxygen supply.

What Is Limiting the Oxygen Supply in Exercise?

Certainly the demand for oxygen in the skeletal muscles is determined by the number of cross bridges formed between actin and myosin in the muscles and the rate of these interactions. Eventually, the aerobic metabolism will not cover the energy demand and anaerobic glycolysis will support the mitochondrial "power plants" in their efforts to rephosphorylate ADP to ATP. Beyond this stage, the oxygen transport chain is stressed to its maximum. Which of the conductance steps in the cascade of oxygen from air to mitochondria can potentially limit the overall oxygen flow and thus the oxygen available for aerobic metabolism in the muscle cell? I will briefly discuss (1) the convective conductance of oxygen from air to the alveoli, the pulmonary ventilation, (2) the diffusion of oxygen between air and blood in the lungs, (3) the next convective step, i.e., the cardiac output, and (4) the diffusion of oxygen from the capillary blood to its targets, the mitochondria.

Pulmonary Ventilation

There are data which indicate that ventilation is normally not limiting the oxygen uptake. (1) During exercise when the maximal oxygen uptake is reached, it is still possible for the subject to exercise at a higher intensity because of the anaerobic processes. However, the pulmonary ventilation continues to increase without any distinct ceiling being reached. (2) At maximal exercise, it is possible voluntarily to increase the ventilation further, showing that the ability of the respiratory muscles to ventilate the lungs evidently is not exhausted during spontaneous respiration. (3) At heavy exercise, the alveolar oxygen tension increases and the carbon dioxide tension decreases, facts that indicate an effective gas exchange in the lungs.

Oxygen Diffusion from Alveolar Air to Blood

During maximal exercise, there is only a slight reduction in the oxygen tension of the arterial blood and due to hemoconcentration the oxygen content of the arterial blood is increased as compared with resting conditions.

Central Circulation

The relationship between the oxygen consumption during maximal exercise and the oxygen content of the arterial blood has been analyzed by several investigators (Åstrand and Rodahl, 1977, pp. 184–186). (1) An increase in the oxygen tension in the inspired air will significantly increase the maximal oxygen uptake and improve the performance. (2) During acute exposure to hypoxia (a low barometric pressure) the maximal oxygen uptake is reduced in parallel to the decrease in the arterial blood's O_2 content. (3) With part of the hemoglobin blocked by carbon monoxide (up to 20%), the oxygen transport at a given submaximal rate of work can be maintained. The heart rate is increased and the cardiac output is at control levels or somewhat higher. During maximal work, the oxygen uptake is reduced more or less in proportion to the reduction in oxygen content of the arterial blood. However, with 15% HbCO the cardiac output averages 5% lower than in the control experiments. (4) With controlled blood loss and reinfusion of red cells, the effect of acute variations in hematocrit can be studied. The effect of blood loss is a deterioration of physical performance which is related to a reduced maximal oxygen uptake. One of the earlier studies of the effect of blood loss on physical performance was conducted by Luft and coworkers (Balke et al., 1954). A reinfusion of red cells (equivalent to 800 ml of blood) in subjects who had recovered after blood loss could dramatically, "over a night," improve the maximal oxygen uptake and the performance to supernormal values (an average increase in max $\dot{V}O_2$ of 9%). In 5 subjects running at a speed which could be maintained for about 5 min, the oxygen content of the arterial blood averaged 13% higher after reinfusion of red cells compared with the values after blood loss. The difference in maximal oxygen uptake was actually about 13% but the individual variations were rather large (Figure 1). The maximal heart rate and stroke volume, were similar in the different experiments.

Oxygen Diffusion from Blood to Skeletal Muscles

The purpose of this brief summary is to illustrate that the maximal oxygen uptake in exercise engaging large muscle groups is apparently not limited by the capacity of the muscle mitochondria to consume oxygen. Slight variations in the volume of O_2 offered to maximally activated skeletal muscles will produce almost proportional changes in the volume of oxygen consumed by the mitochondria. At least there are enzymes with the potential to yield energy aerobically if extra oxygen is available Gollnick et al. (1972) have concluded that the metabolic potential of both conditioned and unconditioned muscles normally exceeds the actual O_2 uptake of the muscles. This agrees with the more recent findings of Henriksson and Reitman (1977). Newsholme et al. (1980) have pointed out that the maximal activities *in vitro* of enzymes that catalyze near-equilibrium reactions *in vivo* are probably considerably higher

Figure 1. Maximal oxygen uptake after venesection and after reinfusion of an equivalent volume of red cells approximately 4 months later compared with the control values.

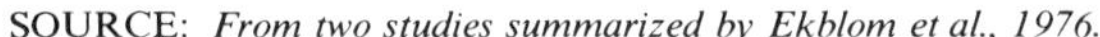
SOURCE: *From two studies summarized by Ekblom et al., 1976.*

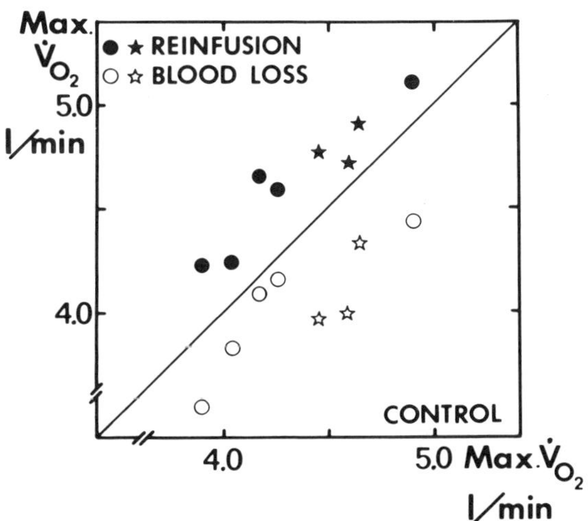

than the maximal flow through that particular pathway. Their potentials are never fully utilized. In contrast, the maximal activity of an enzyme that catalyzes a nonequilibrium reaction *in vivo* may provide useful quantitative information. They present a few enzymes which may be useful as flux indicators. Thus, 2-oxoglutarate dehydrogenase activity provides a quantitative indication of the maximal flux through the citric acid cycle (but succinate dehydrogenase activity does not). In many studies, enzymes have been analyzed "on the basis of the ease of assay rather than quantitative relevance of the activity to the *in vivo* flux."

I think that it is still an open question to what extent the enzyme activity in skeletal muscle cells can limit their aerobic energy yield. At this stage it is logical to give some thoughts to the "composition" of the skeletal muscle.

Fiber Types and Arrangement

From a functional point of view, most muscles are built up of muscle fibers with different mechanical properties. There is presently a debate about classification and nomenclature. *Slow twitch fibers* or Type I fibers have a relatively slow contraction time but have a high mitochondrial density and thereby a high potential for aerobic enzyme activities. They are well-adapted for prolonged exercise as they have a relatively low activity of myosin ATPase. The *fast twitch fibers* (Type II fibers) have a relatively short contraction time and a well-developed glycolytic enzyme system. The mitochondrial density and oxidative activity are lower and the fibers fatigue more rapidly. However, Type II fibers may be divided into several subgroups. The IIa fibers have a relatively high oxidative (aerobic) potential and are more resistant to fatigue. Type IIb are the "typical" fast twitch fiber with a low aerobic potential. A few percent of the muscle fibers may be of Type IIc which is relatively undifferentiated.

It may well be that the oxygen diffusion from the capillaries to the mitochondria is a critical factor for aerobic metabolism. The capillaries generally occupy the corners of the polygonal muscle fibers. That means that several fibers, e.g., Type I and Type II, share a common capillary. Mitochondria are more numerous and larger in the fiber regions close to the capillaries (Weibel and Taylor, 1981) which will reduce the distance for diffusion. Hoppeler et al. (1981) point out that in the skeletal muscle the exchange of gases and metabolites through the very thin blood-tissue barrier is favored by the arrangement of the capillary network in close spatial relationship with the muscle fibers, with the capillaries running mainly parallel to the fibers, with some anastomoses. It seems as if the O_2 supply unit is not cylindrical but cone-shaped, i.e., the density of capillary branches increases towards the venular end of the vascular bed (Hoppeler et al., 1981). The total surface area of the capillary network has been estimated to about 200 m^2 in 30 kg of muscle. How will the fiber type modify the oxygen flux within a muscle? It has been pointed out that the highest volume of oxygen that can be offered to exercising skeletal muscles may be decisive for their aerobic power. From a teleological viewpoint, it is very efficient that low-threshold slow twitch fibers are recruited during exercise of moderate intensity. They have the enzyme potentials for aerobic metabolism, and the myoglobin enchances the oxygen diffusion within the cells (Åstrand and Rodahl, 1977, pp. 245 and 418). Their capillary density is also relatively high. During very severe exercise, the high-threshold fast twitch fibers also become activated, but at this stage the oxygen supply is deficient. The myoglobin in the slow twitch fibers will direct the oxygen to those fibers thus preventing the fast twitch fibers from "stealing" oxygen. On the other hand, the fast twitch fibers are well-equipped for anaerobic energy yield. In other words, when the fast twitch fibers are recruited, a limited volume of oxygen is available for them (at the beginning of exercise and during very vigorous exercise). It would be somewhat of a waste of resources to have their metabolic repertoire developed as replicas of the slow twitch fibers. However, with training, the potential of the central circulation to transport oxygen out to the tissues is improved and there is an increased capillary density in the trained muscle (Åstrand and Rodahl, 1977, pp. 394 and 416–418). With more O_2 available, it makes sense that fast twitch fibers can increase their aerobic potential; they will not be competing for oxygen with the slow twitch fibers, and in fact the maximal oxygen consumption during exercise will increase. There are data indicating that Type IIb fibers can, by training, be transformed to Type IIa fibers which have a higher aerobic potential.

It is presently a hot issue whether or not a transformation between Type I and Type II fibers can occur. When subjecting an animal to cross-innervation or prolonged electrical stimulation of the skeletal muscles, a transformation of a fast twitch fiber to a slow twitch fiber is possible by all histochemical criteria which have so far been applied. Whether such a transformation is possible under normal conditions is presently disputed (Salmons and Henriksson, 1981). It is an interesting observation that the density of mitochondria and activity of enzymes are similar in longitudinal sections of a muscle fiber. Therefore the aerobic potential of a single muscle fiber is relatively constant over its length (Hoppeler et al., 1981). The muscle fibers within a motor unit seem to be "identical twins" in their morphology and function but neighboring fibers which belong to other motor units can differ markedly. Most likely the motoneuron has a very strong trophic effect on its slaves, the muscle fibers.

Training

There is ample evidence that the number of fibers in the skeletal muscle cannot increase but the individual fiber diameter can be modified by prolonged training or inactivity. As mentioned, the capillary density can increase during a period of training as well as the volume and number of mitochondria and the activity of many enzymes in the aerobic metabolic pathways (Åstrand and Rodahl, 1977, pp. 394, 433–434, 503–504).

A very important effect of training is certainly the induced increase in maximal cardiac output and therefore in maximal aerobic power. Often a widening of the arteriovenous O_2 difference also contributes to the improved aerobic performance. Another positive effect is the increase in oxidation of free fatty acids and the reduced energy requirement from glycogen. This change in fuel utilization is not only evident at a given metabolic rate but also when exercising at a given percentage of the maximal aerobic power. The modifications at a cellular level mentioned above may be essential for these metabolic events. All this means that the endurance-trained individual can exercise closer to her or his maximal aerobic power for longer periods of time than the untrained person. One still unsettled question is how to explain the specificity in training. For instance, a good swimmer can only after intensive swim training reach the same peak oxygen uptake during swimming as attained when running.

The stimuli triggering the adaptive changes in the skeletal muscles' oxidative potential to different levels of physical activity are so far unknown. Henriksson et al. (1980) showed that one candidate, a specific activation of beta-receptors on the muscle fibers could be ruled out. In sympathectomized rats (with or without destruction of the adrenal medulla), there was a training induced increase in activity of several enzymes irrespective of whether the sympathetic-adrenal system was intact or not.

Summary and Conclusions

Weibel and Taylor (1981) and coworkers have recently analyzed whether or not we have a regulated morphogenesis resulting in a state of structural design of the mammalian respiratory system where all parts are balanced to each other and matched to the functional needs. It would be a sound and economical principle that no more structure is formed and maintained than is required to secure the maximal O_2 flow rate from air to mitochondria when the system is pushed to its limit, perhaps with some minimal safety factor. For instance, a superfluous mitochondrial mass would be wasteful. In animals ranging in body weight (M_b) from 7 g to 260 kg, they noted that the maximal oxygen uptake measured when the animals were running on a treadmill scaled approximately to $M_b^{0.75}$. The estimated diffusing capacity of the lung, however, scaled, approximately to $M_b^{1.0}$. The conclusion was that the larger animals required a larger pulmonary diffusing capacity to transfer O_2 at a given rate from air to blood than smaller animals. Similarly, they did not find an agreement between the scaling factors for mitochondria volume and capillary density and for maximal oxygen uptake. They ended the discussion with, "But the situation is less simple than one could think––," and indicated that the study of scaling relationships is useful to improve understanding of how structure may affect function.

It was mentioned that the maximal activity of some enzymes evidently exceeds the functional need. That holds true for enzymes active in glycolysis, the Krebs cycle, and the respiratory chain. This luxuriance is apparently more obvious in the trained individual. The situation may have been different in species living hundreds of millions of years ago but specific instructions remain in our genetic code for the production of these enzymes.

There is a definite limit in the individual's maximal oxygen uptake during exercise but we cannot precisely define the limiting factor(s). Of prime importance is the natural endowment. That explains why most women have a lower maximal aerobic power than the average man of the same age. Top athletes in endurance events are only partly products of a tough training program. Fortunately the skeletal muscles do remember the anaerobic glycolysis developed billions of years ago when the concentration of molecular oxygen in the atmosphere was very sparse. It should be emphasized that the formation of lactate from pyruvate does not yield any energy for ATP regeneration, but it is essential for the reoxidation of NADH (or $NADH_2$). The capillary network around the fast twitch muscle fibers becomes very important to remove the lactate produced and the blood can distribute the lactate to the large water pool in the body. Its accumulation in the muscle fiber is delayed which evidently facilitates the anaerobic machinery. Lactate is also an excellent substrate and it can easily diffuse into the adjacent muscle fibers which may be active slow twitch fibers. There may be those who regret that the skeletal muscles do not know the alternative route to reduce pyruvate, that is by producing ethyl alcohol and CO_2!

References

Åstrand, P.-O. and Rodahl, K. 1977. *Textbook of Work Physiology*. New York: McGraw-Hill.

Balke, B., Grillo, G.P., Konecci, E.B. and Luft, U.C. 1954. Work capacity after blood donation. *J. Appl. Physiol.* 7:231–238.

Ekblom, B., Wilson, G., and Åstrand, P.-O. 1976. Central circulation during exercise after venesection and reinfusion of red blood cells. *J. Appl. Physiol.* 40:379–383.

Gollnick, P.D., Armstrong, R.B., Saubert, IV, C.W., Piehl, K., and Saltin, B. 1972. Enzyme activity and fiber composition in skeletal muscle of untrained and trained men. *J. Appl. Physiol.* 33:312–319.

Henriksson, J. and Reitman, J.S. 1977. Time-course of changes in human skeletal muscle succinate dehydrogenase and cytochrome oxidase activities and maximal oxygen uptake with physical activity and inactivity. *Acta Physiol. Scand.* 99:91–97.

Henriksson, J., Svedenhag, J., Richter, E.A., and Galbo, H. 1980. Significance of the sympathetic-adrenal system for the exercise-induced enzymatic adaptation of skeletal muscle. *Muscle and Nerve* 3:277–278.

Hoppeler, H., Mathieu, O., Weibel, E.R., Krauer, R., Lindstedt, S.L., and Taylor, C.R. 1981. Design of the mammalian respiratory system. VIII. Capillaries in skeletal muscles. *Respir. Physiol.* 44:129–150.

Newsholme, E.A., Crabtree, B., and Zammit, V.A. 1980. Use of enzyme activities as indices of maximum rates of fuel utilization. In *Trends in Enzyme Histochemistry and Cytochemistry*. Ciba Foundation Symposium 73. New York: Elsevier North Holland. pp. 245–248.

Salmons, S. and Henriksson, J. 1981. The adaptive response of skeletal muscle to increased use. *Muscle and Nerve* 4:94–105.

Weibel, E.R. and Taylor, C.R. (guest editors). 1981. Design of the mammalian respiratory system. *Respir. Physiol.* 44:1–164.

SECTION IV:

Effects of Altitude on Oxygen Transport

J.A. Loeppky and M.L. Riedesel, editors
OXYGEN TRANSPORT TO HUMAN TISSUES

Limitations to Work at Altitude

Bruno Balke

The effect of high altitude on man's physical performance capacity has been the subject of several national and international symposia in recent years. The 1968 Olympic Games in Mexico City provided a great stimulus for researchers in all countries to investigate the potential inhibition of athletic performance at the moderate altitude of 2300 m, especially in sports events that require maximal aerobic endurance. The results of the Games concurred with the predictions that short-duration and explosive events were rather favorably affected by the reduced air density but that world record performances were not achievable in competitions that lasted longer than 2 or 3 min. "Aerohypoxia" (Luft, 1972) was certainly to blame for the reduction of maximal aerobic work capacity (max $\dot{V}O_2$).

Numerous investigations have shown that a period of acclimatization helps in restoring some but not all of the sea level performance, depending on the duration and intensity of training at altitude. As an example, we might consider the Tarahumara Indians of Mexico who live at altitudes between 2000 to 2700 m and have become well-known for their endurance in kickball races over distances far in excess of 60 miles. Despite their phenomenal endurance (authentically 500 miles have been covered within 5 days), no Tarahumara has ever been successful in an international marathon race over "only" 26 miles. In the practice of running many consecutive hours, they have adapted to a relatively slow pace for energy saving and cannot successfully compete with those who have trained to run at the fastest possible speed for slightly more than 2 hr. It would be interesting to induce a gifted altitude-adapted Tarahumara to train more adequately and see whether or not he could reach the performance level of the famous runners from Kenya who train according to modern principles at various elevations.

There is still controversy on what factors limit max $\dot{V}O_2$ at sea level. Is it the oxidative capacity of the muscles or limitations in the oxygen transport system? Gollnick et al. (1972) estimated that the oxidative capacity of muscles is in excess of the observed maximal oxygen delivery/kg of muscle mass. They suggested that maximal cardiac output would have to be doubled in order to satisfy the oxidizing capacity of muscle. On the other hand, Holloszy (1973) reported adaptation in muscle enzymes and mitochondria as the result of physical conditioning that would permit muscles to work at a lower oxygen tension. Thus, the increased aerobic capacity may not depend solely on increased oxygen transport.

Great differences exist in maximal aerobic power between highly trained endurance athletes, people who exercise very regularly for enjoyment or for the purpose of staying fit, sedentary individuals, and patients with cardiorespiratory problems. For all of them, max $\dot{V}O_2$ determines the length of time anyone in these groups can work at given levels of submaximal exercise intensity. According to Saltin (1973), work at 90, 80, and 70% of max $\dot{V}O_2$ can be performed for approximately 30, 120, and 240 min, respectively. Naturally, the better conditioned individual could perform more total work during such time periods. For example, a person with a max $\dot{V}O_2$ of 4.0 liter/min would, theoretically, climb the vertical 1800 m from Albuquerque to Sandia Peak in approximately 2 hr when working at 80% of max $\dot{V}O_2$ while the less trained person of equal body weight with a max $\dot{V}O_2$ of 3.9 liter/min would arrive at least one hr later, exerting the same relative effort. This estimation does not take into consideration the slowest possible pace in ascending the peak of 3300 m.

The controversy over what factors limit maximal aerobic metabolism under atmospheric conditions at or near sea level might subside somewhat if one were to consider the limitations for maximum work at altitude in temporarily exposed sojourners. Instantaneous biochemical changes that would favor increased oxidative capacity of the muscle are then not to be expected. Possibly such changes might occur during long periods of training at altitude or most likely in altitude natives (Hurtado et al., 1956). Thus, the overwhelming reason for work limitations in recent newcomers to altitude might be seen in factors affecting the oxygen transport system.

Pulmonary Limitations

West (1966) found that the oxygen diffusing ability of the lung was reduced at high altitude when the level of exercise was relatively high. Since oxygen diffusing capacity in the lung is affected by the area and thickness of the alveolar-capillary membrane, the volume and velocity of blood flowing through the capillaries, and the alveolar-capillary oxygen pressure gradient, one should try to evaluate the significance of each of these factors for oxygen diffusion separately. The alveolar surface area increases when tidal volume becomes greater with higher demands on pulmonary ventilation, along with a thinning of the alveolar-capillary membrane. These mechanisms should favor the oxygen diffusion until tidal volume tends to decrease again because of inefficient high respiratory frequencies.

Vital capacity, although per se not an indicator of functional capacity, is nevertheless an important factor of maximal ventilation. Within its limits, it allows for gradual adaptation of the tidal volume during progressive exercise. At slow breathing rates, almost the entire vital capacity can be utilized but at higher frequencies the tidal volume begins to decrease. Apparently, optimal efficiency of pulmonary ventilation is found at a rate of 50 to 60 breaths/min, permitting a 66% utilization of the vital capacity. In addition to such functional and anatomical limitations, the high energy cost of maximal breathing sets a limit to work capacity. Riley (1960) presented a diagram according to which the oxygen cost of breathing during work requiring a pulmonary ventilation of 150 liter/min might attain a value of 1.5 to 2.0 liter/min. However, he considered the probability that in a well-trained athlete the oxygen cost of ventilating at high rates would not be that enormously high. An elite marathon runner, requiring a steady oxygen intake of about 4.5 liter/min with a ventilation of nearly 150 liter/min (BTPS) would scarcely go very far if the oxygen required by the respiratory muscles would amount to one-third of the total oxygen uptake. Nevertheless, the extreme ventilatory demands at altitudes above 4500 m limit performance capacity (Christensen, 1937). As every mountaineer at such altitudes has experienced, painful dyspnea slows uphill progress to a snail's pace.

Maximal oxygen intake decreases about 10% for every 1000 m of altitude gain (Buskirk et al., 1967). When studying 6 middle-distance athletes in Mexico City, Pugh (1972) concluded that at 2300 m a number of factors caused the reduction of max $\dot{V}O_2$. Among these were respiratory muscle fatigue, myocardial hypoxia, reduced blood volume, and insufficient pulmonary diffusing capacity. Similar work-limiting factors have been observed by Pugh et al. (1964) during the 1960–61 Himalayan scientific and mountaineering expedition to Makalu. Using progressive work on the cycle ergometer at elevations of 4600, 5800, 6400, and 7300 m, limitations occurred sooner at the higher altitudes. Oxygen intakes for the same submaximal work intensities were practically identical but pulmonary ventilation (STPD) was actually lower during the first few weeks at altitude than at sea level, a fact also reported by Balke (1972). The ability for maximal ventilation to be increased with altitude up to the higher altitudes seemed apparent, with hypoxic limitations then becoming evident. Despite the excessive ventilation and the concomitant rise of alveolar oxygen tension, the arterial oxygen saturation fell from a value of 67% at rest to 46% during work requiring an oxygen consumption of 2.0 liter/min. The authors concluded that strenuous exercise at such high altitude resulted in arterial hypoxemia. One could speculate that perhaps excessive hyperventilation during exercise could result in the symptoms of hypocapnia similar to those observed in military aviation (Balke et al., 1957).

Cardiac Limitations

Maximal cardiac output was considerably reduced on Makalu along with the maximal heart rate (Pugh et al., 1964). The resting ECG showed the signs of right ventricular strain. A greater stress on the right than on the left ventricle during work on the cycle ergometer has also been observed by Gurtner et al. (1966) even at sea level, but aerohypoxia of altitude actually affects the entire heart. Grover et al. (1970) measured coronary blood flow at rest and during light work in subjects after 10 days at 3100 m and found a marked decrease. That, of course, restricts cardiac working capacity and sets limits to cardiac output. Consequently, pulmonary capillary blood flow must also be curtailed. That should be reflected in a reduction of alveolar-capillary oxygen diffusion, thereby contributing to failing oxygen transport.

Maximal cardiac output appears to be mainly affected by a lower maximal heart rate, as reported by many investigators (Christensen, 1937; Åstrand and Åstrand, 1958; Balke, 1960; Pugh et al., 1964; Biersteker and Van Leeuwen, 1966; Hartley et al., 1967; Consolazio, 1967). Differences in age of subjects, in altitude and duration of altitude sojourn might partly explain the findings by others (Kellogg, 1962; Buskirk et al., 1967; Grover and Reeves, 1967; Vogel and Hansen, 1967; Faulkner, 1967) that maximal heart rates at altitude did not differ from sea level values. However, the results of exercise tests in Aspen, Colorado (2400 m) suggest that maximal heart rates of all age groups were below the level one would expect at sea level.

Adequate oxygen supply to the myocardium depends almost entirely on the adaptability of coronary blood flow. Unlike the skeletal muscle, cardiac muscle cannot work properly below a tissue oxygen tension of about 20 mm Hg. Thus any decrease in the oxygen content of the arterial blood necessitates an increase of coronary blood flow to satisfy myocardial oxygen needs (Balke, 1964). Coronary blood flow depends largely on the recoil pressure of the aorta during ventricular diastole and on the duration of diastolic filling. The limitation of cardiac work during extreme exercise becomes evident by a decrease of the arterial blood pressure, usually when the heart rate becomes "critical." Critical in so far as the left ventricular filling time is becoming so short that even the increase in right ventricular pressure cannot sustain an adequate stroke volume. The relationship of systolic tension time (Q-T interval) to diastolic filling time (T-Q interval) reveals that in almost all exercise experiments the work capacity of the heart approaches limitations when diastolic filling time is shortened to below 50% of systolic tension time. It seems a miracle that the left ventricle can be filled to a volume of 100 ml or more within 0.1 sec.

Nielsen and Hansen (1937) pointed out that inadequate oxygen supply to the myocardium during maximal work prevents the heart from further increasing cardiac output. An unexpected incident during one of our gradual exercise tests at an altitude of 3000 m in the Tyrolian Alps underscored the validity of this statement. One experimental subject (the one we honor here with this symposium) proceeded normally to a work intensity requiring an oxygen consumption of 2.75 liter/min with a heart rate of 156 bpm and a systolic pressure of 190 mm Hg. When the work intensity was increased by another 10 W on the cycle ergometer, the systolic blood pressure suddenly dropped about 40 mm Hg and the heart rate fell to 126 bpm. This was accompanied by severe facial cyanosis. Recovery at rest was quick and there were no further complications during the remainder of the altitude sojourn.

Recently, Robertson and Robertson (1981) reported the case of a patient who had repeated episodes of chest discomfort with concomitant S-T segment elevation. Frequently the episodes were ended with sudden bradycardia and normalization of the electrocardiogram. According to Frink and James (1971), this Bezold-Jarisch reflex originates predominantly in the left ventricle, proceeds toward the origin of the main left coronary artery and ultimately results in activation of the vagus nerve (Fox, 1977). Left ventricular receptors are activated by inadequate myocardial oxygen supply as can occur following obstruction of coronary blood flow (Thorén, 1972).

I have experienced what seemed to be cardiac limitations during a 2-hr training run at an altitude of 3200 m. Without symptoms of muscular or respiratory difficulties, the extra effort of an uphill slope suddenly caused an intense burning sensation in the upper left chest which only disappeared after a few minutes of walking. Unmistakingly, this was a somewhat frightening anginal event. Apparently, coronary blood flow had become insufficient for the amount of cardiac work required. "Increased cardiac activity requires additional energy and reduces the cardiac reserves for increased physical activity," as stated by Luft (1972).

It seems possible that "hardening" of coronary arteries with age limits maximum cardiac performance and thus affects pulmonary oxygen diffusing capacity. Scherrer (1966) observed a significant difference in the arterial oxygen tension in men of 20 and 50 yr of age during ergometer exercise at a simulated altitude of 2750 m. Arterial O_2 tension declined from 86 to 64 mm Hg in the 20-yr-olds and from 82 to 54 mm Hg in the 50-yr age group. But Dill et al. (1964) found considerable differences in the adaptability of older men for maximum work in their studies on White Mountain, California.

Conclusions

It should be clear that not only one single factor limits maximal aerobic power at altitude. Anatomical lung volumes and their functional dependence on respiratory frequency curtail pulmonary ventilation. Likewise, there are definite limitations for cardiac output determined by the size of the heart and the most efficient stroke volume and heart rate adjustments. Furthermore, the blood supply to the myocardium eventually encounters restrictions, thereby limiting the work capacity of the heart. By physical training, an optimal synergism of all contributing factors might be attained, making it difficult to separate the contribution of each toward maximal aerobic performance. The achievements in climbing the highest mountains on earth on difficult routes without the aid of supplementary oxygen underscores man's ability to attain such maximum functional harmony of all organ systems under conditions of strenuous physical work at extreme altitudes.

References

Åstrand, P.-O. and Åstrand, I., 1958. Heart rate during muscular work in man exposed to prolonged hypoxia. *J. Appl. Physiol.* 13:75–80.

Balke, B. 1960. Work capacity at altitude. In *Science and Medicine of Exercise and Sports*. Johnson, W.R. ed. New York: Harper and Brothers. pp. 339–347.

Balke, B. 1964. Cardiac performance in relation to altitude. *Am. J. Cardiol.* 14:796–810.

Balke, B. 1972. Physiology of respiration at altitude. In *Physiological Adaptations: Desert and Mountain*. Yousef, M.K., Horvath, S.M., and Bullard, R.W., eds. New York: Academic Press. pp. 195–208.

Balke, B., Wells, J.G., and Clark, Jr. R.T., 1957. In-flight hyperventilation during jet pilot training. *J. Aviat. Med.* 28:241–248.

Biersteker, P.A. and Van Leeuwen, A.M. 1966. *Physiological Effects of Medium Altitude*. Report by the Netherlands Olympic Committee. Asten: Schricks Drukkerij.

Buskirk, E.R., Kollias, J. Picon-Reatigue, E., Akers, R. Prokop, E., and Baker, P. 1967. Physiology and performance of track athletes at various altitudes in the United States and Peru. In *International Symposium on the Effects of Altitude on Physical Performance*. R.F. Goddard, ed. Chicago: Athletic Institute. pp. 65–71.

Christensen, E.H. 1937. Sauerstoffaufnahme und respiratorische Funktionen in grossen Höhen. *Skandinav. Arch. Physiol.* 76:88–100.

Consolazio, C.F. 1967. Submaximal and maximal performance at high altitude. In *International Symposium on the Effects of Altitude on Physical Performance*. R.F. Goddard, ed. Chicago: Athletic Institute. pp. 91–95.

Dill, D.B., Robinson, S., Balke, B., and Newton, J.L. 1964. Work tolerance: age and altitude. *J. Appl. Physiol.* 19:483–488.

Faulkner, J.A. 1967. Training for maximum performance at altitude. In *International Symposium on the Effects of Altitude on Physical Performance*. R.F. Goddard, ed. Chicago: Athletic Institute. pp. 88–90.

Fox, I.J. 1977. Left ventricular mechanoreceptors: a hemodynamic study. *J. Physiol. (London)* 273:405–425.

Frink, R.J. and James, T.N. 1971. Intracardiac route of the Bezold-Jarisch reflex. *Am. J. Physiol.* 221:1464–1469.

Gollnick, P.D., Armstrong, R.B., Saubert, C.W., IV, Peihl, K., and Saltin, B. 1972. Enzyme activity and fiber composition in skeletal muscle of untrained and trained men. *J. Appl. Physiol.* 33:312–319.

Grover, R.F., Lufschanowski, R., and Alexander, J.K. 1970. Decreased coronary blood flow in man following ascent to high altitude. In *Hypoxia, High Altitude and the Heart*. Vogel, J.H., ed. Basel: S. Karger. pp. 72–79.

Grover, R.F. and Reeves, J.T. 1967. Exercise performance of athletes at sea level and 3,100 m altitude. In *International Symposium on the Effects of Altitude on Physical Performance*. R. F. Goddard, ed. Chicago: Athletic Institute. pp. 80–85.

Gurtner, H.P., Keller, M.F., and Salzmann, C. 1966. Die Haemodynamik gesunder Studenten in Ruhe und bei abgestufter Belastung. *Schweiz. Z. Sportmed.* 14:70–80.

Hartley, L.H., Alexander, J.K., Modelski, M., and Grover, R.F. 1967. Subnormal cardiac output at rest and during exercise in residents at 3,100 m altitude. *J. App. Physiol.* 23:839–848.

Holloszy, J.O. 1973. Biochemical adaptations to exercise. In *Reviews in Exercise and Sports Science*. Wilmore, J.H., ed. New York: Academic Press. p. 45.

Hurtado, A., Velasquez, T., Reynafarje, C., Lozano, R., Chavez, R., Aste-Salazar, H., Reynafarje, B., Sanchez, C., and Muñoz, J. 1956. *Mechanisms of Natural Acclimatization*. USAF Report No. 56-1. School of Aviation Medicine, Randolph AFB, Texas.

Kellogg, R.H. 1964. Heart rate and alveolar gas in exercise during acclimatization to altitude. In *The Physiological Effect of High Altitude*. Weihe, W.H., ed. Oxford: Pergamon Press. pp. 191–198.

Luft, U.C. 1972. Principles of adaptation to altitude. In *Physiological Adaptations: Desert and Mountain*. Yousef, M.K., Horvath, S.M., and Bullard, R.W., eds. New York: Academic Press. pp. 143–154.

Neilsen, M. and Hansen, O. 1937. Maximale körperliche Arbeit bei Atmung O_2-reicher. *Skandinav. Arch. Physiol.* 76:37–59.

Pugh, L.G. 1972. Athletes at altitude. In *Environmental Effects on Work Performance*. Cumming, G.R., Snidal, D., and Taylor, A.W., eds. The Canadian Association of Sports Sciences, University of Alberta, Edmonton: Printing Services. pp. 87–99.

Pugh, L.G., Gill, M.B., Lahiri, S., Milledge, J.S., Ward, M.P., and West, J.B. 1964. Muscular exercise at great altitudes. *J. Appl. Physiol.* 19:431–440.

Riley, R.L. 1960. Pulmonary function in relation to exercise. In *Science and Medicine of Exercise and Sports*. Johnson, W.R., ed. New York: Harper and Brothers. pp. 162–177.

Robertson, R.M. and Robertson, D. 1981. The Bezold-Jarisch reflex: possible role in limiting myocardial ischemia. *Clin. Cardiol.* 4:75–79.

Saltin, B. 1973. Oxygen transport by the circulatory system during exercise in man. In *Limiting Factors of Physical Performance*. Keul, J., ed. Stuttgart: Georg Thieme. pp. 235–252.

Scherrer, M. 1966. Altersabhängigkeit des alveolo-arteriellen PO_2-Gradienten während Schwerarbeit in akuter, leichter Hypoxie, entsprechend 2750 m. *Schweiz. Z. Sportmed.* 14:61–69.

Thorén, P. 1972. Left ventricular receptors activated by severe asphyxia and by coronary artery occlusion. *Acta Physiol. Scand.* 85:455–463.

Vogel, J.A. and Hansen, J.E. 1967. Cardiovascular function during exercise at high altitude. In *International Symposium on the Effects of Altitude on Physical Performance*. R.F. Goddard, ed. Chicago: Athletic Institute. pp. 47–50.

West, J.B. 1966. Exercise limitations at increased altitudes. *Schweiz. Z. Sportsmed.* 14:149–154.

J.A. Loeppky and M.L. Riedesel, editors
OXYGEN TRANSPORT TO HUMAN TISSUES

Gas Exchange at Altitude

John B. West

Pulmonary gas exchange under the severely hypoxic conditions of high altitude has long been an interest of Dr. Luft and it is a pleasure to discuss some aspects of the topic in this symposium in his honor. There has recently been a resurgence of interest in gas exchange at extreme altitude stimulated in part by the remarkable ascent of Mt. Everest, altitude 8848 m, without supplementary oxygen by Messner and Habeler in 1978. The physiological significance of this feat is emphasized by Figure 1A, which shows maximal oxygen consumption (max $\dot{V}O_2$) of acclimatized subjects plotted against barometric pressure using the data of Pugh (1964a). The barometric pressure axis has been transformed so that available data lie on a straight line and it can be seen that extrapolation indicates a max $\dot{V}O_2$ on the summit which is very close to the basal level. The same data are shown in Figure 1B, which emphasizes the extreme sensitivity of predicted max $\dot{V}O_2$ to barometric pressure at these extreme altitudes.

The colorful history of climbing Mt. Everest is consistent with these predictions. As long ago as 1924, Norton and Somervell climbed to within 300 m of the summit without supplementary oxygen. The last 300 m therefore took 54 years! Various explanations were offered for the lack of success of the intervening expeditions, such as early monsoon conditions. However, such excuses are hardly necessary when we appreciate that the summit of Everest is right at the limit of human activity breathing ambient air. What evolutionary pressures have been responsible for this critical relationship between the world's highest point and man's minimal activity are obscure and it is presumably yet another cosmic coincidence.

The relationship between barometric pressure and altitude is clearly critical in this context. However, this link is not as clear as some would think. The

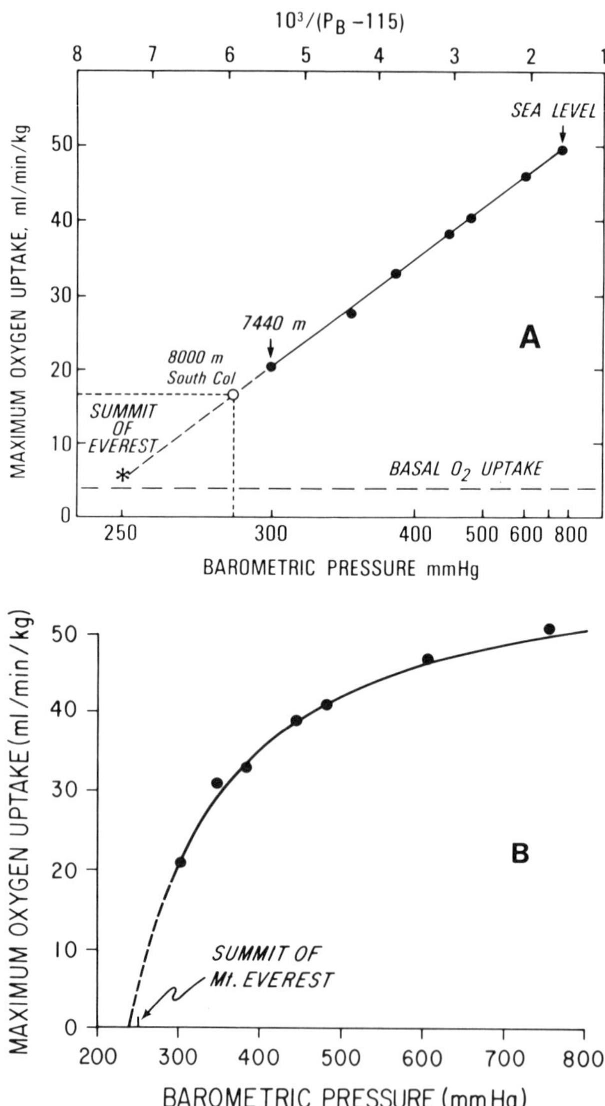

Figure 1. Maximal oxygen consumption of acclimatized subjects plotted against barometric pressure using the data of Pugh (1964a). In A, the barometric pressure axis has been transformed to give a linear relationship. Also note the low max $\dot{V}O_2$ predicted for the South Col of Everest (8000 m, P_B: 280 Torr).

SOURCE: *West and Wagner, 1980.*

introduction of the ICAO Standard Atmosphere (1968) was perhaps something of a disservice because it has been used by physiologists to predict barometric pressures under conditions that it was not designed for. It transpires that the relationship between barometric pressure and altitude differs considerably with latitude. Fortunately the pressure at a given altitude is higher in the Himalayas (latitude of Everest is 28 degrees N) than in regions further from the equator. The reason is that the higher temperatures near the equator expand the atmosphere causing a higher atmospheric pressure. The net result is that the barometric pressure on the summit of Mt. Everest is approximately 250 Torr, whereas that predicted from the ICAO (or U.S.) Standard Atmosphere for the same altitude is only 235 Torr. The difference is of great physiological significance because it certainly would be impossible to reach the summit without supplementary oxygen if the pressure were as low as suggested by the Standard Atmosphere (West and Wagner 1980). The figure of 250 Torr is based on Radiosonde measurements and on measurements made at somewhat lower altitudes in neighboring areas (Figure 2).

An interesting facet is that whether a climber will be able to reach the summit of Mt. Everest without supplementary oxygen probably depends on which month he chooses for the attempt. Figure 3 shows that the pressure is highest in the summer and lowest in the winter, the difference being more than 10 Torr. This is sufficient to alter the predicted max $\dot{V}O_2$ by about 25%. Even the day-by-day variations caused by changes of weather are probably important at these extreme altitudes. The standard deviation of the daily pressure is about 2 Torr and a decrease of 4 Torr (that is twice the standard deviation) results in a fall in calculated maximal oxygen consumption of about 10%. Thus a climber who plans to make his summit bid might be wise to consult his barometer first.

Why is max $\dot{V}O_2$ so sensitive to the inspired PO_2 and therefore barometric pressure? The answer is that work rate under these conditions is limited by the delivery of oxygen to the exercising muscles and that the transfer of oxygen from the air into the blood is strikingly limited by the diffusion properties of the lung. It is this phenomenon of diffusion limitation which results in the markedly nonlinear relationship between max $\dot{V}O_2$ and barometric pressure (Figure 1B). Pulmonary gas exchange under these conditions has been carefully analyzed elsewhere (West and Wagner, 1980) and there is not space to go into the details here. However, Figure 4 shows a typical plot of PO_2 in the blood as it passes along the pulmonary capillary for a climber on the summit of Mt. Everest (P_B: 250 Torr). Note that the PO_2 rises very slowly and that there is a very large alveolar-end capillary PO_2 difference which is the hallmark of diffusion limitation. It is this phenomenon that results in a relentless fall in the PO_2 of arterial and mixed venous blood as the oxygen consumption is increased, and these factors soon put a stop to any further increase in work rate.

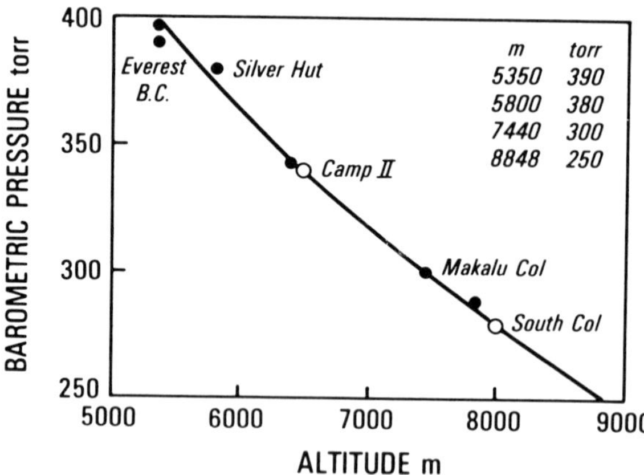

Figure 2. Relationship between barometric pressure and altitude in the vicinity of Mt. Everest. The solid data points are from previous expeditions. The open circles show expected barometric pressures for two laboratory camps on the forthcoming American Medical Research Expedition to Everest.

How can we improve max $\dot{V}O_2$ under these extraordinary conditions? One way is to shift the oxygen dissociation curve to the left, that is increase the affinity of hemoglobin for oxygen. The relationship between shifts of the oxygen dissociation curve and work capacity at high altitude is an interesting topic in its own right. Several studies (Aste-Salazar and Hurtado, 1944; Lenfant et al., 1968) have shown that a rightward shift of the oxygen dissociation curve occurs in man as a result of acclimatization to high altitude, and it has been argued that this is advantageous. However, a leftward shift of the curve is commonly seen in animals living at high altitude (Bullard et al., 1966; Petschow et al., 1977), and rats with leftshifted curves have been shown to have increased survival breathing air at a barometric pressure of 233 Torr (Eaton et al., 1974). Of particular interest was the study of Hebbel et al. (1978) who showed that two subjects with a higher oxygen affinity hemoglobin (hemoglobin Andrew-Minneapolis, P_{50}: 17.1 Torr) had a better exercise tolerance at an altitude of 3100 m than their two normal siblings.

To examine this paradox, we recently made a theoretical study of the role of shifts in the oxygen dissociation curve on exercise tolerance at different altitudes (Bencowitz et al., 1981). The results showed that whether a leftward or rightward shift of the curve is advantageous depends on the presence or absence of diffusion limitation in the pulmonary capillary. If diffusion equilibration for oxygen within the lung is complete, a rightshifted curve is advantageous at all but extreme altitudes. On the other hand, if oxygen consumption is increased to such an extent that diffusion limitation occurs, a leftshifted oxygen dissociation curve is advantageous (that is, results in a higher PO_2 in mixed venous blood) at any altitude.

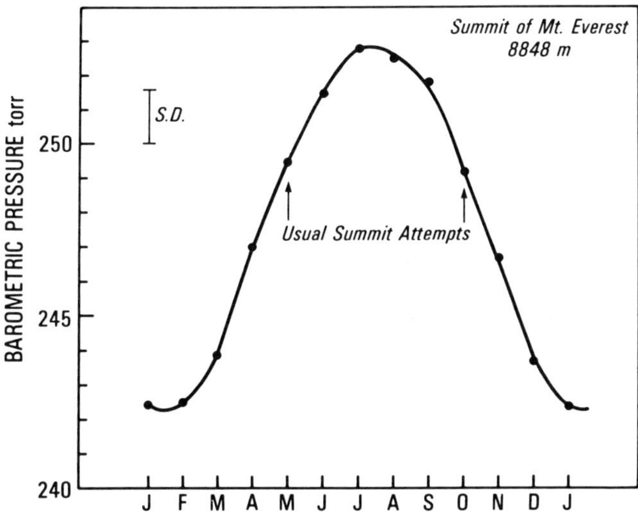

Figure 3. Predicted barometric pressure on the summit of Mt. Everest plotted against the month of the year. The data were obtained from over 7,000 Radiosonde observations from New Delhi. The preferred months for climbing (May and October) are indicated by arrows. The approximate monthly standard deviation is also shown.

Figure 4. Calculated time course of the PO_2 in the pulmonary capillary of a climber on the summit of Mt. Everest. Note the slow rate of rise of PO_2 and the large alveolar-end capillary PO_2 difference.

SOURCE: *West and Wagner, 1980.*

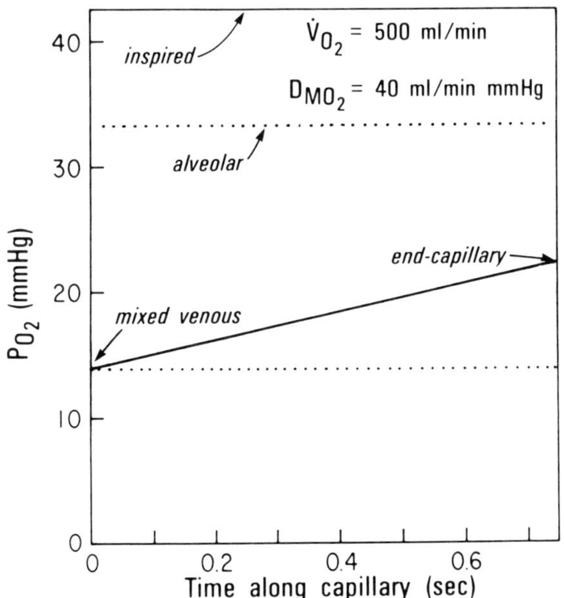

Are there any other options available to increase maximal work levels under these conditions of extreme altitude? Figure 5 shows an analysis of factors limiting max $\dot{V}O_2$ at a barometric pressure of 250 Torr (West and Wagner, 1980). To prepare this graph, calculations were made by changing only one variable at a time, all others being kept the same for the appropriate work level. Max $\dot{V}O_2$ was assumed to occur when the PO_2 of mixed venous blood fell to 15 Torr. First the sensitivity of max $\dot{V}O_2$ to barometric pressure is clearly shown. Next it is obvious that improving the membrane diffusing capacity (D_M) of the lung would result in an improvement. This is expected because oxygen transfer is diffusion limited as indicated earlier. Note also that a reduction of P_{50} improved max $\dot{V}O_2$ to some extent, as discussed above. The righthand panel shows that increases in either alveolar ventilation or cardiac output also improve predicted max $\dot{V}O_2$.

An interesting question is why ventilation and cardiac output do not increase more than they do. Figure 6 shows that maximal exercise ventilation increases as barometric pressure falls with increasing altitude, but only up to the altitude where the barometric pressure is about 350 Torr (about 6300 m). At lower barometric pressures (higher altitudes), maximal ventilation falls off and is predicted to be less than 60 liter/min BTPS on the Everest summit. Of course, work rate decreases to very low levels at these extreme altitudes as Figure 6 also shows. But why the body does not take advantage of the higher alveolar PO_2 that would result from an increased ventilation is not clear. Perhaps the respiratory muscles themselves are limited by hypoxia, or the increased oxygen consumption caused by the greater activity of the respiratory muscles steals more oxygen than is gained.

Figure 5. Analysis of factors limiting max $\dot{V}O_2$ at a barometric pressure of 250 Torr. Note the extreme sensitivity to barometric pressure. The membrane diffusing capacity (D_M) also plays an important role. Other variables studied are capillary transit time (T_T), P_{50} of the O_2 dissociation curve, alveolar ventilation ($\dot{V}_A$) and cardiac output ($\dot{Q}$).
SOURCE: *West and Wagner, 1980.*

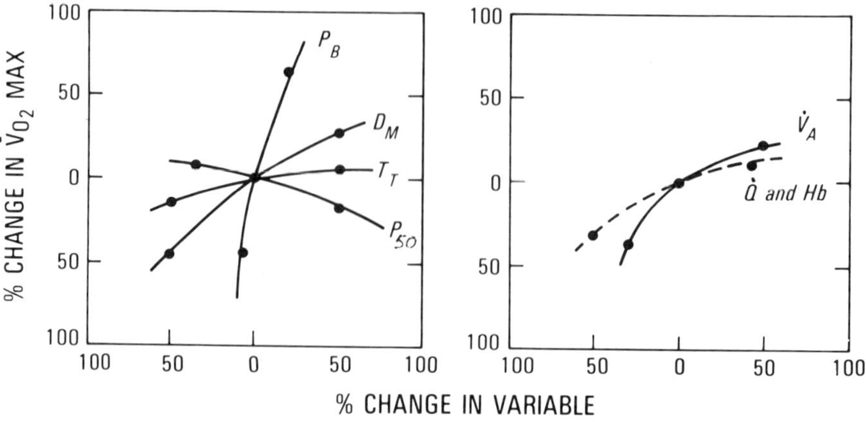

The situation with cardiac output is equally puzzling. Pugh (1964b) showed that the relationship between cardiac output and work rate was the same at an altitude of 5800 m (P_B: 380 Torr) in acclimatized subjects as at sea level. It is known that acute exposure to altitude increases cardiac output at a given work level (Alexander et al., 1967) but apparently with acclimatization, the relationship reverts to that seen at sea level. Why this should be when an increase in cardiac output would improve oxygen delivery to the exercising muscles is obscure. However, the answer to this paradox may have to wait until we understand the control of cardiac output at sea level which, as far as I can determine, is far from the case at the present moment.

We hope to test some of these predictions during the American Medical Research Expedition to Everest in the summer and fall of 1981. For example, Figure 1B shows the predicted max $\dot{V}O_2$ on the South Col where we hope to have a bicycle ergometer. We expect the barometric pressure at this altitude (8000 m) to be about 280 Torr and the max $\dot{V}O_2$ approximately 17 ml/min/Kg or in the region of 1,200 ml/min. We hope that this very ambitious expedition will continue the traditions of physiology in the natural laboratory of high mountains, including the work done by Dr. Luft on Nanga Parbat in 1937.

Figure 6. Maximal oxygen consumption and maximal exercise ventilation against barometric pressure (compare Figure 1A). Note that maximal ventilation increases with falling barometric pressure up to a certain point and then decreases strikingly.

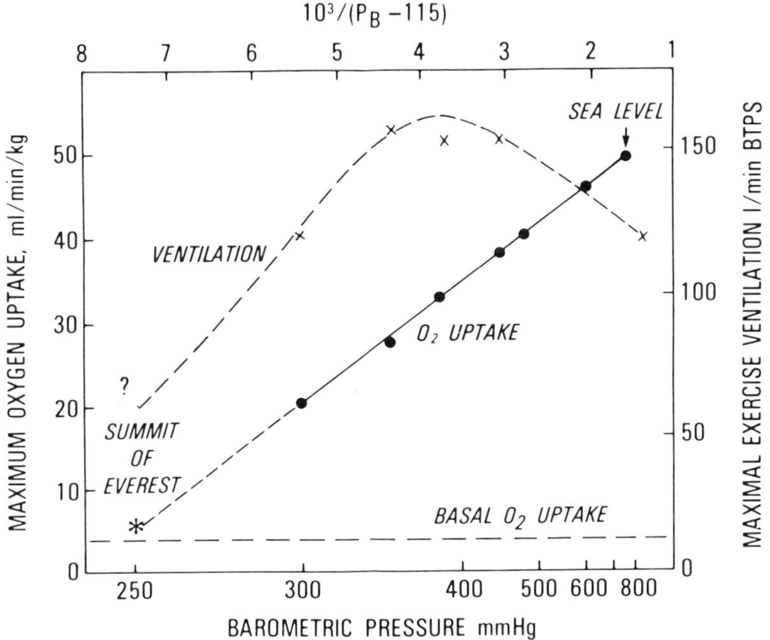

ACKNOWLEDGMENTS
This work was supported by PHS Grants HL 17731 and HL 24335.

References

Alexander, J.K., Hartley, L.H., Modelski, M. and Grover, R.F., 1967. Reduction of stroke volume during exercise in man following ascent to 3,100 m altitude. *J. Appl. Physiol.* 23:849–858.

Aste-Salazar, H. and Hurtado, A. 1944. The affinity of hemoglobin for oxygen at sea level and at high altitudes. *Am. J. Physiol.* 142:733–743.

Bencowitz, H.Z., Wagner, P.D., and West, J.B. 1981. Effect of change in P_{50} on exercise tolerance at high altitude: a theoretical study. *J. Appl. Physiol.*, in press.

Bullard, R.W., Broumand, C., and Meyer, F.R. 1966. Blood characteristics and volume in two rodents native to high altitude. *J. Appl. Physiol.* 21:994–998.

Eaton, J.W., Skelton, T.D., and Berger, E. 1974. Survival at extreme altitude: protective effect of increased hemoglobin-oxygen affinity. *Science* 183:743–744.

Hebbel, R.P., Eaton, J.W., Kronenberg, R.S., Zanjani, E.D., Moore, L.G., and Berger, E.M. 1978. Human llamas: adaptation to altitude in subjects with high hemoglobin oxygen affinity. *J. Clin. Invest.* 62:593–600.

ICAO. *Manual of the ICAO Standard Atmosphere.* 1968. 2nd edition. Montreal: International Civil Aviation Organization.

Lenfant, C., Torrance, J., English, E., Finch, C.A., Reynafarje, C., Ramos, J., and Faura, J. 1968. Effect of altitude on oxygen binding by hemoglobin and on organic phosphate levels. *J. Clin. Invest.* 47:2652–2656.

Petschow, D., Wurdinger, I., Baumann, R., Duhm, J., Braunitzer, G., and Bauer, C. 1977. Causes of high blood O_2 affinity of animals living at high altitude. *J. Appl. Physiol.* 42:139–143.

Pugh, L.G. 1964a. Animals in high altitudes: man above 5000 meters—mountain exploration. In *Handbook of Physiology. Section 4. Adaptations to the Environment.* Dill, D.B., ed. Washington, D.C.: American Physiological Society. pp. 861–868.

Pugh, L.G. 1964b. Cardiac output in muscular exercise at 5800 m (19,000 feet). *J. Appl. Physiol.* 19:441–447.

West, J.B. and Wagner, P.D., 1980. Predicted gas exchange on the summit of Mt. Everest. *Respir. Physiol.* 42:1–16.

J.A. Loeppky and M.L. Riedesel, editors
OXYGEN TRANSPORT TO HUMAN TISSUES

The Role of Gas-Phase Diffusion at Altitude

Herman Rahn and Charles V. Paganelli

Introduction

According to the calculations of Gomez (1965), a *critical zone* exists in the conducting airways where convective transfer of inspired O_2 equals the molecular transfer rate by diffusion. Beyond the critical zone, diffusion becomes the dominant transport mechanism as shown in Figure 1, adapted from Gomez. Since that time many studies have been directed toward the role diffusion plays in the phenomenon of stratified inhomogeneity (residual gas tension gradients during the respiratory cycle), a topic which recently received an excellent review by Scheid and Piiper (1980). As inspired gas travels down the conducting airways, it begins to mix by convection with gas in the functional residual capacity. This mixing, however, is never complete, and the rate at which a homogeneous alveolar gas concentration is approached depends upon the rate of gas diffusion and the convection induced by the contracting heart. This incomplete mixing or stratification reduces the efficiency of gas exchange, giving rise to a partial pressure difference between alveolar gas and arterial blood. One may visualize this stratification as a gas-phase diffusion barrier between the gas completely mixed by convective flow in the upper airways and the gas in contact with the alveolar wall, as shown in Figure 2. Such a concept suggests a total diffusing capacity of the lung consisting of a gas-phase conductance, D_{gas}, and the classical tissue conductance, D_L, or I/D_L total$=$ $I/D_{gas} + I/D_L$. Various experimental data interpreted by Scheid and Piiper (1980) suggest that the gas-phase diffusing capacity, D_{gas}, is 2 to 10 times greater than that measured for the tissue phase, D_L.

If one accepts the existence of a gas barrier to the transport of O_2, then the magnitude of the barrier depends in part on the binary diffusion coefficient of

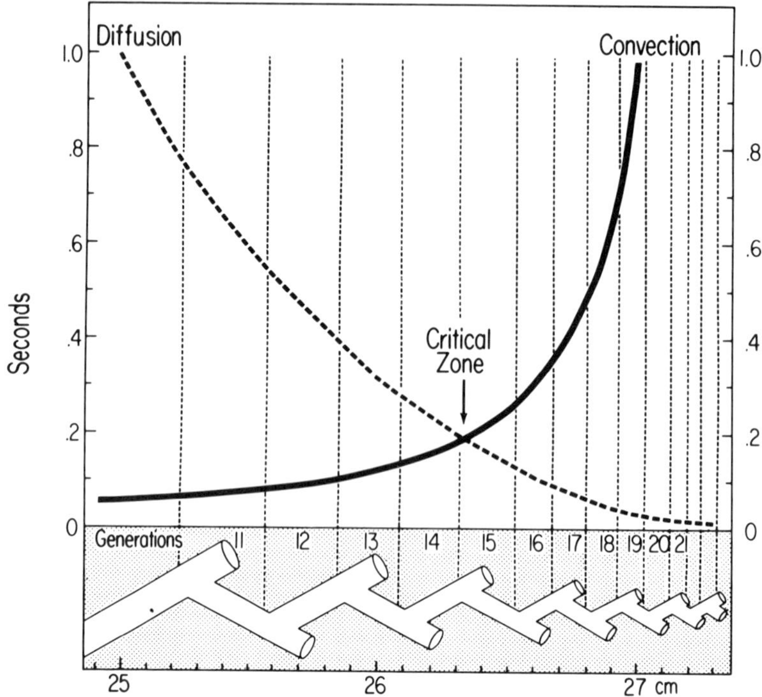

Figure 1. Time of molecular transfer through a given generation for convective and diffusive transport from generation 10 to 23. Redrawn from Gomez (1965) using the Weibel lung model as the abscissa.

$O_2\mathcal{D}_{O_2}$). One must then ask to what extent this conductance is increased at altitude since the diffusion coefficient for gases is theoretically inversely related to barometric pressure. For example, at 5500 m (0.5 atm) the diffusivity should be twice that at sea level, and at the top of Mt. Everest where $P_B = 250$ (West and Wagner, 1980), $\mathcal{D}_{O_2}$ should be increased by a factor of 3 over its sea level value. Thus, it is worthwhile to explore in more detail the evidence for the inverse relationship between pressure and binary diffusivity as given by the Chapman-Enskog equation (Reid and Sherwood, 1966), and to ask whether animals that depend entirely upon diffusive gas exchange exhibit adaptations to altitude.

The Chapman-Enskog Equation

It is important at the outset to realize that alveolar gas, although it contains O_2, N_2, CO_2, and water vapor, behaves approximately like a binary gas mixture because of the similar diffusion properties of its two main constituent molecules, O_2 and N_2, (Chang, 1980; Worth and Piiper, 1978). Therefore, in

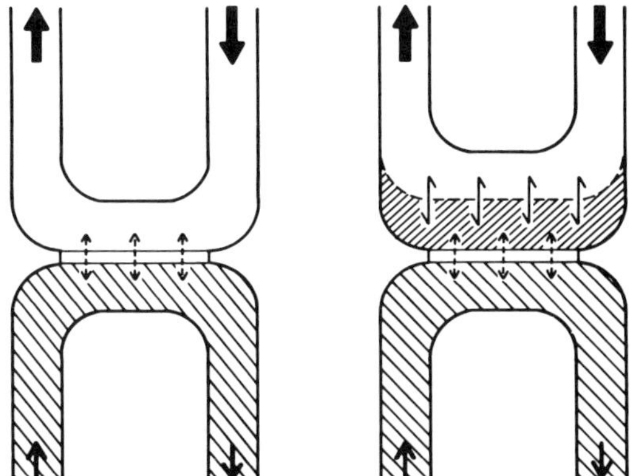

Figure 2. The left hand figure shows the conventional analog of gas and blood convection of the lung. In this model, gas convection carries the O_2 molecule to the alveolar surface. The small arrows depict the tissue-phase conductance expressed as the diffusing capacity of the lung. On the right hand, gas convection carries the O_2 to the mixing zone. From here, O_2 diffuses to the alveolar wall. The larger arrows represent the gas-phase resistance of the diffusing capacity.

the discussion which follows, we shall assume that diffusion in air or alveolar gas takes place according to the laws of binary diffusion.

Binary diffusion depends on the molecular weights and energies of interaction of the gas pair involved and on the total ambient pressure. These relations are given quantitative expression by the semi-empirical Chapman-Enskog equation for dilute gases (Reid and Sherwood, 1966), which allows calculation of binary diffusion coefficients:

$$\mathcal{D}_{1,2} = 0.00186\ T^{3/2} \frac{760}{P_B} \left[\frac{1}{M_1} + \frac{1}{M_2} \right]^{1/2} \frac{1}{\sigma_{1,2}^{\ 2}} \frac{1}{\Omega_D} \qquad (21.1)$$

where $\mathcal{D}_{1,2}$ = binary diffusion coefficient, cm^2/sec, T = absolute temperature, °K; P_B = barometric pressure, Torr; M_1, M_2 = molecular weights of gases 1,2; $\sigma_{1,2}$ = Lennard-Jones characteristic distance of the gas pair, Ω_D = collision integral, a dimensionless function of temperature and the intermolecular potential field for a single molecule of gas 1 interacting with a single molecule of gas 2.

Experimental values of $\mathcal{D}$ for respiratory gases in air or N_2 at 37°C and one atmosphere in units of cm^2/sec are 0.25 for O_2, 0.18 for CO_2, and 0.27 for H_2O (Paganelli and Kurata, 1977; Worth et al., 1978). The $\mathcal{D}$ values predicted from the Chapman-Enskog equation agree reasonably well with those experimentally measured, although for gas pairs containing water vapor, He and SF_6, predicted values do not agree as well.

It is particularly important for our discussion to note that $\mathcal{D}$ is inversely proportional to barometric pressure, i.e., as gas density increases, diffusivity is reduced in a reciprocal fashion. There are experimentally determined values of $\mathcal{D}$ at various pressures which in general support the reciprocal relation between $\mathcal{D}$ and P_B, but these data also show deviation from the ideal (Berry and Koeller, 1960; Durbin and Kobayashi, 1962; Paganelli and Kurata, 1977). On the other hand, the reciprocal relation between $\mathcal{D}$ and P_B should become closer to ideal at ambient pressures below one atmosphere, but experimental data in this pressure range are lacking.

Measurement of Gas-Phase Conductance

To determine changes in relative diffusivity of gases as a function of barometric pressure, one can measure a gas flux and its partial pressure difference across a porous barrier. Dividing the former by the latter yields by definition the conductance (or diffusing capacity) of the barrier:

$$\dot{M}_x/\Delta P_x = G_x \tag{21.2}$$

where $\dot{M}_x$ = flux rate of gas x (cm^3/sec); P_x = partial pressure difference of gas x across the barrier (Torr); and G_x = barrier conductance ($cm^3/sec/Torr$). According to Fick's first law of diffusion, conductance can be further defined (Paganelli, 1980) as

$$G_x = (A_p/L)(\mathcal{D}_x/RT) \tag{21.3}$$

where A_p = total area of the pores (cm^2); L = length of pores or thickness of the barrier (cm); $\mathcal{D}_x$ = diffusion coefficient of gas x (cm^2/sec); and $1/RT$ = capacitance coefficient ($Torr^{-1}$). For any given porous barrier A_p, L, and RT are constants and therefore

$$G_x = k\mathcal{D}_x \tag{21.4}$$

Thus any change in $\mathcal{D}_x$ will produce a directly proportional change in G.

For making measurements of the effect of pressure on diffusion, we chose a porous barrier with a surface of about 70 cm^2 and a thickness of about 0.3 mm. This was perforated by about 10,000 holes spaced 1 mm apart. The functional radius of each hole was 8 μm. Thus the total pore area available for diffusion is 2 mm^2. The conductance of such a barrier is low enough so that the boundary layer of relatively stagnant air adhering to the surface of the barrier offers negligible diffusive resistance, and gas transport is unaffected by convection currents (Spotila et al., 1981). Thus gas transport through the barrier is limited by diffusion alone.

When such a barrier separates a reservoir of liquid water from a relatively dry environment, the water vapor flux escaping from the reservoir can be measured gravimetrically. At constant humidity and temperature in the environment, the water vapor pressure difference across the barrier is also known, and one may now calculate its conductance from Equation (21.2), and its total effective pore area from Equation (21.3).

Such a porous barrier is easily obtained from the hen's egg. Not only does its shell have the dimensions described above, but it also encloses a reservoir which contains 75% water. There is a gas space between the fibers of the inner and outer membranes which separates the egg contents from the inner surface of the shell. Placing an egg in a desiccator at 25°C and weighing periodically enables one to determine the water vapor flux. The vapor pressure inside the egg is 23.8 Torr (saturation vapor pressure at 25°C) which represents the vapor pressure difference across the pores. The flux rate divided by the vapor pressure difference defines the shell conductance or its diffusing capacity.

Relative Diffusivity Changes at Altitude

With this technique, we attempted to demonstrate the validity of the Chapman-Enskog equation of increased diffusivity of gas molecules at low barometric pressures. By placing fresh eggs in a desiccator at constant temperature and exposing them to pressures below one atmosphere, we were able to determine the increase in conductance. For example, exposure to $P_B = 304$ Torr (equivalent to an altitude of 7100 m) caused these eggs to lose 2.5 times more water than at sea level. Since the vapor pressure difference across the shell was identical at both 304 Torr and sea level, the conductance had also increased by 2.5 times, and by Equation (21.4), so had the relative diffusivity. This value is shown as a square symbol in Figure 3, the average value and S.E. for 11 eggs, and fits on the theoretical curve. The two other points (circles) show the increased diffusivity of O_2 in N_2. They were obtained by measurement of the O_2 flux across the half-shell of an egg by the technique described by Wangensteen et al. (1970/71). These and additional values at higher simulated altitudes, not shown, all fall on the theoretical curve. Such data provide evidence in the pressure range studied that diffusivity does indeed increase in inverse proportion to pressure; this principle should be taken into account when one considers the problem of pulmonary gas mixing and stratified inhomogeneity at altitude.

Increased Diffusivity at Altitude and the Pore Structure of Bird Eggs

How does the increased diffusivity at altitude alter the shell porosity of bird eggs that are laid and develop at altitude? Many birds are known to reside at altitude and at least 21 species nest above 4000 m. The highest reported nesting site is for a jackdaw at 6500 m, where gas diffusivity is increased 2.2 times over sea level values. While this would obviously benefit O_2 transport, it would also mean that under normal conditions of nest humidity an egg with a porosity designed for sea level would lose 2.2 times more water. It turns out that bird eggs are designed with water conservation as a first priority. It is well-known

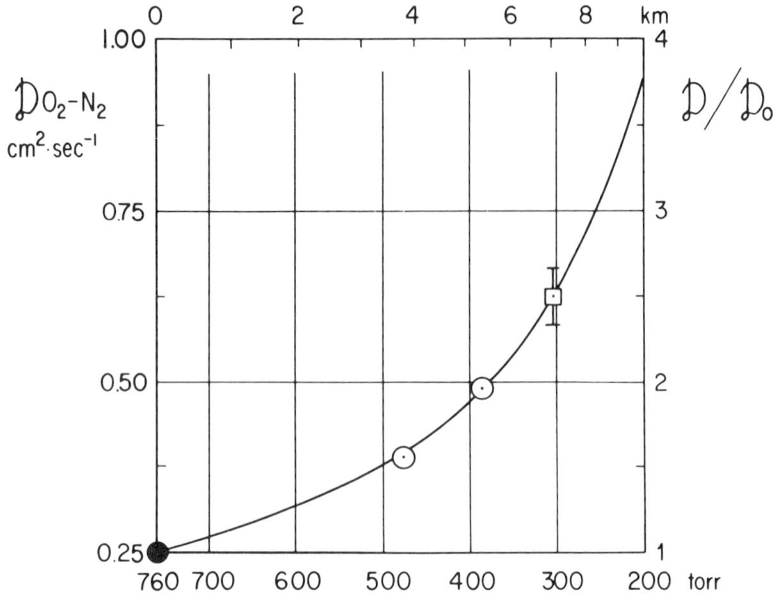

Figure 3. Changes in the binary diffusion coefficient for O_2 in N_2($\mathcal{D}_{O_2}$-N_2) as a function of barometric pressure according to the theoretical Chapman-Enskog equation. Equivalent altitudes are shown at the top. Experimental evidence for the relative increase in diffusivity ($\mathcal{D}/\mathcal{D}_O$-right ordinate) at reduced barometric pressures is shown for O_2 in N_2 by the two open circles and for water vapor in air by the square, ±S.E. The black circle at $P_B = 760$ represents the control values.

SOURCE: *Paganelli et al., 1975.*

that during normal incubation most bird eggs lose about 15% of their initial mass, regardless of egg size or duration of incubation (Ar and Rahn, 1980). In fact, it appears that this water loss is a mandatory prerequisite for normal development since hatchability is reduced not only when more, but also when less water is lost (Landauer, 1967). According to the recent work of Ar and Rahn (1980), the reason for this precise regulation is to assure an optimal water content at the time of hatching.

With a mandatory water loss of 15%, one can argue that shell conductance should be reduced in eggs that are incubated at altitude in order to avoid dehydration. If nest humidity at altitude is similar to that at sea level, (ca. 40 to 50% relative humidity), then the conductance should be reduced in direct proportion.

The first evidence of such acclimation came from our studies of hen's eggs at the Barcroft Laboratory of the White Mountain Research Station (Wangensteen et al., 1974). Fifteen years prior to our measurements, A.H. Smith at the University of California, Davis, had introduced a strain of White Leghorn hens to this Laboratory at 3800 m (P_B: 480 Torr). When these eggs were placed in an incubator at constant humidity together with sea level eggs brought up from Davis, California, the ratio of water loss of the high altitude to the sea level eggs was 0.68, while the barometric pressure change was 480/760, or 0.63. Similar changes were recorded by B. Bhatia when he compared water loss of eggs from native chickens of the Himalayas with those in New Delhi, and by C. Carey when she compared conductances of eggs of the Red-Winged Blackbird collected near sea level and at 2400 m in the Rocky Mountains (Rahn et al., 1977). Packard et al. (1977) and Sotherland et al. (1980) have observed altitude-related changes in shell conductance in the Barn Swallow and the Cliff Swallow, respectively. Carey (1980) has recently reviewed the effect of altitude on shell conductance.

If shell thickness is known, water loss measurements in a desiccator permit one to calculate not only shell conductance but also total effective pore area (Ap) from Equation (21.3). In Figure 4, we have plotted reduction in relative pore area against barometric pressure at which these eggs were collected. The straight line is calculated on the assumption that pore area is reduced in direct proportion to the increase in diffusivity as shown by the dotted curve and the

Figure 4. Reduction in pore area at altitude as percent of pore area at sea level (black circle) plotted against barometric pressure at which these eggs were collected. Bars indicate S.E. The solid line indicates the expected change in relative pore area if this reduction is directly proportional to the increase in diffusivity as shown by the dotted line and the right ordinate.

SOURCE: *Data from Rahn et al., (1977) and Wangensteen et al. (1974).*

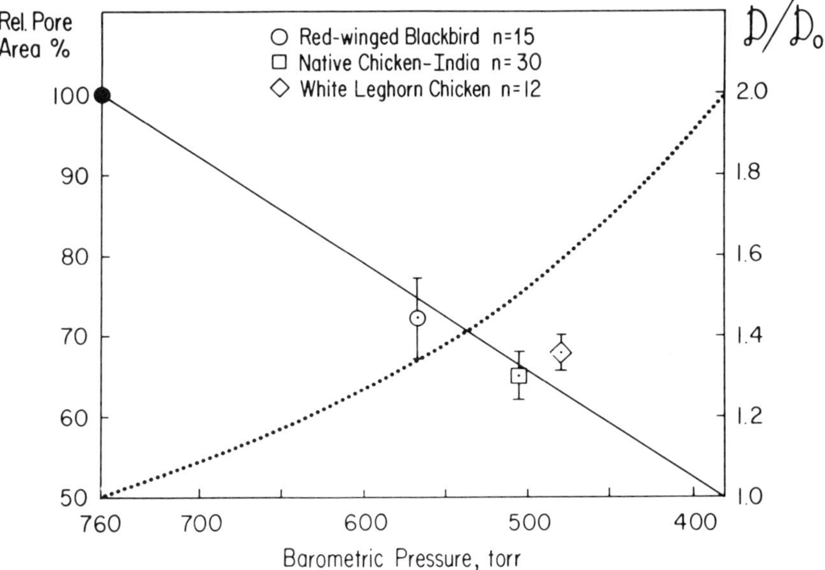

right-hand ordinate. The reasonably good fit of these data suggests that at these altitudes the conductance of the eggshell is proportional to the product of the pore area and the diffusivity, or $G_x = kA_p \cdot \mathcal{D}_x$. As diffusivity increases, the pore area is reduced proportionally so that the conductance at altitude remains the same as at sea level. This can be viewed as an adaptation to altitude which prevents undue water loss during incubation.

These observations raise many questions. How is the change in barometric pressure sensed and what mechanism in the hen's uterus responds to reduce the total pore area of the shell? One may further ask whether the increased diffusivity at altitude affects the stomatal structure of plants and the tracheolar dimensions of insects. These organisms have successfully colonized our highest mountain ranges, depend upon diffusivity gas transport and place their priorities on conservation of water.

References

Ar, A. and Rahn, H. 1980. Water in the avian egg: overall budget of incubation. *Amer. Zool.* 20:373–384.

Berry, V.J., Jr. and Koeller, R.C. 1960. Diffusion in compressed binary gaseous systems. *A.I. Ch. E.J.* 6:274–280.

Carey, C. 1980. Adaptation of the avian egg to altitude. *Amer. Zool.* 20:449–459.

Chang, H.K. 1980. Multicomponent diffusion in the lung. *Fed. Proc.* 39:2759–2764.

Durbin, L. and Kobayashi, R. 1962. Diffusion of Krypton-85 in dense gases. *J. Chem. Phys.* 37:1643–1654.

Gomez, D.M. 1965. A physicomathematical study of lung function in normal subjects and in patients with obstructive pulmonary diseases. *Med. Thorac.* 22:275–294.

Landauer, W. 1967. The hatchability of chicken eggs as influenced by environment and heredity. *Conn. Agr. Exp. Stat. Monogr.* 1:1–315 (revised).

Packard, C.C., Sotherland, P.R., and Packard, M.J. 1977. Adaptive reduction in permeability of avian eggshells to water vapor at high altitudes. *Nature* 266:255–256.

Paganelli, C.V. 1980. The physics of gas exchange across the avian eggshell. *Amer. Zool.* 20:329–338.

Paganelli, C.V., Ar, A., Rahn, H., and Wangensteen, O.D. 1975. Diffusion in the gas phase: the effect of ambient pressure and gas composition. *Respir. Physiol.* 25:247–258.

Paganelli, C.V. and Kurata, F.K. 1977. Diffusion of water vapor in binary and ternary gas mixtures at increased pressure. *Respir. Physiol.* 30:15–26.

Rahn, H., Carey, C., Balmas, K., Bhatia, B., and Paganelli, C.V. 1977. Reduction of pore area of the avian eggshell as an adaptation to altitude. *Proc. Natl. Acad. Sci. U.S.A.* 74:3095–3098.

Reid, R.C. and Sherwood, T.K. 1966. *The Properties of Gases and Liquids. 2nd edition*. New York: McGraw Hill.

Scheid, P. and Piiper, J. 1980. Intrapulmonary gas mixing and stratification. In *Pulmonary Gas Exchange, Vol. I, Ventilation, Blood Flow, and Diffusion*. West, J.B., ed. New York: Academic Press. pp. 87–130.

Sotherland, P.R., Packard, G.C., Taigen, T.L., and Boardman, T.J. 1980. An altitudinal cline in conductance of Cliff Swallow eggs to water vapor. *Auk* 97:177–185.

Spotila, J.R., Weinheimer, C.J., and Paganelli, C.V. 1981. Shell resistance and evaporative water loss from bird eggs: effects of wind speed and egg size. *Physiol. Zool.* 54:195–202.

Wangensteen, O.D., Rahn, H., Burton, R.R., and Smith, A.H. 1974. Respiratory gas exchange of high altitude adapted chick embryos. *Respir. Physiol.* 21:61–70.

Wangensteen, O.D., Wilson, D., and Rahn, H. 1970/71. Respiratory gas exchange by the avian embryo. *Respir. Physiol.* 11:31–45.

West, J.B. and Wagner, P.D., 1980. Predicted gas exchange on the summit of Mt. Everest. *Respir. Physiol.* 42:1–16.

Worth, H., Nüsse, W. and Piiper, J. 1978. Determination of binary diffusion coefficients of various gas species used in respiratory physiology. *Respir. Physiol.* 32:15–26.

Worth, H. and Piiper, J. 1978. Diffusion of helium, carbon monoxide, and sulfur hexafluoride in gas mixtures similar to alveolar gas. *Respir. Physiol.* 32:155–166.

J.A. Loeppky and M.L. Riedesel, editors
OXYGEN TRANSPORT TO HUMAN TISSUES

Hypobaria: An Etiologic Factor in Acute Mountain Sickness?

Robert F. Grover, Alan Tucker, and John T. Reeves

Headache, lethargy, nausea, vomiting, and impaired mental function constitute the symptom complex known as acute mountain sickness (AMS). These distressing symptoms appear within hours of fairly rapid ascent to mountainous regions above 2800 m. With the advent of exploration of the atmosphere using balloons, much greater heights were attained in a matter of hours, and this added to the list of high altitude effects the blurring of vision, loss of consciousness, coma, and death.

What causes AMS? Since it was known from balloon ascents that barometric pressure falls with increasing altitude, this decrease in the pressure of air on the body (hypobaria) was a proposed mechanism for AMS, and a "relaxation of blood vessels" was suggested by De Saussure in 1786. However, when Paul Bert (1877) demonstrated that the symptons of AMS could be prevented or relieved by oxygen breathing, this established that it was the decrease in the partial pressure of inspired oxygen, i.e., hypoxia, rather than the decrease in total atmospheric pressure, which caused the symptoms of AMS.

But was it really hypoxia per se? Mosso (1897) argued that one of the usual responses to high altitude is an increase in ventilation which lowers carbon dioxide tension. He believed that the resulting "acapnia" was the direct cause of AMS.

Thus, over the years all three of the consequences of ascent to high altitude—hypobaria per se, hypoxia, and hypocapnic alkalosis—have been implicated in the etiology of AMS. As is so often the case, there is probably some truth in all three factors, even though hypoxia is by far the dominant one. In this discussion, we would like to present evidence that a fairly rapid reduction in atmospheric pressure per se may have physiological effects which relate to the symptomatology of AMS.

In the conventional approach to research, a hypothesis is formulated, and experiments are designed to test that hypothesis. However, in real life, those experiments may yield unanticipated results. This poses a problem when it comes to publication, because the apparent logic behind the investigation has been lost. Hence, after the fact, a new hypothesis is formulated from which the results now appear to follow in a more logical fashion. Such research is called "doing the right thing for the wrong reason." However, such a mistake is far better than doing no experiment and learning nothing. Unfortunately, published reports almost never reveal these fortuitous discoveries. Rather, they read as if the investigator has remarkable insight prior to entering the laboratory.

We had such a fortuitous experience in 1974. Our laboratory had developed a keen interest in the chemical control of breathing, which includes the sensitivity of the carotid body to hypoxia. This is measured by having the subject breathe from a system in which the end-tidal oxygen tension (PAO_2) is lowered progressively from 140 to 40 Torr over 8 to 10 min. In response to this progressive hypoxia, ventilation increases. End-tidal carbon dioxide is held constant by adding CO_2 to the inspired air as needed. Since the hypoxic ventilatory response (HVR) is hyperbolic, it can be described by the equation (Weil et al., 1970):

$$\dot{V}_E = \dot{V}_0 + A/(PAO_2 - 32) \qquad (22.1)$$

Hence, the overall HVR may be quantitated by the parameter "A," such that the greater the HVR, the larger the value of A.

We wished to determine the effect of ascent to high altitude on the HVR, i.e., to measure HVR at different levels of barometric pressure (P_B). This led to a controversy over the terms by which to express HVR. We took this problem to our bioengineers who reasoned that the purpose of ventilation is to bring a quantity of oxygen into the lungs, and to remove a similar quantity of carbon dioxide from the lungs. In that context, it is the number of molecules of oxygen moved which is important. Hence, ventilatory volume should be expressed as "STPD." In contrast, when we took our problem to the respiratory physiologists, they reasoned that the body cannot meter the flow of oxygen molecules. The respiratory center can only activate the thoracic bellows, producing a volume change expressed as "BTPS."

The implications of these contrasting concepts are as follows. If ventilation is to transport a given molecular quantity of oxygen, i.e., STPD volume, then in response to a reduction in P_B, HVR expressed as "STPD" should remain constant, whereas HVR expressed as "BTPS" should increase in proportion to the decrease in P_B. On the other hand, if BTPS ventilatory volume, i.e., the excursion of the thoracic bellows, is determined by PAO_2, then HVR should be independent of P_B and remain constant, whereas HVR expressed "STPD" should decrease as P_B is decreased (Table 1).

Table 1. Theoretical Change in Hypoxic Ventilatory Response (HVR) with Decrease in Barometric Pressure (P_B).

P_B (Torr)	HVR (STPD) 750 to 480	HVR (BTPS) 750 to 480
"STPD" concept	0	+
"BTPS" concept	—	0

To examine the validity of these concepts, 9 healthy young men were tested at sea level sitting in a hypobaric chamber. First, with the chamber door open, HVR was measured with P_B at 750 Torr. To avoid any possible influence of atmospheric hypoxia, each subject then began breathing 40% O_2 by mask. Next, the chamber door was closed and P_B lowered to 480 Torr over 15 min. Breathing of 40% O_2 was continued up to the HVR measurements. Only then was the PAO_2 lowered from 140 to 40 Torr, as described above.

The results were not as predicted by either concept. In every subject, HVR was markedly reduced, whether expressed as "BTPS" or "STPD" (Table 2). Normoxic hypobaria reduced HVR by 60% BTPS and by 73% STPD, and in half the subjects, HVR was virtually abolished!

After these measurements of HVR, the subjects removed their masks, thereby discontinuing the breathing of 40% oxygen and exposing themselves for the first time to the hypoxic chamber atmosphere where P_B was 480 Torr. After 4 hr of continuous hypoxia, the measurements of HVR were repeated again. The HVR had now increased; expressed "BTPS," it had returned to the sea level values, but expressed STPD, it remained reduced (Table 2). In those subjects in whom HVR had almost disappeared during normoxic hypobaria, it had now returned. These results now supported the "BTPS" Concept of Table 1. Returning to the observations made during normoxic hypobaria, how do we explain the markedly depressed values of HVR in Table 2? It appears that fortuitously we demonstrated a physiological effect of hypobaria per se, an

Table 2. Observed Change in Hypoxic Ventilatory Response (HVR) with Decrease in P_B.

P_B (Torr)	Sea level normoxia 750	Normoxic hypobaria (0.5 hr) 480	Hypoxic hypobaria (4.0 hr) 480
HVR, STPD	111	30	62
HVR, BTPS	133	53	124

NOTE: Values are for "A" in Equation (22.1), mean of 9 subjects.

effect which was transient and had essentially disappeared after 4 hr of hypobaric hypoxia. Furthermore, this effect on respiratory chemosensitivity was selective for the ventilatory response to hypoxia, since no such depression after 30 min was observed in the ventilatory response to hypercapnia (Table 3). Although intriguing, these observations have not been published before because we are at a loss to explain the mechanism responsible. Nevertheless, they support the concept that hypobaria per se may alter respiratory chemosensitivity, and this in turn could modify the ventilatory adaptions to high altitude which we believe plays an important role in the pathogenesis of AMS (Hackett et al, 1981).

In addition to hypobaria, ascent to high altitude involves exposure to a reduction in inspired oxygen tension, but the resulting arterial hypoxemia is not simply a reflection of this atmospheric hypoxia. It is well-known that on arrival at high altitude the arterial oxygen tension (PaO_2) is significantly lower than after several days of adaptation to that altitude. Multiple factors are involved. Although minute ventilation (BTPS) increases, the mass of air (STPD) moved is actually less than prior to ascent (Grover, 1965). Hence, relative hypoventilation accentuates the initial alveolar hypoxia. Over succeeding days, there is a progressive increase in ventilation (BTPS) which raises, PaO_2. In this process of adaptation, the initial relative hypoventilation probably reflects respiratory alkalosis, since this early phase is avoided if hypocapnia is prevented (Cruz et al., 1980). Once ventilation adaptation is complete, the increase in ventilation (BTPS) offsets the decrease in P_B, so that the mass of air moved (STPD) is virtually the same at all altitudes. Christensen (1937), perhaps fortuitously, found this to be exactly true. This also supports the "BTPS" concept in Table 1. A second factor contributing to the exaggerated arterial hypoxemia during the initial phase of exposure to high altitude is a widening of the difference in oxygen tension between alveolar gas and arterial blood (A-a gradient) as reported by Reeves et al. (1969) and Reeves and Daoud (1970). Although the mechanism involved is not known, this probably reflects a disturbance of the matching of local ventilation (V_A) to local perfusion (Q). Uneven hypoxic pulmonary vasoconstriction would disrupt V_A/Q, but just why vasoconstriction should be uneven is not obvious.

Table 3. Effect of a Decrease in P_B on the Ventilatory Response to Hypercapnia.

	Sea level normoxia	**Normoxic hypobaria 0.5 hr**	**Hypoxic hypobaria 4.0 hr**
P_B (Torr)	**750**	**480**	**480**
S, STPD	1.54	1.29	0.71
S, BTPS	1.85	2.60	1.44

NOTE: Values are for the Slope (S) in liter/min/mm Hg, mean of 8 subjects.

Recently, Reeves (Tucker et al., 1981) proposed an alternative explanation, namely that this disturbance of V_A/Q might be a consequence of pulmonary microembolism caused by micro-bubble formation analagous to decompression sickness in divers (Luft, 1965). He speculated that the nitrogen normally dissolved in all tissues would come out of solution as the ambient pressure was reduced. Upon entering the venous circulation, microbubbles of nitrogen would form and act as the stimulus for activating leukocytes, or as the nidus for clumping of platelets, as Gray et al. (1975) suggested. These leukocytes or platelet microemboli would then be carried to the lung and be trapped in the pulmonary microcirculation causing vasoconstriction and/or endothelial injury. By this means, lung perfusion would be disturbed.

To test the hypothesis that hypobaria is an etiologic factor in AMS by causing the formation of nitrogen bubbles, we decided to denitrogenate subjects prior to decompression. This was accomplished by having the subjects breathe 100% oxygen by mask for 1.5 hr prior to and during decompression from 625 to 430 Torr. Upon arrival at simulated high altitude, the oxygen masks were removed, thereby initiating exposure to hypoxia which was then maintained for 2 to 4 hr. In control experiments, the same subjects were exposed to the same reduction in P_B without oxygen breathing to lower nitrogen stores. The results showed that prior oxygen breathing diminished the ventilatory response to high altitude. Minute ventilation increased less with less tachypnea, producing less alkalosis. From arterialized venous blood, $PaCO_2$ was higher, and presumably PAO_2 was lower. In spite of this relative hypoventilation, hypoxemia was not exaggerated; the fall in saturation (ear oximeter) was about 15% with or without denitrogenation. However, the further fall in saturation during exercise at altitude was prevented. In one subject, saturation fell from 83 to 74% with exercise following decompression breathing air. However, when he was decompressed breathing oxygen and then remained hypoxic at rest for 2 hr, his saturation remained at 83% during subsequent exercise. We interpret these observations to indicate less disturbance of V_A/Q (smaller increase in the A-a oxygen gradient both at rest and during exercise) if the subject is denitrogenated prior to decompression.

Cardiovascular responses to simulated high altitude were also modified by prior oxygen breathing. Heart rate increased less both at rest and during exercise. Systemic blood pressure remained unchanged during decompression on air, but following decompression with oxygen breathing, both systolic and diastolic pressure decreased.

Since antidiuresis is often reported by persons developing AMS, we examined the effects of decompression on urine output. To establish a stable baseline of urine production, the subjects were water-loaded until urine volume reached 5 to 6 ml/min. Then each half hour, the subjects drank a volume of water equal to the volume of urine voided. Following decompression with air breathing, many subjects experienced antidiuresis and the mean urine output fell to half the control level. This antidiuresis was prevented by prior oxygen breathing. The increase in urine osmolarity associated with the antidiuresis was also prevented.

In summary, the breathing of 100% oxygen for 1.5 hr prior to and during decompression significantly modified the physiological responses to the subsequent hypobaric hypoxia. Most impressive was an improvement in pulmonary gas exchange implying less disruption of V_A/Q matching. Antidiuresis was prevented, and there was less tachycardia, particularly during exercise (Tucker et al., 1981).

How are we to explain these observations? In both these latter studies, as well as the former investigation of respiratory chemosensitivity, decompression to simulated high altitude was modified by oxygen breathing prior to and during ascent; supplemental oxygen was then discontinued. Since the body cannot store oxygen, it is not obvious how the prior breathing of oxygen could modify the subsequent responses to hypoxia, particularly after several hours. Nevertheless, delayed effects of a period of hyperoxia must be excluded.

The rationale for breathing 100% oxygen was to deplete the normal body stores of dissolved nitrogen. Although total denitrogenation requires more than 5 hr, over two-thirds of the dissolved nitrogen is washed out during the first hr of oxygen breathing (Luft, 1965) which comes mainly from blood, muscles, and well-perfused viscera. Removal from fatty tissue takes much longer. Hence, our use of 1.5 hr of oxygen breathing should have been effective in removing much of the dissolved nitrogen prior to decompression.

Could decompression cause microbubbles to appear in the venous blood? We employed a decompression rate of 1000 ft/min, so P_B was reduced from 630 to 430 Torr in 10 min. When one of our bioengineers, Al Micco, placed a Doppler ultrasonic probe over the subclavian vein or the pulmonary artery following decompression, he was able to detect an occasional, discrete bubble. Hence, bubble formation does occur but their size and number are unknown.

Assuming that significant numbers of microbubbles do appear in the venous blood, could they alter lung function? Recently, Staub et al., (1981) reported that when air bubbles 1.0 mm in diameter were injected intravenously in sheep neutrophils collected at the air-blood interface and the neutrophils accumulated in the lung microcirculation, causing lung injury and increased vascular permeability (Craddock et al., 1977; Flick et al., 1981). Similarly, Gray et al. (1975) reported that decompression resulted in platelet accumulation in the lungs. Platelets play a significant role in the altered pulmonary hemodynamics in pulmonary microembolization through the release of vasoactive substances (Mlczoch et al., 1978). Therefore, microbubbles could alter lung function by means of activating either neutrophils or platelets. However, if the bubbles are trapped in the lung, it is difficult to explain how they could alter renal function unless the renal effects were indirect.

Thus far, we have considered physiological effects of decompression which might be mediated by microbubble formation. Could hypobaria exert influences unrelated to bubbles? Early in thc U.S. manned flight space program, normoxic hypobaric atmospheres were employed. To study the effects of such atmospheres, Epstein and Saruta (1972) exposed 8 men to 258 Torr with PIO_2 and PIN_2 at 181 and 65 Torr, respectively, for 9 days. Following dietary sodium restriction, hypobaria caused a progressive fall of 40% in creatinine clearance not seen under normobaric conditions, and the decrease in body weight was significantly less. Although the mechanism involved was not clear, they concluded that the results were due to hypobaria per se.

Finally, do these observations made over 2 to 4 hr following fairly rapid decompression permit any conclusions regarding the role of hypobaria in the etiology of AMS? Probably not. However, in the treatment of high altitude pulmonary edema, a severe manifestation of AMS, an increase in P_B by descent has proven to be far more effective than simple relief of hypoxia by oxygen breathing (Hackett 1980). Perhaps the role of hypobaria in the physiology of high altitude has been underestimated. At the very least, it is clear that if one wished to study the physiological adaptations involved in climbing to great altitudes such as Mt. Everest, the use of supplemental oxygen during ascent may well modify respiratory function measured soon after the oxygen mask is removed.

References

Bert, P. 1943. *Barometric Pressure: Researches in Experimental Physiology*. Hitchcock, M.A. and Hitchcock, F.A., translators. Columbus, Ohio: College Book Co.

Christensen, E.H. 1937. Sauerstoffaufnahme und Respiratorische Funktionen in grossen Hohen. *Skand. Arch. Physiol.* 76:88–100.

Craddock, P.R., Fehr, J., Brigham, K.L., Kronenberg, R.S., Jacob, H.S. 1977. Complement and leukocyte-mediated pulmonary dysfunction in hemodialysis. *N. Engl. J. Med.* 296:769–774.

Cruz, J.C., Reeves, J.T., Grover, R.F., Maher, J.T., McCullough, R.E., Cymerman, A., and Denniston, J.C. 1980. Ventilatory acclimatization to high altitude is prevented by CO_2 breathing. *Respiration* 39:121–130.

Epstein, M. and Saruta, T. 1972. Effects of simulated high altitude on renin-aldosterone and Na homeostasis in normal man. *J. Appl. Physiol.* 33:204–210.

Flick, M.R., Perel, A., and Staub, N.C. 1981. Leukocytes are required for increased lung microvascular permeability after microembolization in sheep. *Circ. Res.* 48:344–351.

Gray, G. W., Bryan, A.C., Freedman, M.H., Houston, C.S., Lewis, W.F., McFadden, D.M., and Newell, G. 1975. Effect of altitude exposure on platelets. *J. Appl. Physiol.* 39:648–651.

Grover, R.F. 1965. Effects of hypoxia on ventilation and cardiac output. *Ann. N.Y. Acad. Sci.* 121:662–673.

Hackett, P.H. 1980. Acute mountain sickness—the clinical approach. *Adv. Cardiol.* 27:6–10.

Hackett, P.H., Rennie, D., Hofmeister, S.E., Grover, R.F., and Reeves, J.T. 1981. Relative hypoventilation and fluid retention in acute mountain sickness. *J. Appl. Physiol.*, in press.

Luft, U.C. 1965. Aviation physiology—the effects of altitude. In *Handbook of Physiology. Section 3: Respiration, Vol. II.* Fenn, W.O. and Rahn, H. eds. Washington D.C.: American Physiological Society. pp. 1099–1145.

Mlczock, J., Tucker, A., Weir, E.K., Reeves, J.T., and Grover, R.F. 1978. Platelet-mediated pulmonary hypertension and hypoxemia during pulmonary microembolism: reduction by platelet inhibition. *Chest* 74:648–653.

Mosso, A. 1897. *Der Mensch auf den Hochalpen*. Leipzig: S. Hirzel.

Reeves, J.T. and Daoud, F. 1970. Increased alveolar-arterial oxygen gradients during treadmill walking at simulated high altitude. *Adv. Cardiol.* 5:41–48.

Reeves, J.T., Halpin, J., Cohn, J.E., and Daoud, F. 1969. Increased alveolar-arterial oxygen difference during simulated high-altitude exposure. *J. Appl. Physiol.* 27:658–661.

Staub, N.C., Schultz, E.L., and Albertine, K.H. 1981. Number and distribution of neutrophils (PMNs) in sheep lungs after air embolization. *Am. Rev. Respir. Dis.* 123 (No. 4, Part 2):235.

Tucker, A., Reeves, J.T., Busch, M.A., Russel, B.E., Robertshaw, D. and Grover, R.F. 1981. Improved ventilatory, hemodynamic, and renal responses to acute altitude exposure in denitrogenated subjects. *Fed. Proc.* 40:609.

Weil, J.V., Byrne-Quinn, E., Sodal, I.E., Friesen, W.O., Underhill, B., Filley, G.F., and Grover R.F. 1970. Hypoxic ventilatory drive in normal man. *J. Clin. Invest.* 49:1061–1072.

J.A. Loeppky and M.L. Riedesel, editors
OXYGEN TRANSPORT TO HUMAN TISSUES

Regulation of Respiration and CSF Acid-Base Balance

John W. Severinghaus

As my part of this delightful festival honoring Ulrich Luft, I plan to summarize the role of high altitude physiological studies in our understanding of the regulation of respiration and CSF acid-base balance. These are not technical climbing experiments, like those of Ulrich Luft, but rather comfortable well-heated high altitude laboratory games. I will discuss primarily the work conducted in the Cardiovascular Research Institute and the Anesthesia Research Center at the University of California in San Francisco since 1958. During this period, a large number of our colleagues elsewhere have made significant contributions, and I only regret that I will not have time to do justice to all of them.

Acclimatization Theories Before 1962

The story concerns central respiratory chemoreceptors, the blood-brain barrier and active transport of hydrogen ions. The role of the hydrogen ion in controlling ventilation began to be understood about 1910 through Winterstein's reaction theory and the Danish studies of CO_2 responses. However, by about 1930, the theory had been faulted by the discovery of the carotid body by Heyman. To explain acclimatization, it was then postulated that the kidney excreted bicarbonate in response to the alkalosis produced by the hypoxic hyperventilation originating in the carotid body. That was the story when I was in medical school and it persisted well through the 1950s. The first evidence of trouble with that theory, however, came from a study done by Dick Riley and Charlie Houston called "Operation Everest" (Houston and Riley, 1947). It is delightful to have both of them participating in this symposium some 35 years later! Their critical observation was this: when a subject who had been made very hypoxic in a chamber for several weeks was brought out of the chamber back to sea level, blood pH was found to be 7.53 at rest and 7.50 on exercise. There remained no obvious stimulus to explain his continued hyperventilation. Their experiment was crucial in stimulating my interest in high altitude.

Altitude and the CSF Chemoreceptors

In 1960, Hans Loeschke came to San Francisco to join Bob Mitchell in locating CO_2 central chemoreceptors within the CSF compartment on the ventral medullary surface, where they "taste" the extracellular fluid pH (Mitchell et al., 1963). As a result of that localization, and discussions with Ralph Kellogg, we decided to determine whether both the process of acclimatization and Houston and Riley's mysterious drive after returning from high altitude might be explained by acidosis in the CSF at a time when the blood was alkaline. This would suggest that CSF pH was somehow better regulated than was blood pH. Kellogg introduced us to the White Mountain Laboratory, east of the Sierras, which was built in the 1950's by University of California (Berkeley) physiology graduate students under Nello Pace's direction. The first human CSF study at altitude was done in 1962 (Severinghaus et al., 1963).

If you can imagine yourself transported suddenly to the Barcroft laboratory at 3810 m altitude, you would experience about a 3 Torr fall of PCO_2 within minutes, and after an hour or so, PCO_2 would begin to fall further, reaching 29 to 30 Torr after a few days at 3800 m. As hyperventilation occurs, blood HCO_3^- falls, primarily due to hemoglobin buffering, without much change of base excess during the first few days. Blood pH rises about 0.05 units. We found that CSF pH, even at 8 hr, had risen by about 0.02 units. The CSF HCO_3^- cannot be reduced by hypocapnia through chemical buffering in itself, since CSF has almost no buffers. Figure 1 illustrates the central idea of the 1962 CSF study. These are mean CO_2 response curves of 4 subjects at sea level and after 8 days at altitude, expressing the stimulus as blood and CSF pH rather than as PCO_2. A single determination of pH in CSF at the start of each study was done in order to determine the relation between arterial and CSF PCO_2, and to determine the level of CSF HCO_3^- during the study. We assumed that CSF HCO_3^- did not change during a CO_2 response test, and that CSF PCO_2 changed by 0.9 of the change of end-tidal PCO_2. Figure 1 also shows the effects of acutely changing PO_2. The CSF was alkaline until PO_2 was normalized, but less alkaline after 8 days than initially. The CSF pH response curve was not significantly altered by acclimatization, while blood pH response was shifted to an alkaline position. This supported the idea that acclimatization was due to alteration of CSF HCO_3^-. The results indicated that CSF HCO_3^- fell by some mechanism other than renal HCO_3^- excretion. If the CSF HCO_3^- had not fallen, we computed that CSF pH would have risen by 0.08 units due to the fall of PCO_2 during the first few days. We postulated the blood-brain

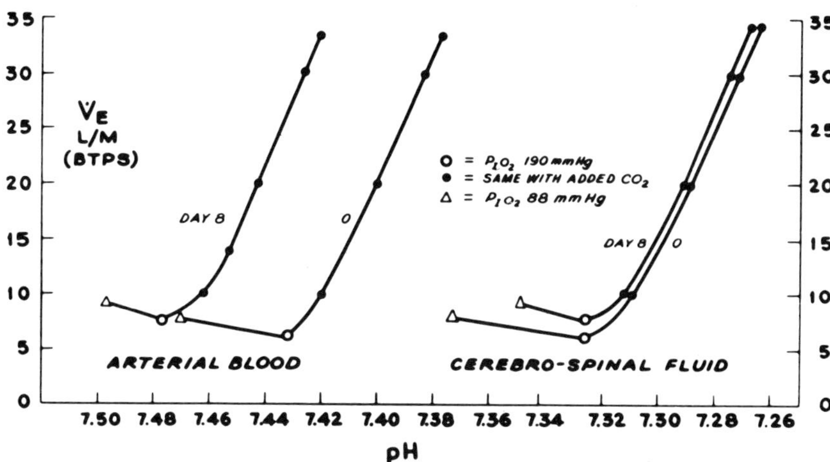

Figure 1. The effect of altitude acclimatization on the CO_2 response when plotted as a function of the induced variations of arterial and CSF pH. See text for assumptions and calculations. At sea level, the open circles represent the chronic steady state, the triangles the acute change with hypoxia. At altitude, the open triangles are the steady state, the open circles the acute effect of hyperoxia.

barrier regulated CSF pH by active transport, and hypothesized that pH would be found to gradually return to or toward normal during acclimatization.

Persisting CSF Alkalosis at Altitude

The role of CSF in regulating respiration was studied in many laboratories during the following decade. A discrepancy soon appeared between theory and observation. Dempsey, Forster, Orr, Bisgard, and others at Wisconsin, and Weiskopf, Gabel, and Fencl in Boston reported that CSF became more alkaline than we had found, and remained alkaline at altitude indefinitely, showing no evidence of the postulated correction. Four years ago at an Aspen conference, I confessed my error and admitted that our data had not actually shown a return toward control but rather a persistent, although insignificant, elevation. In the words of the Danish poet philosopher Piet Hein:

"The noble art of losing face
May one day save the human race
And turn into eternal merit
What weaker minds would call disgrace."

Role of Hypoxia in Sustaining CSF Alkalosis

However, 4 years ago, neither we nor anyone had measured CSF pH after normalizing PO_2 in acclimatized man at altitude. We had predicted that normoxia would restore medullary chemoreceptor pH to its normal value, while Dempsey and his colleagues believed that there must be some other missing factor keeping CSF alkaline. In order to answer that question, Bob Crawford and I organized another study of CSF in volunteers at White Mountain (Crawford and Severinghaus, 1978). This time, each subject's CO_2 response was determined at both high and low PO_2 at each stage of acclimatization, in conjunction with CSF sampling directly into a pH electrode by a gas-impermeable Kel-F catheter. The effects of acute hypoxia and hyperoxia on PCO_2 were documented continuously during the first 45 min. The CSF pH was not found significantly different from the sea level control when the PO_2 had been restored to normal for 45 min at altitude. This was long enough to permit the PCO_2 in lumbar spinal fluid to equilibrate with the 3.7 Torr rise of arterial PCO_2. Analysis of the central chemoreceptor response suggested that the continued hyperventilation after acute normalization of PO_2 would require that CSF pH be about 0.006 units more acid than at sea level, well within the limits of accuracy of the method. The mean altitude CSF pH was 7.307, compared with the sea level mean of 7.312.

Acid-Base Effects on Acclimatization

In 4 subjects, we studied whether altitude acclimatization (the reduction of blood and CSF HCO_3^-) could be augmented by NH_4Cl ingestion, or inhibited by $NaHCO_3$ ingestion (Severinghaus, 1965). Each subject served as his own control a month later on a second ascent. Acidification marginally accelerated acclimatization, while keeping bicarbonate constant in the plasma did not prevent acclimatization (Figure 2). This study was subsequently confirmed by Dempsey and his colleagues.

Acid-Base Imbalance and Respiratory Drive

Mitchell had shown that metabolic acidosis stimulated ventilation primarily via carotid body chemoreceptors in dogs, since denervation prevented the ventilatory response to an acid load. This had also been contested during the subsequent decade. Accordingly, Irsigler et al. (1980) used the same methods of testing ventilatory responses to hypoxia and CO_2, together with CSF samples, to repeat the investigation earlier reported by Fencl et al. (1969). Four subjects ingested ammonium chloride for 3 days and then switched to sodium bicarbonate. With NH_4Cl for 48 hr, to a base excess of -10.6 ± 1.1 meq/liter, the CO_2 response curve shifted 9.0 ± 1.4 Torr to the left, CSF HCO_3^- fell 4.4 meq/liter (46% of the fall of arterial HCO_3^-) and CSF pH rose 0.033 ± 0.020, a

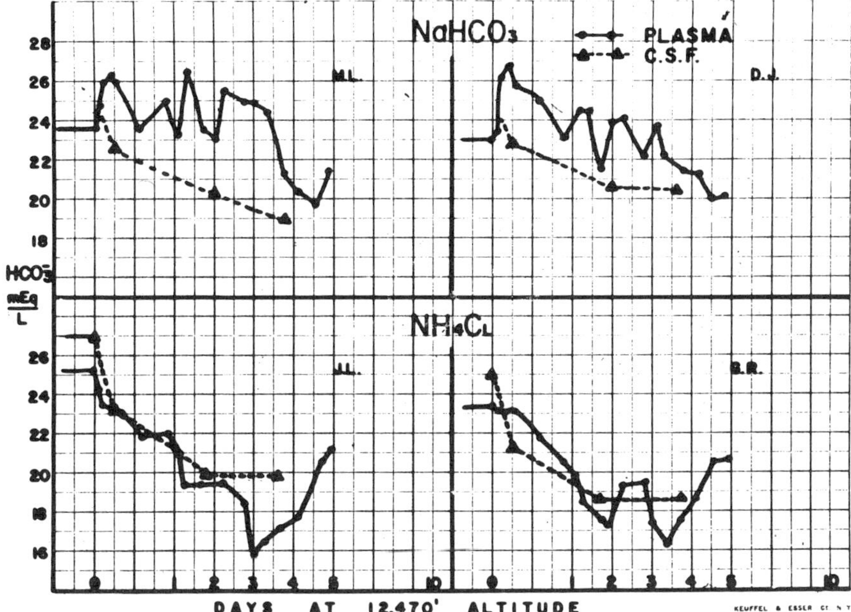

Figure 2. The acclimatization of two subjects to altitude was not significantly inhibited by elevation of their plasma HCO_3^- to sea level values during the first 3 days at altitude. Two other subjects showed small but nonsignificant acceleration in acclimatization when given NH_4Cl during the first 3 days.

paradoxic alkalosis in the presence of moderate, sustained blood acidosis. The CSF HCO_3^- reduction therefore could not have caused the hyperventilation. The carotid body response to arterial acidemia remains as the most likely source of the incremental respiratory stimuli.

With ingestion of $NaHCO_3$, CSF pH was found unchanged, while PCO_2 and HCO_3^- rose proportionately. The implication is that arterial alkalosis depressed peripheral chemoreceptor drive, while having little effect on central drive.

CSF pH Regulation and Blood-Brain Barrier

We found that if we kept the plasma bicarbonate constant while hyperventilating dogs to a PCO_2 of 20 Torr, CSF HCO_3^- fell 2.3 ± 1.0 in 3.7 hr, and 2.0 ± 1.9 after 7.2 hr. This could have been due to lactic acid generated in brain by vasoconstriction induced by extreme hypocapnic alkalemia (pH = 7.68), or by some active transport across the blood-brain barrier. The CSF ions are not in electrochemical equilibrium with brain capillary blood plasma water, HCO_3^- being about 77% of equilibrium, or −7 mV. After the 7.2-hr hyperventilation, CSF HCO_3^- was −11.6 mV, or 64.7% of the electrochemical equilibrium value.

Infusion of $NaHCO_3$ into dogs, ventilated at constant PCO_2, was found to raise CSF HCO_3^-, but again the changes did not restore electrochemical equilibrium. After 9 hr of normocapneic alkalosis, at arterial pH=7.70, CSF HCO_3^- was −14 mV, or 59% of equilibrium. Bledsoe and Hornbein carefully tested each of the 4 acid-base states, and initially concluded that changes could be explained by passive permeability of the blood-brain barrier. They recently found that this was not the case when transbarrier electrical potential was altered by K^+ elevation, and altered their conclusion in favor of active transport (personal communication).

Brain surface ECF pH in rabbits subjected to severe metabolic acidosis and alkalosis was compared to arterial pH. In the acid direction, ECF pH followed blood closely. In the alkaline direction it did not. One likely reason is that the alkalinity is limited by its effect on cerebral blood flow, such that tissue hypoxia resulting from reduced flow generates lactic acid, titrating whatever HCO_3^- ion migrates across the blood-brain barrier.

Role of Hypoxic Lactacidosis on Brain ECF pH

Hypoxia plays a very significant role in brain acid-base balance. Cullen et al. (1970) mounted flat pH electrodes on dog cortex and showed that brain ECF H^+ fell 10 to 15 meq/liter in 30 min at an arterial PO_2 of 27 Torr. The fall was faster if the dogs were permitted to hyperventilate in response to the hypoxia than when PCO_2 was controlled, but both showed large reductions due to brain lactic acid production. Eger et al. (1968) tested CSF HCO_3^- changes in normal subjects by an indirect method, by studying the "acclimatization" as a shift in position of the CO_2 response curve. They showed that after 8 hr of normoxic hyperventilation the CO_2 response curve was shifted left by 18% of the imposed (8-hr) PCO_2 shift. With hypoxic hyperventilation (acclimatization), the CO_2 response curve shifted left by 36% of the PCO_2 shift. Eight hours of hypoxia without a fall of PCO_2 caused a 3.9 Torr left shift. Their study then established that acclimatization as defined by leftward shift in the CO_2 response curve is about half due to the hypoxia, half to the associated hypocapnia.

Carbonic Anhydrase Inhibition

Acetazolamide administration (25 mg/kg) caused an immediate fall of the pH of brain extracellular fluid of 0.13±07 units in 15 dogs, when brain PCO_2 was kept at its normal level by hyperventilation (Figure 3). This produces cerebral vasodilitation. Cerebral blood flow was increased 69% by 25 mg/kg in dogs (Cotev et al., 1968) and 31.5% by 0.5 g total i.v. in 20 tests in 5 normal human males. This vasodilation is presumably responsible for the amelioration by acetazolamide of the cerebral symptoms of hypoxia at altitude. We found this

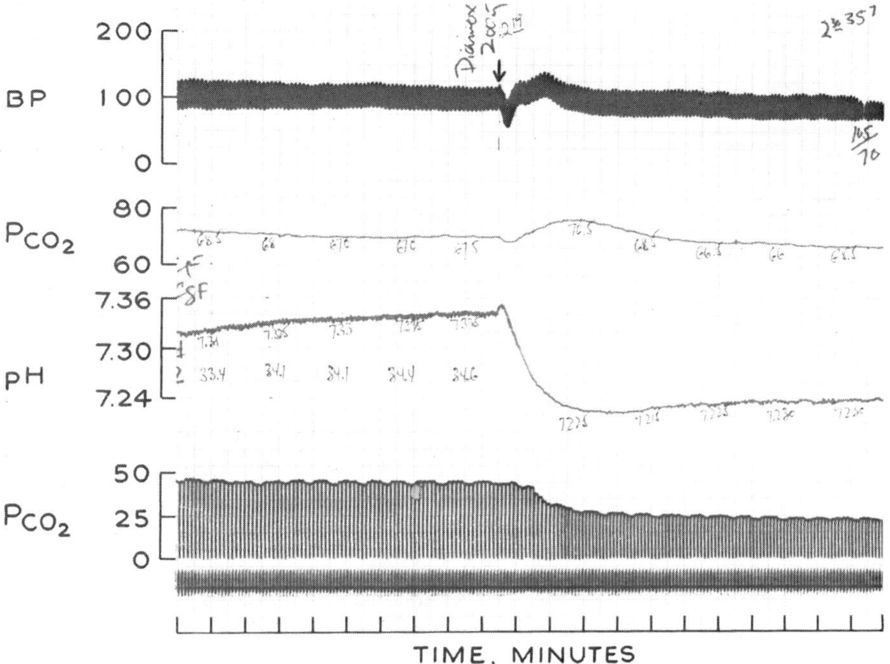

Figure 3. The inhibition of brain carbonic anhydrase by i.v. injection of 25 mg/kg acetazolamide in a dog leads to prompt acidification of brain ECF as recorded by a flat, brain surface pH electrode. Surface PCO_2 (2nd trace) was held constant by adjustment of ventilation, and reduction of end-tidal PCO_2 (bottom line).

vasodilation to be due to carbonic acidosis in brain, in which both H^+ and HCO_3^- are elevated (Severinghaus et al., 1969). Brain metabolism generates H^+ and HCO_3^-, not CO_2 gas, and the ions must be dehydrated to CO_2 to be carried away by blood.

Medullary Chemoreceptor Blood Flow

Feustel has recently determined blood flow in the central chemoreceptors with implanted hydrogen clearance electrodes (Feustel et al., 1981). At normal PCO_2 (in cats), flow averaged 60 (ml/100 g/min) in the chemoreceptor (at less than 0.5 mm depth). In adjacent white matter, flow was 30, while in cortex it averaged 100 ml/100 g/min. The chemoreceptor tissue histologically appears similar to the surrounding white matter, particularly in terms of numbers of mitochondria, and thus is believed to have a low metabolism in relation to its blood flow. Such an over perfusion should establish a tissue PCO_2 rather near that of arterial blood.

Central and Peripheral Chemoreceptor Interaction

We now understand that as peripheral drive increases, whether by hypoxia, acid, drugs or other drive, ventilation rises, PCO_2 falls, CSF pH becomes alkaline, and central chemoreceptor ventilatory drive decreases. The CSF HCO_3^- changes about half the amount required to correct the resulting CSF alkalosis. As peripheral drive fades way with residence at high altitude, CSF pH falls. High altitude natives have lost most of their ventilatory response to peripheral chemoreceptor stimuli and their CSF pH has been variously found normal or slightly acid (Sorensen and Milledge, 1971). Animals or patients with denervated peripheral chemoreceptors hypoventilate and show an acid CSF shift in pH of about 0.03 units (Bisgard et al., 1976). This extra central chemoreceptor drive should have the effect of driving ventilation upwards by about 6 to 9 liter/min, depending upon the slope of the CO_2 response. Since ventilation is slightly reduced, one may estimate that at least 6 to 9 liters of drive have been lost by denervation of the cartoid bodies.

Subthreshold Ventilatory Drive

The total respiratory drive thus seems to be far more than the 6 liter/min of actual ventilation. This paradox may be resolved if there exists substantial drive below the apneic threshold. The Oxford fan of CO_2 response curves determined at several PO_2 isopleths, in our subjects usually originates from a common point whose coordinates are at an average ventilation of about −20 liter/min and a PCO_2 of about 30 Torr (Crawford and Severinghaus, 1978; Irsigler et al., 1980). Were this point to accurately represent zero drive, the total resting ventilatory drive would approximate 26 liter/min. However, there are reasons for believing a linear extrapolation downward is inappropriate, because of the so called "dog leg" curvature often seen at the foot of CO_2 response curves. At present, we have no way of estimating accurately how much of a subthreshold drive exists.

Hypoxic Ventilatory Depression

When one induces hypoxia at constant end-tidal PCO_2, ventilation immediately rises but, after 5 to 15 min, it falls back towards normal (Figure 4). This is hypoxic ventilatory depression. Kagawa et al. (1980) showed that this depression was not reversed by naloxone and accordingly was not an endorphin effect. This depression was not included when we modeled the medullary chemoreceptor's role in altitude acclimatization, and thus the subject of chemical control is again in trouble. Two hypotheses of the mechanism of hypoxic depression are under consideration: (1) Increased chemoreceptor blood flow, reducing its tissue PCO_2 at constant $PaCO_2$. This mechanism would have limited effect and could not explain apnea or severe depression. (2)

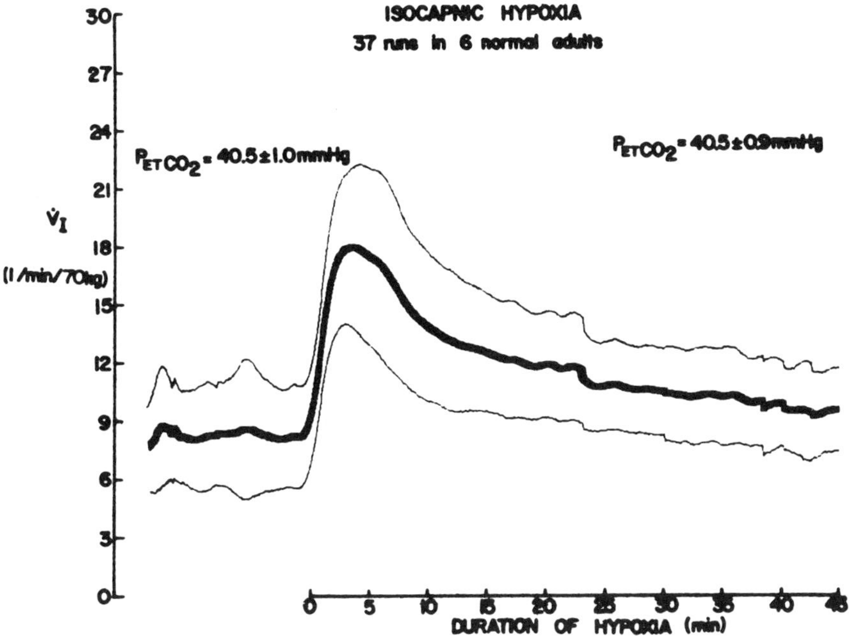

Figure 4. Hypoxic ventilatory depression during isocapneic hypoxia in 30 runs in 5 normal adults at an alveolar PO_2 of 45 Torr. Naloxone given at about 15 min of hypoxia failed to alter ventilation.

SOURCE: *Kagawa et al., (1980.)*

Intracellular acidosis in chemoreceptor sensors could be due to lactacidosis. In this hypothesis, chemoreceptors act like glass pH electrodes, such that intracellular acidosis would act in the same direction as extracellular acidosis, by making the ICF potential more negative.

Summary

The CSF acid-base regulation appears to depend primarily upon respiratory chemoreceptors on the ventral medullary surface, in which an alteration of 0.01 pH units induce about a 3 liter/min change of ventilation. At rest, such an increase would reduce arterial PCO_2 more than 10 Torr, which would increase CSF pH about 0.10 units. This suggests that the regulator has a 10-fold gain. Peripheral chemoreceptor drive to ventilation results in brain ECF alkalosis (typically 0.03 units at 3800 m altitude) which persists as long as the drive persists. This suggests that the total respiratory drive contains substantial subthreshold drive. The blood-brain barrier probably is capable of some active transport regulation of brain ECF acid-base balance, and is relatively impermeable to blood-borne acidosis and alkalosis over small ranges. Hypoxia in brain generates lactacidosis which contributes about half of the HCO_3^- reduction of acclimatization. However, there appear to be other mechanisms by which CSF HCO_3^- is altered or maintained, and they remain obscure. The difficulty of understanding the behavior of the CSF and brain ECF and ICF compartments reminds me of a Piet Hein grook:

"A bit beyond perception's reach I sometimes believe I see
That life is two locked boxes, each containing the other's key."

Ulrich Luft and Bruce Dill have had life-long love affairs with their mountains—affairs that seem to have kept them out of trouble for a long time. Perhaps I may be forgiven if I close with another grook of a philosophic nature probing into these love affairs:

"The human spirit sublimates the impulses it thwarts.
A healthy sex life mitigates the lust for other sports."

References

Bisgard, G.E., Forster, H.V., Orr, J.A., Buss, D.D., Rawlings, C.A., and Rasmussen, B. 1976. Hypoventilation in ponies after cartoid body denervation. *J. Appl. Physiol.* 40:184–190.

Cotev, S., Lee, J., and Severinghaus, J.W. 1968. Effect of acetazolamide on cerebral blood flow and cerebral tissue PO_2. *Anesthesiology* 29:471–477.

Crawford, R.D. and Severinghaus, J.W. 1978. CSF pH and ventilatory acclimatization to altitude. *J. Appl. Physiol.* 45:275–283.

Cullen, D.J., Cotev, S., Severinghaus, J.W., and Eger, II, E.I. 1970. The effects of hypoxia and isovolemic anemia on the halothane requirement (MAC) of dogs. II. The effects of acute hypoxia on halothane requirement and cerebral-surface PO_2, PCO_2, pH, and HCO_3^-. *Anesthesiology* 32:35–45.

Eger, E.I. II, Kellog, R.H., Mines, A.H., Lima-Ostos, M., Morrill, C.G., and Kent, D.W. 1968. Influence of CO_2 on ventilatory acclimatization to altitude. *J. Appl. Physiol.* 24:607–615.

Fencl, V., Vale, J.R., and Broch, J.A. 1969. Respiration and cerebral blood flow in metabolic acidosis and alkalosis in humans. *J. Appl. Physiol.* 27:67–76.

Feustel, P., Stafford, M.J., Allen, J., and Severinghaus, J.W. 1981. Central chemoreceptor blood flow estimated by hydrogen clearance. *Physiologist*, 24(4):115.

Houston, C.S. and Riley, R.L. 1947. Respiratory and circulatory changes during acclimatization to high altitude. *Am. J. Physiol.* 149:565–588.

Irsigler, G.B., Stafford, M.J., and Severinghaus, J.W. 1980. Relationship of CSF pH, O_2, and CO_2 responses in metabolic acidosis and alkalosis in humans. *J. Appl. Physiol.* 48:355–361.

Kagawa, S., Stafford, M.J., Waggener, T.B., and Severinghaus, J.W. 1980. No effect of naloxone on hypoxic ventilatory depression in adults. *Physiologist* 23(4):139.

Mitchell, R.A., Loeschcke, H.H., Massion, W.H., and Severinghaus, J.W. 1963. Respiratory responses mediated through superficial chemosensitive areas on the medulla. *J. Appl. Physiol.* 18:523–533.

Severinghaus, J.W. 1965. Electrochemical gradients for hydrogen and bicarbonate ions across the blood-CSF barrier in response to acid-base changes. In *Cerebrospinal Fluid and the Regulation of Ventilation*. Brooks, C., Kao, F., and Lloyd, B., eds. Oxford: Blackwell. pp. 247–259.

Severinghaus, J.W., Hamilton, F.N., and Cotev, S. 1969. Carbonic acid production and the role of carbonic anhydrase in decarboxylation in brain. *Biochem. J.* 114:703–705.

Severinghaus, J.W., Mitchell, R.A., Richardson, B.W., and Singer, M.M. 1963. Respiratory control at high altitude suggesting active transport regulation of CSF pH. *J. Appl. Physiol.* 18:1155–1166.

Sørensen, S. and Milledge, J.S. 1971. Cerebrospinal fluid acid-base composition at high altitude. *J. Appl. Physiol.* 31:28–30.

J.A. Loeppky and M.L. Riedesel, editors
OXYGEN TRANSPORT TO HUMAN TISSUES

Pulmonary Hypertension and Pulmonary Edema

Herbert N. Hultgren

The etiology of high altitude pulmonary edema (HAPE) remains uncertain. Rapid exposure to an altitude exceeding 8000 ft by an unacclimatized individual will result in HAPE in approximately 0.5% of ascents by adult males. Heavy exercise during the first few days after arrival will result in a higher incidence. The incidence of HAPE is about 5 to 10 times more common in children and adolescents. Subclinical HAPE with only minimal disability may occur in a larger number of individuals. The signs and symptoms of HAPE rapidly resolve upon descent, bed rest, and with the administration of oxygen (Hultgren et al., 1961; Hultgren, 1978). Some individuals appear to be susceptible to recurrent episodes of HAPE and one rare congenital abnormality of the pulmonary circulation (absence of one pulmonary artery) may predispose individuals to HAPE (Hackett et al., 1980). Further studies of the mechanism of HAPE are clearly needed. It is estimated that over a hundred serious and occasionally fatal cases occur annually in the United States alone.

The incidence is higher in mountaineers but HAPE occurs in skiers and tourists as well. Mechanisms involved in HAPE probably have important sea level analogs particularly with certain forms of the acute respiratory distress syndrome. Pulmonary edema is a common final cause of death in a wide variety of sea level diseases.

This discussion will be directed toward 4 aspects of the mechanism of HAPE with reference to pulmonary hypertension: HAPE studies at high altitude, response of the pulmonary circulation to hypoxia in subjects with a prior history of HAPE, hemodynamic models of HAPE, and the role of high pulmonary blood flow and capillary permeability. Information regarding the pathophysiology of HAPE is limited by the paucity of studies of the acute illness at high altitude, its low incidence in man and the lack of an adequate animal model.

High Altitude Studies

Only 6 published hemodynamic studies have been performed in patients with HAPE during the acute stage, before therapy or descent. The mean altitude where these studies were done was 13,000 ft. The mean pulmonary artery (PA) pressure was 60 mm Hg and the pulmonary wedge (PAW) pressure was 3.0 mm Hg with a mean pulmonary arteriolar resistance (PAR) of 1145 dyne·sec/cm^5. The mean arterial oxygen saturation while breathing ambient air was 66%.

Five studies have been performed in patients with HAPE after removal from an altitude of 13,620 ft to 9,760 ft. In these patients, the mean PA pressure was 29 mm Hg, PAW pressure: 5 mm Hg, PAR: 670 dyne·sec/cm^5, and arterial oxygen saturation: 76%. These data are summarized in Figure 1 and compared with normal values for healthy high altitude residents living at 12,400 ft.

Hemodynamic data clearly indicate that left ventricular failures cannot be implicated in the genesis of HAPE. The PAW pressure accurately reflects the left ventricular filling pressure. In one patient with HAPE, the cardiac catheter fortuitously entered the left atrium via a patent foramen ovale and a normal left atrial pressure was recorded (Fred et al., 1962). The data also indicate that the pulmonary vasoconstriction in HAPE is labile and initiated largely by hypoxia. This would explain the lower pressures with higher arterial oxygen saturations seen in the group of patients studied after descent. Other studies in acute HAPE have shown a rapid fall in PA pressure with oxygen breathing and a rapid further rise in pressure with acute hypoxia (Hultgren et al., 1964).

With the development of alveolar edema, arterial oxygen saturation in HAPE falls to very low levels (Hultgren and Wilson, 1981). In 26 patients with severe and moderate HAPE (7 and 19 patients, respectively) studied upon hospital admission, the mean arterial PO_2 was 42 mm Hg with a range from 23 to 56 mm Hg (Table1). These studies were performed at a substantially lower elevation (sea level to 4100 ft) than that at which HAPE appeared (greater than 8,000 ft). Thus at high altitude, HAPE is associated with a profound decrease in arterial oxygen saturation and a concomitant decrease in mixed venous oxygen saturation. When arterial oxygen saturation is 60%, the mixed venous oxygen saturation may be below 30%. While a reduction in mixed venous oxygen saturation alone does not cause pulmonary vasoconstriction, one must consider its possible role in altering capillary permeability when accompanied by a decrease in alveolar PO_2.

Response of the Pulmonary Circulation to Hypoxia

Is the individual's susceptibility to HAPE related to an abnormal response of the pulmonary circulation to acute hypoxia? In 7 subjects with a history of

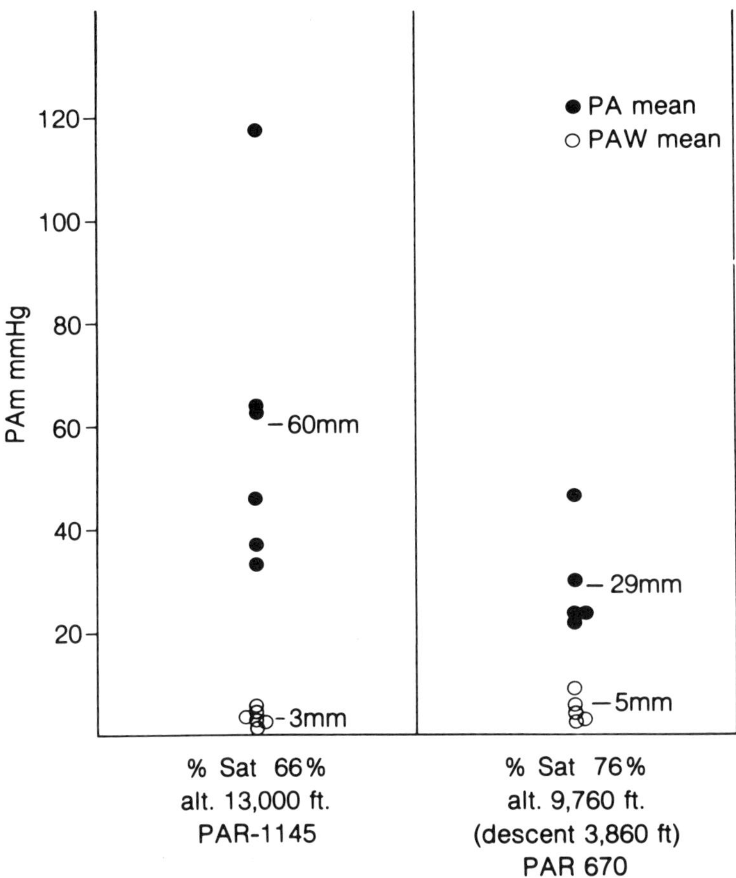

Figure 1. Hemodynamic data from studies during HAPE. On the left are data from 6 patients studied at 13,000 ft. Five patients on the right were studied at 9,760 ft after descent from 13,620 ft (Fred et al., 1962; Hultgren et al., 1964; Penaloza and Sime, 1969; Roy et al., 1969). *Note*: PAR=pulmonary arteriolar resistance (dyne·sec/cm^5).

HAPE studied in our laboratory, the mean PA pressure rose from 15 to 24 mm Hg during 10 min of breathing 11% oxygen. In 30 controls reported in the literature and collected from our files and studied in a similar manner, the PA pressure rose from 13 to 18 mm Hg (Figure 2). Indian researchers (Viswanathan et al., 1969a, b) performed similar studies on a larger number of subjects and concluded that those who had experienced HAPE had a slightly higher rise in PA pressure during hypoxia (15.3 to 24.8 mm Hg) compared to controls (12.8 to 18.6 mm Hg). However, if one calculates the PAR in the Indian study, the increase in PAR in the control group was essentially the same as in the HAPE group (39 versus 26%). Resting PA mean pressures were slightly higher in the HAPE group. It can be concluded from these studies that subjects susceptible

Table 1. Arterial Blood Gases and pH in HAPE.

	Age (yr)	Room air PO_2 (mm Hg)	Oxygen PO_2 (mm Hg)	Room air PCO_2 (mm Hg)	Oxygen PCO_2 (mm Hg)	Room air pH	Oxygen pH
Mean	29	42	57	28	28	7.46	7.41
Range	19–56	23–56	45–115	21–32	27–36	7.40–7.58	7.31–7.52

Blood gas values in 26 patients with severe and moderate HAPE, measured after descent while breathing room air and following the administration of high flow oxygen.

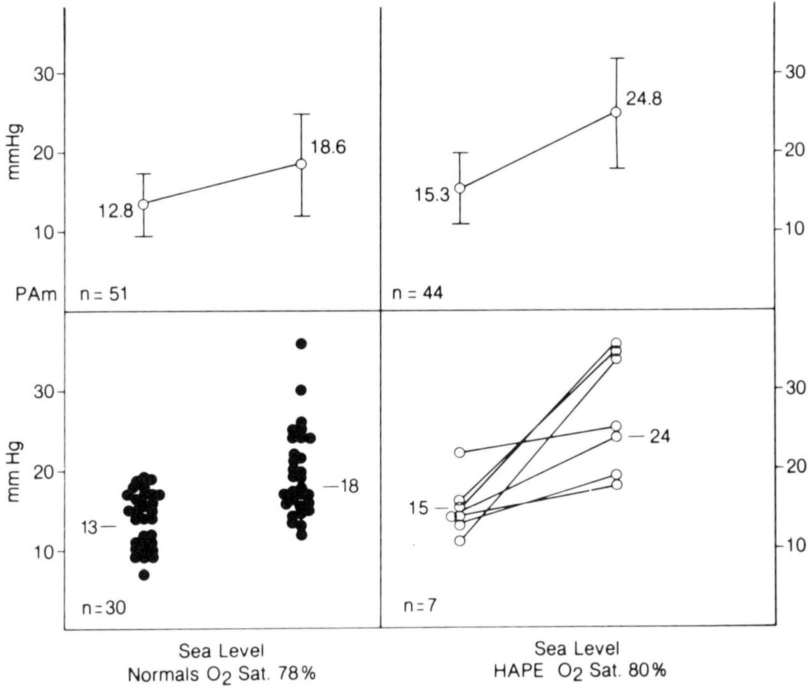

Figure 2. Response of mean PA pressure to 11% oxygen breathing in 7 subjects with a prior history of HAPE compared to 30 normal subjects. Studies performed at sea level (Westcott et al., 1951; Doyle et al., 1952). The upper panels show mean values of similar subjects studied in India (Viswanathan et al., 1969a, b).

to HAPE studied at sea level do not exhibit an abnormal increase in PA pressure or PAR during short periods of hypoxia. However, they may have slightly higher resting PA mean pressures than control subjects.

Different results are obtained if the hypoxia studies are done at high altitude (Hultgren et al., 1964; Penaloza and Sime, 1969). In 11 patients studied at 12,400 ft following recovery from HAPE, the mean PA pressure rose from 33 to 52 mm Hg during acute hypoxia. Normal high altitude residents studied in a similar manner exhibited a PA pressure rise from 21 to 40 mm Hg. The resting pressures again are higher in the subjects susceptible to HAPE but the pressure rise and increase in PAR was actually greater in the control subjects ($p < 0.05$). Four normal subjects studied at 14,200 ft with a more severe degree of acute hypoxia had lower resting PA pressures than the subjects susceptible to HAPE at a lower altitude (Figure 3).

Another method of studying susceptibility is to expose HAPE subjects to high altitude and 24 hr after arrival examine the resting PA pressure and the

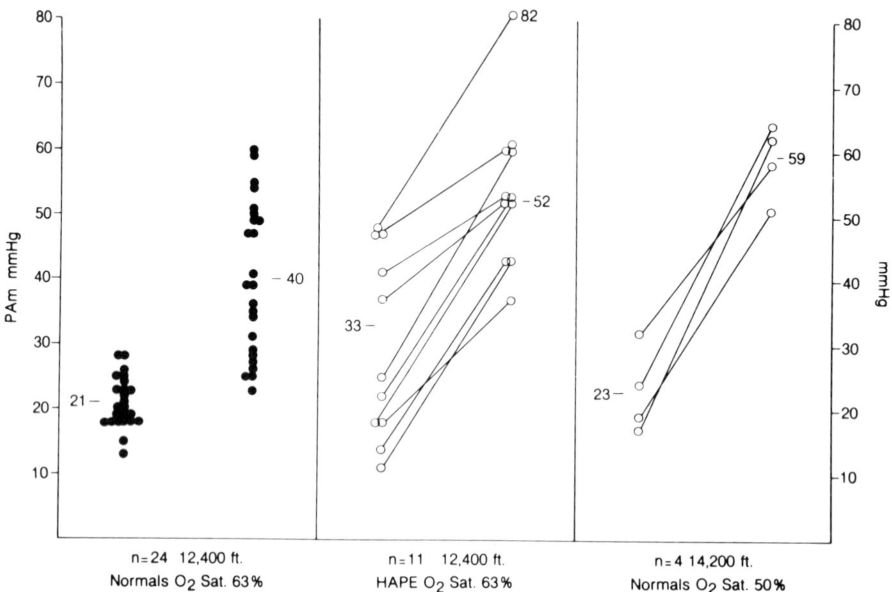

Figure 3. Response of mean PA pressure to acute hypoxia in 11 subjects with a prior history of HAPE compared to 24 normal high altitude residents. These studies were performed at 12,400 ft (Hultgren et al., 1964). On right are results from 4 healthy subjects residing and studied at 14,200 ft.

response to supine exercise (Hultgren et al., 1971). In 5 such subjects brought from sea level to 10,152 ft, the resting PA mean pressure rose from 14.0 to 39.0 mm Hg (Figure 4). During supine exercise, the subjects susceptible to HAPE had a mean pressure rise from 39 (rest) to 53 mm Hg (exercise). At sea level, only one subject had a slightly abnormal pressure rise during exercise. At high altitude, 4 of the 5 subjects had an abnormal elevation of resting PA pressure and all had an abnormal rise during exercise. No data are available regarding the effect of acute hypoxia upon recent arrivals at high altitude.

These studies involved only a small number of subjects but do permit certain tentative conclusions. Subjects susceptible to HAPE do not appear to demonstrate an abnormal PA pressure response to hypoxia at sea level or at high altitude. Resting PA pressures are higher at sea level and high altitude than normal controls. When brought to high altitude, these susceptible subjects show a greater rise in resting and exercise PA pressures than control subjects. It seems unlikely therefore that acute hypoxia *alone* is responsible for HAPE. The development of HAPE must involve factors other than acute hypoxia resulting from ascent to high altitude by an unacclimatized subject and its combination with exercise and a latent period of at least 24 hr. Hopefully the employment of noninvasive methods of studying pulmonary function and the

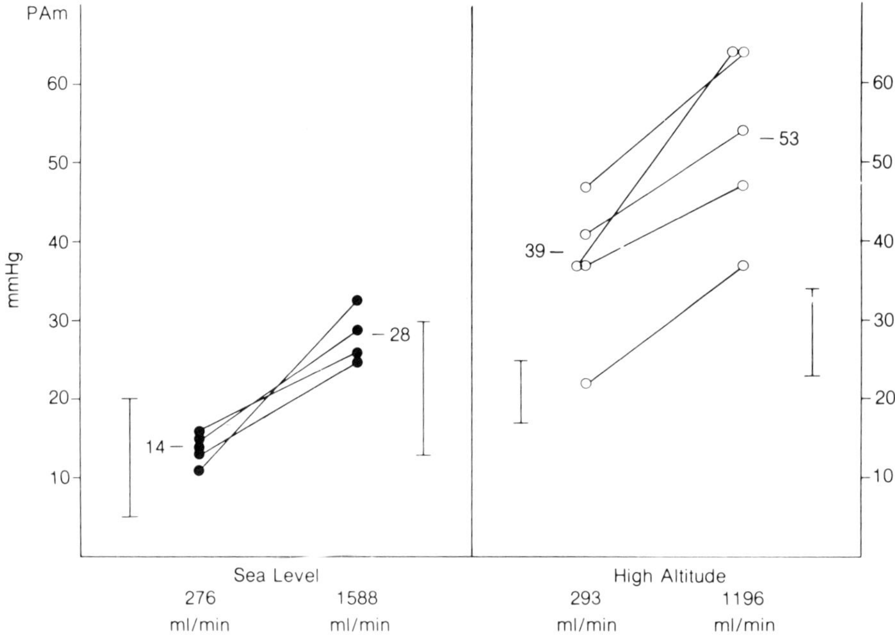

Figure 4. Response to supine exercise at sea level and high altitude (10,152 ft) of 5 subjects with a prior history of HAPE. Altitude studies were performed 24 hr after arrival. Mean ±1.0 S.D. of normal values are indicated by the vertical lines. Mean resting and exercise oxygen consumptions are indicated below each panel.

pulmonary circulation combined with specific pharmacolgic interventions in larger numbers of subjects will provide more information regarding the effect of high altitude upon the pulmonary circulation in HAPE. Studies of the response of the PA pressure to exercise may be more effective in revealing pulmonary circulation abnormalities in subjects susceptible to HAPE than studies performed during acute hypoxia.

Hemodynamic Models of HAPE

The concept of high blood flow (overperfusion) pulmonary edema as it relates to HAPE should be examined in view of the data obtained in man (Hultgren et al., 1956). According to this concept, acute altitude exposure in susceptible subjects results in uneven obstruction of the pulmonary vascular bed. While the major effect may be uneven hypoxic arteriolar constriction, other factors may be involved such as platelet or fibrin deposition with subsequent vascular obstruction. It is possible that the anatomic variations in the thickness of the muscular media of the precapillary arterioles may be involved. Uneven pulmonary vascular constriction and obstruction will result in areas of the lung with greatly increased blood flow and areas where flow is greatly reduced. In areas of high flow, the high pulmonary artery pressure will be transmitted directly to the capillary bed with resultant elevation of capillary pressure and edema formation. The elevated pressure may distend the arterioles thus reducing further the precapillary resistance with the result that the pulmonary venules distal to the capillaries now become the site of the pressure drop. Chest X-rays of patients with HAPE indicate that the edema is patchy in distribution with clear areas between areas of infiltrate. The areas of the lung just above the diaphragm are usually clear. Is this due to more intense vasoconstriction? For some reason not clearly understood, the right middle lung field is most commonly involved in mild or moderate HAPE.

There are two experimental animal models of high blood flow pulmonary edema which mimic the hemodynamics of HAPE, i.e., pulmonary edema with pulmonary hypertension and a normal left atrial pressure. The hemodynamics of these models must be compared to those of clinical HAPE.

Staub and his associates have employed sheep with cannulation of the pulmonary lymphatics to measure lymph flow and lymph protein concentration (Ohkuda et al., 1978; Staub, 1980). Uneven pulmonary vascular occlusion was produced by balloon catheter obstruction or glass bead embolization. Cardiac output was maintained by saline infusions. In these preparations, lung lymph flow increased from 5.7 to 9.3 ml/hr, indicating the development of pulmonary edema. The increase in lymph flow is more significant than it appears since the diffusing surface for fluid exchange had been reduced by 67% due to vascular obstruction. In these preparations, the mean PA pressure rose from 18 to 28 mm Hg. Left atrial pressure remained unchanged (10.8 mm Hg and 10.5 mm Hg) and cardiac output fell from 3.8 to 3.3 liter/min. The protein concentration of the lymph was 72% (lymph/plasma ratio). This indicated that capillary permeability had increased because the usual lymph protein concentration in preparations where left atrial pressure is raised is 58%. The cause of the increase in capillary permeability is unclear since it has previously been shown that neither hypoxia alone or an increase in pressure alone will increase permeability.

Another hemodynamic model of high flow pulmonary edema has been studied in our laboratory (Hultgren et al., 1956; Hultgren, 1978). Open-chest dogs were prepared with a roller pump bypass of the right ventricle to control pulmonary blood flow and to prevent right ventricular failure. Sequential ligation of the right pulmonary artery and the pulmonary arteries to the left middle and left lower pulmonary lobes was then performed at 15-min intervals. This results in the entire cardiac output perfusing one lobe (Figure 5). Under these conditions the perfused lobe becomes swollen, rigid, and a continuous murmur and thrill can be detected over the surface. After 10 to 20 min, pulmonary edema appears, the airways fill with fluid, and the preparation terminates due to asphyxia. The edematous lobe has a specific gravity of 0.93

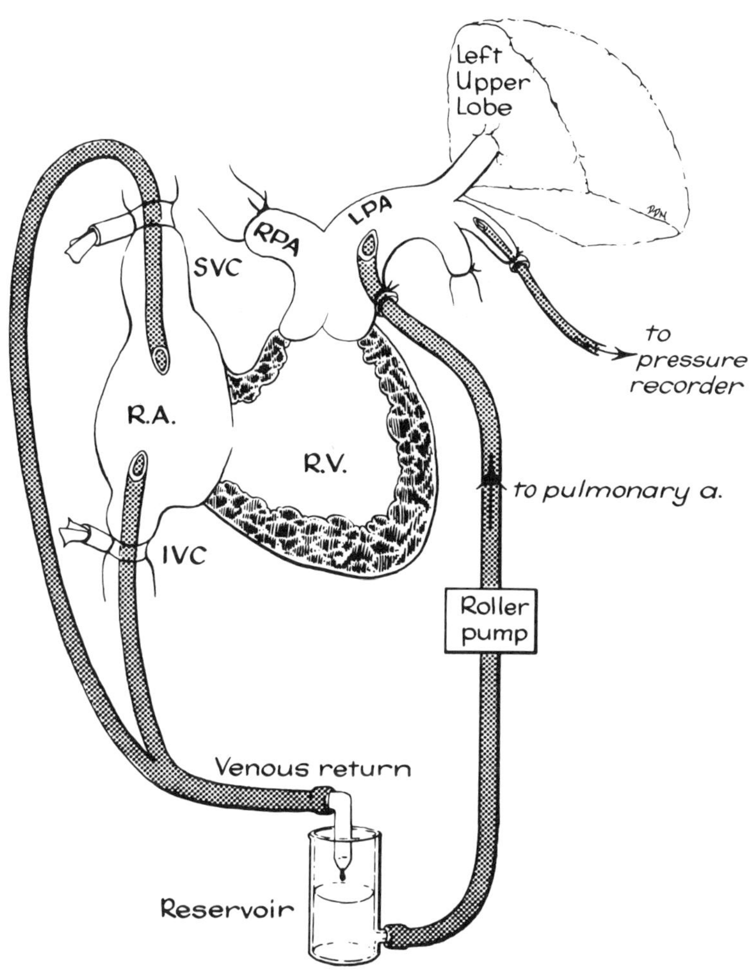

Figure 5. Experimental technique to produce high flow pulmonary edema in the open chest dog preparation. *Note*: SVC and IVC = superior and inferior vena cavae; RA = right atrium; RV = right ventricle; RPA and LPA = right and left pulmonary arteries.

compared to 0.56 for the normal lung. Histologic study reveals diffuse pulmonary edema. At the time of edema formation, the mean PA pressure was 48 mm Hg, the left atrial pressure 4 mm Hg, and the cardiac output 2.0 liter/min. The PA wedge pressure was 6 mm Hg. These pressures are similar to those observed in clinical cases of HAPE (Table 2). The pressures are higher than those observed in Staub's preparation (1980). This is probably due to the fact that right ventricular bypass was employed to prevent right ventricular failure. If a bypass is not employed, right ventricular failure will result with a marked drop in cardiac output and pulmonary edema will not occur. Measure-

Table 2. Hemodynamics of Pulmonary Edema.

	HAPE	Sheep	Dogs
PAm (mm Hg)	45	28	48
PAW (mm Hg)	4	10.5	6
PAR (dyne · sec/cm^5)	908	596	1680
PAR (dyne · sec/cm^5)[a]	1500	320	800
CO (liter/min)	3.0	3.3	2.0
CO (liter/min/50 kg)	2.2	4.4	4.2

Hemodynamics of HAPE in humans (11 clinical studies at high altitude) compared with similar data from the sheep (n = 6) and dog (n = 6) models.
Note: PAm = pulmonary artery mean pressure; PAW = pulmonary artery wedge pressure; PAR = pulmonary arteriolar resistance; CO = cardiac output.
[a]Resistance corrected to CO/50 kg.

ments of the weight of each lobe of the normal dog lung indicated that the left upper lobe constitutes approximately 25% of the total weight of the lung. If we assume that the size of the pulmonary vascular bed is proportional to the weight of each lobe, we can estimate that in the dog model pulmonary flow was increased by 6 times.

High Pulmonary Flow and Capillary Permeability

Protein concentration of edema fluid is probably comparable to the protein concentration of lymph (Vreim et al., 1976). If left atrial pressure is elevated to produce pulmonary edema, the protein concentration of edema fluid and lymph is approximately 58% of the plasma protein concentration. Under these circumstances, capillary permeability is not increased. In preparations where pulmonary edema is associated with an increase in capillary permeability, the lymph protein concentration is usually increased to levels greater than 70%. In Staub's sheep model, high flow pulmonary edema was associated with an increased lymph protein concentration (72%). In the overperfusion dog model, the edema fluid protein concentration was 45% (range: 17 to 76%). In one patient with HAPE edema, fluid removed by tracheal suction revealed an edema fluid/plasma concentration ratio of 58%. This suggests that capillary permeability was not significantly increased.

In view of these studies, the question of altered capillary permeability in HAPE remains open. It seems likely that in mild or moderate cases of short duration capillary permeability is not increased. Rapid clearing of pulmonary infiltrates in 24 to 48 hr during bed rest and oxygen therapy would be compatible with a low protein edema fluid. In severe cases of HAPE, especially when treatment is delayed, slow clearing of infiltrates over a period as long as a week may be observed. In fatal cases, hyaline membranes and red cells may be seen in the alveoli (Arias-Stella and Kruger, 1963; Nayak et al., 1964). These observations suggest a high protein concentration in edema fluid.

Several factors could therefore be responsible for increased capillary permeability in HAPE in view of the above observations: prolonged time-course of the illness, alveolar hypoxia, very low mixed venous oxygen saturation, high shear forces and turbulence due to increased flow, and finally, capillary injury by substances released from the pulmonary vascular bed. Further studies of HAPE in man and in animal models are clearly needed to answer some of these important questions regarding the etiology of this unique form of pulmonary edema.

References

Arias-Stella, J. and Kruger, H. 1963. Pathology of high altitude pulmonary edema. *Arch. Pathol.* 76:147–157.

Doyle, J., Wilson, J.S., and Warren, J.V. 1952. The pulmonary vascular responses to short-term hypoxia in human subjects. *Circulation* 5:263–270.

Fred, H., Schmidt, A.M., Bates, T., and Hecht, H.H. 1962. Acute pulmonary edema of altitude: clinical and physiologic observations. *Circulation* 25:929–937.

Hackett, P.H., Creagh, C.E., Grover, R.F., Honigman, B., Reeves, J.T., Sophocles, A.M., and Hardenbroek, M.V. 1980. High-altitude pulmonary edema in persons without the right pulmonary artery. *N. Engl. J. Med.* 302:1070–1073.

Hultgren, H.N. 1978. High altitude pulmonary edema. In *Lung Water and Solute Exchange*. Staub, N.C., ed. New York: Marcel Dekker, Inc. pp. 437–464.

Hultgren, H.N., Grover, R.F., and Hartley, L.H. 1971. Abnormal circulatory responses to high altitude in subjects with a previous history of high altitude pulmonary edema. *Circulation* 44:759–770.

Hultgren, H.N., Lopez, C., Lundberg, E., and Miller, H. 1964. Physiologic studies of pulmonary edema at high altitude. *Circulation* 29:393–408.

Hultgren, H.N., Robinson, M.C., and Wuerflein, R.D. 1956. Overperfusion pulmonary edema. *Circulation* 33 & 34 (Suppl.):III–132.

Hultgren, H.N., Spickard, W.B., Hellriegel, K. and Houston, C.S. 1961. High altitude pulmonary edema. *Medicine (Baltimore)* 40:289–313.

Hultgren, H.N., and Wilson, R. 1981. Blood gas abnormalities and optimum therapy in high altitude pulmonary edema. *Clin Res.* 29:99A.

Nayak, N.C., Roy, S., and Narayanan, T.K. 1964. Pathologic features of altitude sickness. *Am. J. Pathol.* 45:381–391.

Ohkuda, K., Nakahara, K., Weidner, W.J., Binder, A., and Staub, N.C. 1978. Lung field exchange after uneven pulmonary artery obstruction in sheep. *Circ. Res.* 43:152–161.

Penaloza, D. and Sime, F. 1969. Circulatory dynamics during high altitude pulmonary edema. *Am. J. Cardiol.* 23:369–378.

Roy, S.B., Guleria, J.S., Khanna, P.K., Manchanda, S.C., Pande, J.N., and Subba, P.S. 1969. Hemodynamic studies in high altitude pulmonary edema. *Br. Heart J.* 31:52–58.

Staub, N. 1980. The pathogenesis of pulmonary edema. *Prog Cardiovasc. Dis.* 23:53–80.

Viswanathan, R., Jain, S.K., and Subramanian, S. 1969a. Pulmonary edema of high altitude III. Pathogenesis. *Am. Rev. Respir. Dis.* 100:342–349.

Viswanathan, R., Jain, S.K., Subramanian, S., Subramanian, T.A.V., Dua, G.L., and Giri, J. 1969b. Pulmonary edema of high altitude II. Clinical, aerohemodynamic, and biochemical studies in a group with history of pulmonary edema of high altitude. *Am. Rev. Respir. Dis.* 100:334–341.

Vreim, C.E., Snashall, P.D., and Staub, N.C. 1976. Protein composition of lung fluids in anesthetized dogs with acute cardiogenic edema. *Am. J. Physiol.* 231:1466–1469.

Westcott, R.N., Fowler, N.O., Scott, R.C., Hauenstein, V.D., and McGuire, J. 1951. Anoxia and human pulmonary vascular resistance. *J. Clin. Invest.* 30:957–970.

J.A. Loeppky and M.L. Riedesel, editors
OXYGEN TRANSPORT TO HUMAN TISSUES

Altitude Illness: Manifestations, Etiology, and Management

Charles S. Houston

Altitude Illness

My assignment is to discuss the manifestations and etiology of altitude illness—the clinical counterpart of the elegant and sophisticated studies presented elsewhere in this volume. Emphasis will be on persons who are wise or foolish as they go to altitude, and—if unwise—who fall ill as a result.

Twenty-two years ago, Andre Cournand (1959) wrote:

> "According to reliable authorities it is a sign of age when an investigator chooses to look backward rather than forward... unless I delude myself, a more profound urge guided my choice, a youthful urge if I may say so: to apprehend the progressive conquest of knowledge in its actual state and thereby to give a logical form to intellectual genealogy; to establish a census of epistemological obstacles which have been surmounted; to identify myself with other human beings who have spent a vast deal of energy on matters in which excellence is difficult to achieve and which procure moments of serene satisfaction rarely indeed... and more urgently, to become aware of the impact of philosophy, dogmatism and authority upon the fruits of free inquiry."

Cournand then reviewed beautifully the historical development of our understanding of the pulmonary circulation. In that same spirit, I will mention some of the important historical steps toward understanding altitude and altitude illness.

Appreciation of the pains of reaching high altitude goes back a long way (Houston, 1980). Plutarch wrote that Alexander lost hundreds of his troops as they crossed the Hindu Kush over the Khawak Pass (11,600 ft), but whether from cold or hunger or altitude is unclear. The name Hindu Kush derives from "man" and "to kill." In the first century of the Christian era, Chinese traders described the headache, dizziness, and nausea experienced when crossing the Greater and Lesser Headache Mountains, probably peaks on the high Tibetan plateau. In 1300, Marco Polo noted that the air among the lofty mountains of Yunnan was "so unwholesome and pestilential that it is death to any foreigner," adding that fires did not burn so well there. The most famous account of altitude illness was written by the Jesuit Joseph de Acosta who in 1571 accompanied the Conquistadores into Peru, crossing a pass called Periacaca. Gilbert has shown that this pass, not on modern maps, was 15,890 ft high and understandably described by Acosta as "the highest place in the world." Acosta's vivid description is well-known:

> "...when I went up the highest part of the range, almost immediately I suffered anguish so severe that I had the idea of throwing myself from the cavalcade to the ground...I retched and vomited so violently I thought I was dying...One man had thrown himself on the ground and was screaming from the intense pain which the passage of the Periacaca had caused."

Yet before Acosta some Andean natives ventured much higher and even lived and worked at altitudes thought in later centuries to be insupportable of life. Echevarria (1979) recently summarized archaeological discoveries of the last forty years, showing that the early Incas and their predecessors, as early as 1000 A.D. climbed many high Andean peaks and buried their dead on these summits, often above 19,000 ft. Well-constructed buildings have been found at 20,000 ft, suggesting that these ancients spent more than a little time at altitude. We have no record of their symptoms.

Conway in 1894 wrote: "Mountain sickness was upon me, an agony of helplessness and dispair... a splitting head, and heart and lungs going crazy." His contemporaries were equally graphic:

> "I found myself lying flat on my back... incapable of making the least exertion. We knew the enemy was upon us and that we were experiencing our first attack of mountain sickness. We were feverish, had intense headaches, and were unable to satisfy our desire for air except by breathing with open mouths. Headache for all three of us was intense and rendered us almost frantic or crazy."

And Fitzgerald:

> "I got up and once more tried to go on, but I was only able to advance one or two steps at a time, and then I had to stop, panting for breath, my struggles alternating with violent fits of nausea. At times I would fall down, and each time had greater difficulty rising; black specks swam across my sight; I was like one walking in a dream so dizzy and sick that the whole mountain seemed whirling around with me."

The first detailed medical description of the several forms of altitude illness was written by Ravenhill (1913) who divided his 38 cases into "normal," "cardiac," and "nervous" *puna* (the local name for mountain sickness), a grouping similar to one in use today.

Until the end of the 19th century, the cause of this misery was in doubt; emanations from lead or antimony ores were blamed (the Spanish word for antimony is *soroche*, the term used in parts of the Andes for mountain sickness), and in both the Andes and Himalayas vapors from certain poisonous plants and shrubs were thought responsible. Acosta had been quite specific: "*...there the element of the air is so subtile and delicate as is not proportionable with the breathing of man...*" Barcroft added conclusive evidence in 1919 when he spent ten days in a "glass house" especially built so that the percentage of oxygen inside could be adjusted to simulate any altitude, while the pressure remained that of sea level. He wrote:

> "... on the morning of the 6th day I awoke with typical symptoms of mountain sickness: vomiting, intense headache, and difficulty of vision. There was no cause other than oxygen want to which my sickness could be attributed... the partial pressure of oxygen corresponded to that of 18,000 ft... "

Descriptions of mountain sickness were so common in the 19th century that failure to mention them cast doubt on the climber's veracity. One does not hear similar descriptions today, even though modern transport enables thousands of persons to reach dangerous altitude much more rapidly. Instead more serious problems are being encountered as ill-prepared persons go too high too fast.

Paul Bert's studies in a decompression chamber and those of others in balloons or on mountains, established that lack of oxygen was the primary cause of mountain sickness which could be minimized by slow ascent. Generations of altitude residents were shown to have greater tolerance and work capacity than visiting sea level natives and oxygen was proven to prevent and to relieve symptoms. After a few false leads like the phlogiston theory and belief in the active secretion of oxygen by the lungs, the importance of oxygen to life and health had been proven. Though this is not the place to describe the evolution of knowledge about oxygen and barometric pressure, a few less well-known historic persons should be mentioned.

Berti in 1639 built the first crude barometer, a tall lead pipe appropriately closed with stop-cocks, filled with water and fastened to the outer wall of his house. He showed that water stood only 34 ft high in the tube, and above it was a vacuum—previously denied by many scientists and by the Church. Torricelli, who probably originated the idea for this experiment, soon realized that by using mercury instead of water the tube could be much shorter; from this prototype came the mercurial barometer.

Berti's experiment confirmed Balliani's earlier letter to Galileo, and firmly established the weight of air and existence of a vacuum. Perier, probably inspired by Pascal, carried a mercury barometer to the top of a small mountain and showed that the weight or pressure of the atmosphere decreased with increasing altitude. His was the precursor of many measurements which produced the familiar pressure altitude curves. Air was shown to be compressible, to have weight, and to be thinner at higher altitude, just as Acosta had described.

Meanwhile the composition of air was being studied throughout Europe by Von Helmont, Boyle, Hooke, and others. Less known is John Mayow who in 1674 showed that a candle would soon be extinguished and a mouse would die if either were confined in a closed jar. Of this he wrote:

> "I take it for granted that the air contains certain particles termed by us elsewhere nitro-aerial which are absolutely indispensible for the product of fire... that nitro-aerial spirit is by means of respiration transmitted into the mass of blood and the fermentation and heating of the blood are produced by it."

Carl Scheele generated oxygen, and on September 30th, 1774 wrote Lavoisier describing its importance and exactly how it could be made, two years before the latter's announcement.

So much for the history of air. Berti, Perier, Mayow, and Scheele laid foundations on which others have built, and they deserved honor along with better known figures who refined and publicized their work. What we know about hypoxia and altitude illness depends on them.

Classification

Different ways of classifying hypoxic illness have been offered. Classification by etiology is not particularly useful since all forms are due to lack of oxygen. A purely clinical classification is imprecise because manifestations and symptoms vary so widely. The same is true for divisions by organ systems or by functions. Dickinson (1981) separates hypoxia from mountain sickness and divides the latter into benign or malignant forms. This approach leaves hanging the matter of a common biochemical cause and disregards the diversity of the clinical picture over time and between individuals, and the influence of speed of ascent and altitude reached. Dickinson's analogy to hypertension seems far-fetched for similar reasons.

A simple and widely used classification (Houston, 1980) is based on the concept that hypoxic illness is a continuum or spectrum of signs, symptoms, and biochemical aberrations, any or many of which dominate the clinical picture at different times and in different circumstances (Table 1).

Classifications are important because they help to ensure that different observers are not confusing apples with oranges. Lacking specific pathophysiological categories, this simple classification is general and yet useful.

Incidence

Because there have been many different definitions and because of the wide range in speed of ascent and altitude reached, and different methods of

Table 1. Classification of Altitude Illness.

Acute hypoxia	Mental impairment and usually, collapse after rapid exposure, above 18,000 ft. Rare on mountains.
Acute mountain sickness (AMS)	Headache, nausea, vomiting, sleep disturbance, dyspnea. Above 7–8,000 ft. Self-limited. Common.
High altitude pulmonary edema (HAPE)	Dyspnea, cough, weakness, headache, stupor, and rarely death. Above 9–10,000 ft. Requires rapid descent or treatment early.
High altitude cerebral edema (HACE)	Severe headache, hallucinations, ataxia, weakness, impaired mentation, stupor, and death. Above 10–12,000 ft. Uncommon. Descent mandatory.
Subacute and chronic mountain sickness (CMS)	Failure to recover from AMS may necessitate descent. Some develop dyspnea, fatigue, plethora, and heart failure, after years of asymptomatic residence, at altitude. Rare.
Altitude related problems	Retinal hemorrhage, edema, thrombo-phlebitis and embolism, cold injury.
Chronic conditions made worse at altitude	Sickle trait, chronic cardiac, or pulmonary disease.

collecting and analyzing information, firm data on incidence is lacking. Reports by Hackett et al. (1976) near Everest, Snyder in Kenya, Gerhard on McKinley, Singh in the Himalayas (Singh et al., 1969), Houston on Rainier and Anholm in Colorado, it appears that 25 to 30% of persons going rapidly to 10,000 ft will experience headache, nausea, excessive fatigue, and dyspnea in some combination. Five or 10% will show evidence of fluid in the lungs (early pulmonary edema) and/or brain malfunction, and a few otherwise healthy persons will die from altitude illness. Some deaths are attributable to a complication of hypoxia by a problem such as a congenital circulatory defect, sickle trait, respiratory infection, coronary artery disease, myocardial weakness, or chronic pulmonary disease. Thromboembolism, a common concomitant of dehydration and altitude polycythemia, is a significant hazard.

Above 14,000 ft, the incidence of all forms of altitude illness doubles, and at 18,000 ft practically everyone who goes up too rapidly is affected; mortality is as high as 1 to 2%. The risk is increased by the impaired judgment and perception caused by hypoxia, and by hallucinations which are often suppressed or denied. For example, a competent internist climber had 3 episodes of altitude illness and hallucinated, denied the severity of his condition, and later erased his memory. He probably survived only because his companions clearly appreciated how impaired he was and overruled his objections to descend.

Dickinson (1981) has made a good point in separating acute hypoxic illness from mountain sickness. Healthy persons who become abruptly hypoxic in aircraft, during anesthesia, or from carbon monoxide poisoning, trauma, respiratory obstruction, or respiratory muscle paralysis are at much greater risk and show somewhat different signs and symptoms then climbers. Though this is not the place to discuss such causes of acute hypoxia, it may be considered the extreme end of the spectrum of signs and symptoms which we call altitude illness.

Acute mountain sickness (AMS) begins a few hours after arrival, grows worse during the night and early morning, and usually improves in 36 to 72 hr leaving no residuals. It has been described as a bad hangover. Symptoms experienced most frequently on going above 7 to 8,000 ft in a few hours or above 11 to 12,000 ft in a day or two are: impaired night vision, headache, anorexia and nausea, dyspnea, cardiac palpitations, easy fatigue, disturbed sleep, mental sluggishness, impaired judgment and inability to do complex mental or physical tasks, and fluid retention. Tremor, ataxia for fine motions, and hematemesis are uncommon. It is strange that the bleeding from nose, ears, and even eyes, so prominently described by climbers in the 19th century are rare today.

High altitude pulmonary edema (HAPE) is more severe, less frequent, and seldom occurs below 9 to 10,000 ft. Dyspnea, irritative cough becoming productive of frothy and later blood-tinged sputum, and excessive fatigue are obvious warning signals. Curiously, some victims are more comfortable when lying flat while others are orthopneic. The first signs and symptoms of HAPE appear within 12 to 36 hr of arrival at altitude, although in some cases the picture does not develop for several days. The HAPE is aggravated or precipitated by exertion, relieved somewhat by rest, but usually grows worse unless treated. This is a serious disease, because the migration of edema from early traces in the interstitium of the alveolar walls into the alveoli creates a self-reinforcing feedback loop. As edema accumulates, diffusion of oxygen is impaired, hypoxia worsens, and edema accumulates more rapidly. This may explain why breathing oxygen becomes less helpful at later stages in the condition. Less understandable is the often dramatic improvement usually seen with descent of only a few thousand feet, at least in the early stages. Even this slight increase in atmospheric pressure seems to be more beneficial than breathing additional oxygen while at altitude, though there is only anecdotal evidence to support this observation.

High altitude cerebral edema (HACE) or high altitude encephalopathy, or hypoxic brain injury is the least frequent but most serious form. Headache is usually very severe, throbbing and incessant, worse in the morning, and likened by some to migraine. Ataxia is an early, important, and often dramatically obvious sign. The patient staggers with a wide base, the Romberg test is positive, and heel-to-toe straight line walking, or finger-to-nose tests are poorly done if possible at all. Gait is most commonly affected, but fine motions of fingers, hands, or conjugate eye motion are also occasionally impaired. Hallucinations are a frequent and serious sign, often suppressed by the victim whose judgment is warped. The most common hallucination is that of a companion walking and talking beside one, so real that the climber may try to share food with the illusory figure. Others are more dramatic: one party believed they saw palm trees, bull-dozers, and people trying to steal their flashlights near a 22,000 ft summit. In this case, the hallucinations persisted for a day after descent to base.

These signs and symptoms may progress rapidly to stupor, coma, and death in less than a day, while in other cases coma may persist for days or weeks and leave permanent brain damage. One such involved a climber whose only problem was diarrhea at 18,500 ft before he woke one morning unable to see, talk, or walk normally. Despite descent he deteriorated, became comatose for more than a week, and a year later is confined to a wheel-chair with impairment of all motor functions. Curiously, headache is occasionally mild or absent (as in the case just cited) even when other evidence of brain dysfunction is obvious. Papilledema is sometimes seen but more often the disc is not swollen but suffused with blood from increased retinal flow (see below).

Management has been based on the hypothesis that the brain becomes edematous during hypoxia: steroids have been used but their action is slow and only anecdotal evidence of their effectiveness exists in high altitude brain impairment. Oxygen relieves early signs and symptoms, but these return with ferocity when oxygen is stopped; as the condition worsens, oxygen is less helpful. As in the case of HAPE, descent is very beneficial in the early stages. Ataxia, hallucinations, and coma may persist for several days or even weeks if descent is delayed. Dehydration by hypertonic intravenous fluids (mannitol, urea, sucrose, or saline) has not been used enough to prove its worth.

Subcutaneous edema is commonly seen in climbers and trekkers. Swelling of feet and hands and puffiness of face and eyelids in the morning are common, often with weight gain and oliguria. Hackett and Rennie (1979) and Dickinson (1981) include this in the forms of altitude illness and have found it present in many persons going to 15 to 16,000 ft in Nepal. However, Williams and Ward found similar edema and weight gain during a week of strenuous exertion simulating climbing and trekking in the low British hills (Williams et al., 1979; Ward, 1980) in a carefully controlled study. It appears therefore that subcutaneous edema is not a result of altitude hypoxia but of combined stresses. Anecdotal evidence suggests that women in the premenstrual phase are at greater risk at altitude, especially if they normally tend to retain water at this time.

Sub-acute and chronic mountain sickness (CMS or Monge's disease) is a rather vaguely defined group of problems, occasionally seen in individuals who either never fully recover from acute mountain sickness or, after years at altitude, develop progressive polycythemia, dyspnea, and congestive heart failure, but who recover on descent to sea level. Chronic mountain sickness is attributed to failure of adequate ventilation due to blunted respiratory control and is similar to the chronic alveolar hypoventilation (Pickwickian syndrome) seen at sea level. Subacute or persistent mountain sickness is a different problem of which little is understood today.

High altitude retinopathy (HAR) is often seen above 14,000 ft where retinal circulation is increased and veins and arteries are engorged and tortuous. Above 17,000 ft, retinal blood flow is double that at sea level. Retinal hemorrhages appear in 35 to 60% of all persons at 17,500 ft but the incidence is not known at lower altitudes. Hemorrhages are related to exertion, less significantly to altitude illness, and unrelated to the severity of arterial oxygen desaturation. They are believed due to capillary rupture or leakage on the arterial side of retinal vessels, which has raised the question of similar hemorrhages in other less easily observed tissues. Petechial hemorrhages have been found in the brains of persons dying from altitude illness or acute hypoxia, and subungual splinter hemorrhages have been noted in mountaineers at altitude. Except when hemorrhage occurs in the macular region, few cause symptoms or are detectable by visual acuity screening. They disappear within weeks without residual except that macular hemorrhages often leave small scotomata for years. Cotton wool spots have been reported in one individual at 17,500 ft. Only macular hemorrhage and cotton wool spots are considered cause for descent; no specific treatment has been tested (McFadden et al., 1981).

Altitude related problems, in addition to the conditions primarily caused by oxygen lack, should be briefly mentioned. Polycythemia (a normal response to hypoxia) leads to venous thrombosis and embolism, especially when aggravated by dehydration, inactivity, or constricting clothes. Hypoxia increases susceptibility to hypothermia and frostbite. Persons with sickle trait may develop sickle cell crisis with multiple infarctions in various tissues at even moderate altitude. Cardiac or pulmonary insufficiency is likely to be aggravated. Some sedative and psychotropic drugs appear to have stronger and longer action at altitude and sea level dosages may be dangerous. As to alcohol—one drink does the work of two. Carbon monoxide produced by stoves in poorly ventilated shelters is much more dangerous at altitude than at sea level.

Pathology

Disturbed water and electrolyte distribution is considered the basic abnormality in hypoxic illness and is attributed to reversible failure of the intracellular sodium pump. According to this hypothesis, cells whose membranes have been most affected swell as water enters due to sodium retention in the cell. The resulting tissue edema causes signs or symptoms specific to location and magnitude of the swelling. Headache is so common in all forms of altitude illness that it has been suggested that brain edema may be the basic cause of the nausea, vomiting, and headache of AMS and of the ataxia, hallucinations and abnormal reflexes of HACE. Possibly brain edema may contribute a neurogenic stimulus to the development of pulmonary edema.

Hypoxia causes an increase in pulmonary artery pressure in almost everyone. Hultgren (1978) and others have suggested that in some areas of the lungs, arterial constriction may limit perfusion, while other areas are overperfused under high pressure. The flooded areas might then develop interstitial and subsequently alveolar edema and this would produce the typical patchy appearance of edema seen by X-ray. Just how or why the overperfused vessels leak has not been demonstrated in man, though it has been shown in sheep. No good animal model for HAPE has been identified.

Prevention

Altitude illness is most obviously prevented by staying way from mountains, an unlikely approach. Well-established is the fact that slow ascent prevents or minimizes risk. But how fast is slow enough? Much data has accumulated showing that: (1) a comfortably safe rate of climb varies widely between individuals and even in one person at different times; (2) very rapid high climbs with return to low altitude within 24 to 36 hr have enabled climbers to "get in under the wire" as it were, before major illness evolved—the dangers are large and obvious and the practice is feasible only for experts; (3) sleep desaturation contributes significantly to illness risk, and the familiar climbers' advice to "sleep low and climb high" is helpful; (4) other factors such as latitude, ambient temperature, diet, hydration, and efficiency of work play a poorly defined part in influencing occurrence or absence of illness and the optimal rate of ascent.

Various medications have been tried as preventives: ammonium chloride, cytochrome, calcium carbonate, medroxyprogesterone, coramine, scopolamine, ethacrinic acid, furosemide, and acetazolamide. Only the last has been shown to be effective by adequately controlled studies (Forwand et al., 1968). Acetazolamide (250 mg taken 2 or 3 times daily shortly before and for some time after ascent) increases excretion of urinary bicarbonate, off-setting the increase in blood pH due to increased ventilation. It also increases muscular acidosis. Not all agree on mechanism, but its benefits are established.

Treatment

The obvious treatment is to go down hastily when altitude sickness becomes obvious and before it is severe, and early descent is dramatically beneficial. Rest and oxygen are also helpful but on big mountains the risk of staying high and relying on a limited supply of oxygen is considerable. Climbers are best advised to get down, though tourists with easy access to hospital may stay on. Lasix is considered by some to be helpful in HAPE but is not without risk of hypovolemic shock; morphine has been used infrequently but seems of some value. Digitalis gives no benefit since the defect is not cardiac. Dexamethasone is believed helpful—but slow acting—in cerebral altitude illness; mannitol, urea, and other decongestant hypertonics have not been tested.

Summary

Altitude illness is most conveniently, though loosely, described as five portions of a continuous spectrum of morbidity: (1) acute hypoxia, (2) acute mountain sickness, (3) high altitude pulmonary edema, (4) high altitude encephalopathy (edema or brain injury), and (5) subacute or chronic mountain sickness. The first is limited to abrupt exposure rarely encountered on mountains. The basic pathology of altitude illness appears to be abnormal distribution of fluid and electrolytes most likely due to reversible failure of the sodium pump. Signs and symptoms depend to a great extent on the severity and location of tissue swelling; headache, ataxia, hallucinations, dyspnea, cough, rarely coma, and death are the most frequently encountered manifestations. Treatment is by descent or less advisably by steroids, diuretics, oxygen and rest. Prevention is best achieved by slow ascent, by sleeping low while climbing high, and by acetazolamide taken before and during the ascent.

References

Cournand, A. 1959. *Pulmonary Circulation: An International Symposium*. Adams, H.R. and Veith, I., eds. New York: Grune and Stratton. pp. 1–19.

Dickinson, J. 1981. *Acute Mountain Sickness*. Doctoral Thesis, Tribhuvana University, Kathmandu, Nepal.

Echevarria, E. 1979. The Inca mountaineers: 1400–1800. In *The Mountain Spirit*. Tobias, M.C. and Drasdo, H., eds. Woodstock, N.Y.: Overlook Press. pp. 117–124.

Forwand, S.A., Lansdowne, M., Follansbee, J.N., and Hansen, J.E. 1968. Effect of acetazolamide on acute mountain sickness. *N. Engl. J. Med.* 279:839–845.

Hackett, P.H. and Rennie, D.B. 1979. Rales, peripheral edema, retinal hemorrhage, and acute mountain sickness. *Am. J. Med.* 67:214–218.

Hackett, P.H., Rennie, D.B., and Levine, H.D. 1976. The incidence, importance, and prophylaxis of acute mountain sickness. *Lancet* Nov. 27:1149–1155.

Houston, C.S. 1980. *Going High: The Story of Man and Altitude*. Burlington, Vermont: Queen City Press.

Hultgren, H.N. 1978. High altitude pulmonary edema. In *Lung Water and Solute Exchange*. Staub, N.C., ed. New York: Marcel Dekker. pp. 437–464.

McFadden, D.M., Houston, C.S., Sutton, J.R., Powles, A.C., Gray, G.W., and Roberts, R.S. 1981. High altitude retinopathy. *J.A.M.A.* 245:581–586.

Ravenhill, T. 1913. Some experiences of mountain sickness in the Andes. *J. Trop. Med. Hyg.* 20:313–317.

Singh, I., Khanna, P., Srivastara, M.C., Lal, M., Roy, S.B., and Subramanyam, C.S. 1969. Acute mountain sickness. *N. Engl. J. Med.* 280:175–180.

Ward, M. 1980. Exercise edema and mountain sickness—a field investigation. *Alpine Journal* 85:168–175.

Williams, E.S., Ward, M., Milledge, J.S., Withey, W.R., Older, M.W., and Forsling, M.L. 1979. Effect of the exercise of seven continuous days hill-walking on fluid homeostasis. *Clin. Sci.* 56:305–316.

SECTION V:

Oxygen Transport in Special Situations

J.A. Loeppky and M.L. Riedesel, editors
OXYGEN TRANSPORT TO HUMAN TISSUES

Imposed Ventilatory Resistance

Loren G. Myhre

Air flows relatively freely through the normal respiratory tree which, in man, imposes a resistance of only about 0.2 mm H_2O/cc/sec (Zechman et al., 1957). The added respiratory resistance which accompanies many disease states, or that which is imposed by the use of respiratory protective devices, elicits physiological responses which have been the object of considerable research. Studies of resistance breathing, i.e., when external resistance is imposed either independently or simultaneously to inspiration and expiration, are particularly important for determining human performance capabilities in environments which demand the use of masks or respirators.

Effects of Imposed Ventilatory Resistance

Imposing air flow resistances ranging from 0.10 to 0.43 mm H_2O/cc/sec, Zechman et al. (1957) reported that the primary effect in normal man was a reduction in air flow velocity and an increase in duration of the impeded phase. These investigators further noted that the reduction in respiratory rate and the increase in both tidal volume and expiratory reserve observed during resistive breathing were primarily the result of impedance on the expiratory side. Others (Garrard and Lane, 1978; Whitelaw et al., 1979; Gothe and Cherniack, 1980) have observed similar effects when resistive loading was added to either the inspiratory or to the expiratory phase of the respiratory cycle. Zechman et al. (1957) concluded that the net result of air flow impedance was a reduced pulmonary ventilation which was accompanied by rising alveolar carbon dioxide and falling alveolar oxygen tensions. These investigators noted that although the increase in tidal volume does not completely compensate for the reduced respiratory rate with expiratory resistance, it is an economical adjustment because less energy is spent ventilating dead space; consequently, the decrement in alveolar ventilation is not as great as that for pulmonary ventilation.

Maximal inspiratory flow velocity is reduced to a greater extent when added resistance is limited to the inspiratory phase. The greater increase in alveolar CO_2 which occurs when both phases are impeded, or even when resistance is added only to expiration, apparently acts directly on the respiratory center resulting in a greater inspiratory drive than that which occurs when only inspiratory impedance is encountered (Zechman et al., 1957).

It has been shown that for a given level of resistance, expiratory time is increased to a greater extent than that for inspiration. This has been attributed to the more passive nature of expiration. The increase in expiratory reserve with resistance breathing may be an important adjustment which facilitates alveolar gas exchange by (1) buffering fluctuations in alveolar CO_2 and O_2, (2) increasing alveolar surface areas as a result of greater lung expansion, and (3) increasing the length of expiratory muscles which may then perform the work of breathing with greater efficiency (Zechman et al., 1957).

Although the respiratory pump responds to resistance breathing by proportional increases in respiratory work, hypoventilation persists and increases in alveolar CO_2 and decreases in alveolar O_2 are still allowed to occur. This, in spite of the ability of the respiratory muscles to exert even greater effort (Otis et al., 1950), has been described as a balance between respiratory control and biological economy (Zechman et al., 1957). The retention of CO_2 during resistance breathing has been described as a compromise by the body in preference to spending the extra energy required to maintain ventilation at the original level (Cain and Otis, 1949). The rise in alveolar CO_2 as a result of hypoventilation is considered to be the primary stimulating factor supporting observed increases in the respiratory effort. Thus, one would not expect ventilation to increase to a level that would remove this primary stimulus.

The degree to which work performance is compromised by breathing resistance is influenced by both the resulting changes in alveolar gas exchange and the subjective responses to stress. Consequently, threshold values for the initial detection, initial discomfort, and maximal tolerable level of resistance differ markedly.

Detection

There is a wide range of differences in an individual's ability to detect added resistance to breathing. Bennet et al. (1962) concluded that neither pressure, volume, nor flow alone were sufficient for normal man to detect the sensation of a resistive load. Wiley and Zechman (1966) reported that resistive loading reaches the threshold of detection when it exceeds 25% of the background resistance. Since the total pressure generated during breathing is the sum of the pressures related to volume, flow, and acceleration, Killian et al. (1979) have suggested that for one to perceive resistance, the central nervous system must be capable of discriminating resistive pressure from the total pressure generated. These investigators observed that the mean threshold value for resistance detection was 0.40 cm H_2O/liter/sec for normal men at rest, and they found no appreciable change in this threshold value when ventilation and peak inspiratory flow rate were approximately tripled during either CO_2 breathing or with exercise. Hence, the failure of increases in ventilation to enhance the ability to detect resistance despite large increases in pressure and flow support the hypothesis that it is the relationship of pressure to flow that is perceived (Killian et al., 1979).

Comfort

Respiratory filters and demand-type breathing regulators impose varying levels of resistance to inspiration while expiration is impeded to a much lesser extent. In an effort to determine man's ability to accept a respiratory protection device for prolonged periods of work, Bentley et al. (1973) imposed inspiratory resistance only, varying from 4.0 to 35.0 cm H_2O (measured at an air flow of 100 liter/min, during 30 min of treadmill exercise with speed and grade varied to produce a wide range of ventilatory demands. These investigators observed considerable variability in the discomfort experienced by men under apparently similar conditions. Their findings agreed with those of Campbell and Howell (1963) who suggested that the cause of dyspnea with resistance breathing was closely related to the additional work done per liter of air inhaled compared to the ventilation normally obtained by that effort. Bentley et al. (1973) concluded that, when resistance is limited to the inspiratory phase, 90% of the male population (their subjects were all members of a mine rescue service) will not experience respiratory discomfort until the pressure drop at the mouth exceeds 17.0 cm H_2O.

Maximal Tolerance

The study by Bentley et al. (1973) was not designed to measure one's ability to detect an added inspiratory load nor to determine maximal tolerable levels; it was simply an effort to determine the point at which normal men considered an inspiratory load to be uncomfortable. The values observed considered both the physiological mechanism where by the load is detected as well as the individual's motivation and attitude toward stimuli which may be unpleasant. Silverman et al. (1943, 1945, 1951) investigated the effects of breathing against resistance during graded exercise on a bicycle ergometer; work loads of 415, 830, 1107, and 1660 kg·m/min were performed for 15 min and inspiratory resistance ranged from 6 mm to 106 mm H_2O when measured at a flow rate of 85 liter/min. These investigators concluded that most subjects could tolerate these inspiratory resistances provided the external respiratory work during these three levels of work did not exceed 2.5, 6.0, and 13.3 kg·m/min, respectively. Cerretelli et al. (1969) studied two men breathing through resistance during exercise and observed that the only common factor at the limit of respiratory performance was the algebraic difference between peak inspiratory and expiratory intrathoracic pressures. More recently, Craig et al. (1970) suggested that the duration of the expiratory phase of the breathing cycle may be a factor that limits work for subjects breathing through inspiratory resistance. Concerning oxygen regulators, Ernsting (1981) described the magnitude of resistance imposed by a breathing system as the relationship during breathing between peak respiratory flows and corresponding minimum and maximum pressures within the mask cavity. In presenting his view of maximum acceptable resistance to breathing which is allowable in aircraft breathing systems, he cited the values drafted by the Air Standardization Co-ordinating Committee (1979) which are given in Table 1.

The magnitude of the problem of establishing tolerable limits for resistance breathing for working man can be appreciated when it is recalled that, in addition to an imposed impedance to inspiration and/or expiration, resistance breathing leads to increased alveolar CO_2 and reduced O_2 tensions. As a stimulus for respiration, CO_2 sensitivity may be increased by factors related to exercise (Cunningham and O'Riordan, 1957), but Cain and Otis (1949) have shown that inspiratory resistance tends to decrease the respiratory response to CO_2. This is generally observed as a reduction in ventilation, an increased CO_2 retention, and a lower respiratory quotient. Love et al. (1979) observed that when men breathing against an inspiratory resistance of 10 cm H_2O (measured at a flow of 100 liter/min) while working a rate requiring a $\dot{V}O_2$ of 1.6 liter/min, the ventilation response to CO_2 in the inspired air was smaller than

Table 1. Proposed ASCC Limited for Resistance to Breathing Imposed by Aircraft Oxygen Systems.

Peak respiratory flow	**Mask cavity pressures (in. water gauge)**		
(liter/min, ATPD)	**Minimum**	**Maximum**	**Maximum swing**
	Without safety pressure		
30	−1.5	+1.5	2.0
110	−2.5	+3.0	4.0
150	−4.5	+4.0	7.0
200	−7.6	+6.0	12.0
	With safety pressure		
30	+0.1	+3.0	2.0
110	−1.5	+4.0	4.0
150	−3.5	+5.0	7.0
200	−7.0	+6.6	12.0

(Source: Ernsting, 1981.)

that for similar conditions but without breathing resistance. When inspiring CO_2 concentrations of 4 and 5%, most of their subjects complained of headache and/or breathlessness; at these respective CO_2 levels, 10 and 40% of the subjects were distressed enough to stop before the end of the 30-min exercise. Rebuck et al. (1975) and Rebuck and Juniper (1975) emphasized the similarities in ventilation depression resulting from resistance breathing accompanying either hypoxia or hypercapnia. In addition to ventilation responses, Barnett and Rasmussen (1979) measured occlusion pressure for evaluating the neural output to the inspiratory muscles. These investigators concluded that ventilation is better maintained, i.e., less ventilatory depression, with resistive loading during hypoxia than during hypercapnia. They reasoned that this results from a greater force output of inspiratory muscles as reflected by a higher occlusion pressure which, in turn, suggests a greater neural output to these muscles. Whitelaw et al. (1975) have shown that this measurement approximates the force of isometric contraction of inspiratory muscles and, therefore, the neural output to these muscles.

Attempting to understand why some people allow $PACO_2$ to rise to high levels rather than to reduce it by increasing ventilation, Love et al. (1979) suggested that they may already have been ventilating at a sufficiently high proportion of their maximum breathing capacity to have caused breathlessness. Also, these responses may be due to a true variability among individuals with respect to CO_2 sensitivity which has been shown to persist on retesting even over a period of years (Schaefer, 1958). In general, Love et al. (1979) observed that their older subjects exhibited less sensitivity to CO_2 than did others; those having the most difficulty did not respond to the CO_2 stimulus by increasing their breathing rate sufficiently to maintain an acceptable $PACO_2$.

In a more applied sense, certain emergency conditions may elicit workers to exert near maximal effort for relatively short periods of time while wearing a respiratory protective device. We have recently completed a study (Myhre et al., 1979) where 21 men breathed through a standard self-contained breathing apparatus (SCBA) during 10 min of treadmill exercise; speed was held constant at 3.3 mph and the grade was adjusted to levels requiring 50, 65, and 80% of each subject's aerobic capacity. All work loads were performed without complaint when the subjects wore the SCBA on their backs but did not wear the mask (free breathing). The addition of the mask with its accompanying breathing resistance imposed varying degrees of discomfort which was tolerable at the two lower work levels. However, the breathing resistance imposed by the mask during exercise at 80% max $\dot{V}O_2$ was often reported to cause extreme discomfort; indeed, the feeling of suffocation was frequently expressed. Under these latter conditions, only by exerting considerable self-restraint were some of these men able to resist pulling the mask off during the final 5 to 7 min of the 10-min exercise. The resistance to breathing through the SCBA was related to the peak flow rate as shown in Figure 1, and the peak flow rate was highly correlated with $\dot{V}_I$ as shown in Figure 2.

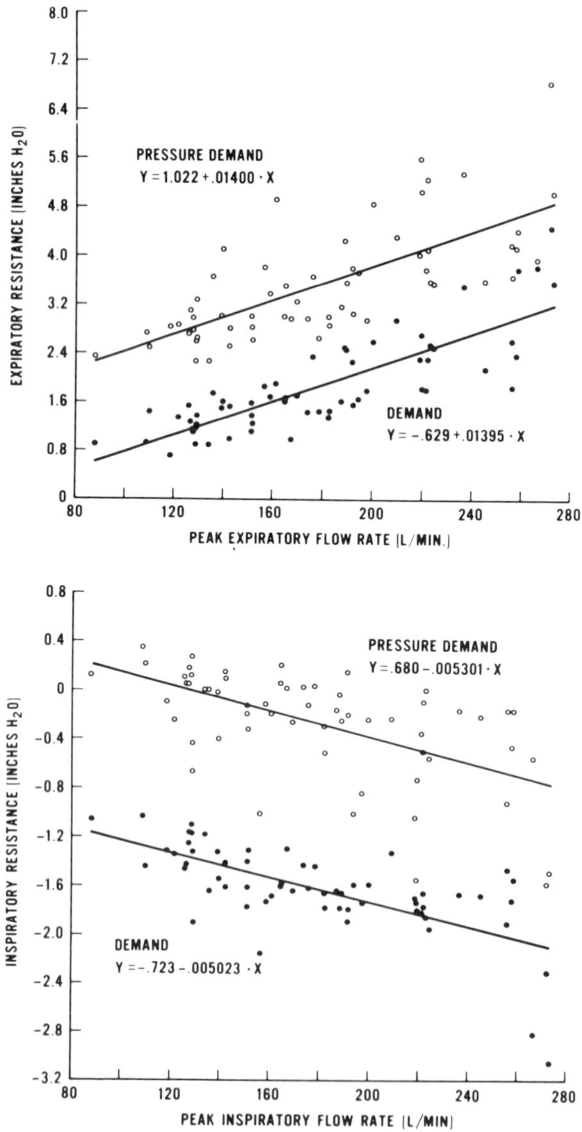

Figure 1. Regression equations derived for predicting breathing resistances from peak inspiratory flow rates when using the Scott Air-Pak II SCBA in Demand and Pressure Demand Modes.

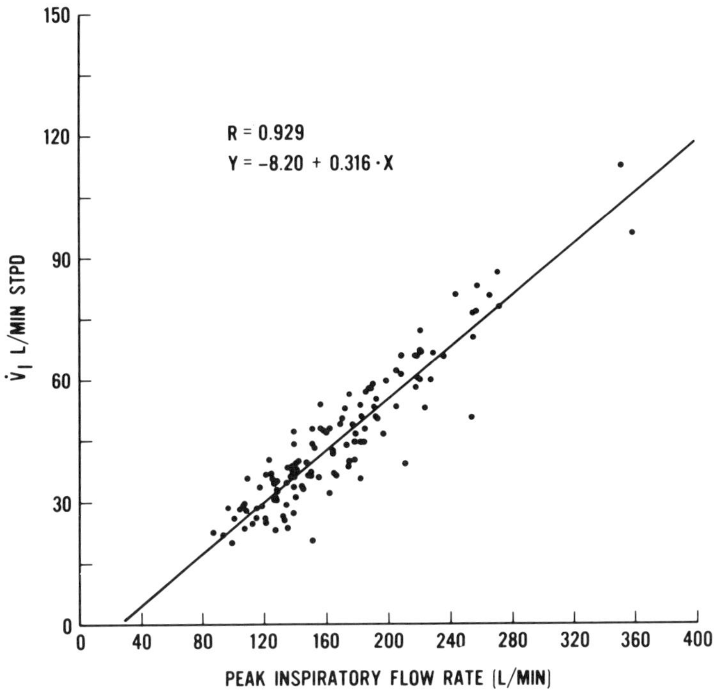

Figure 2. Relationship of peak inspiratory flow rate to ventilation during treadmill exercise requiring 50, 65, and 80% max $\dot{V}O_2$.

Segments of data recorded from one subject during work at 65 and 80% max $\dot{V}O_2$ are presented in Figures 3 and 4, respectively. At the lower work load, $\dot{V}O_2$ and $\dot{V}_I$ averaged 2.5 and 65 liter/min, respectively, and the pressure swing inside the mask cavity was 8.9 cm H_2O. Although not comfortable, this breathing resistance was acceptable for work of this nature. However, at the 80% work load, when $\dot{V}O_2$ and $\dot{V}_I$ had increased to 3.4 and 120 liter/min, respectively, the peak pressure swing inside the mask of 18 cm H_2O approached the subjective limits of tolerance. During the final 2 min of exercise when cylinder pressure had dropped to 375 psi (Figure 5) the SCBA regulator became less efficient and mask pressure swings exceeded 30 cm H_2O. This subject admitted that this resistance was outright intolerable and only a high degree of motivation accompanied by the knowledge that work would be terminated within a few minutes enabled him to complete the 10-min exercise.

In conclusion, several investigators have studied the effects of added resistance to breathing, and some have suggested values which may represent tolerable levels for normal men. Some of these are as follows: (1) The threshold value for detection of inspiratory resistance is about 0.40 and 0.36 cm H_2O/liter/sec during rest and moderate exercise, respectively (Killian et al.,

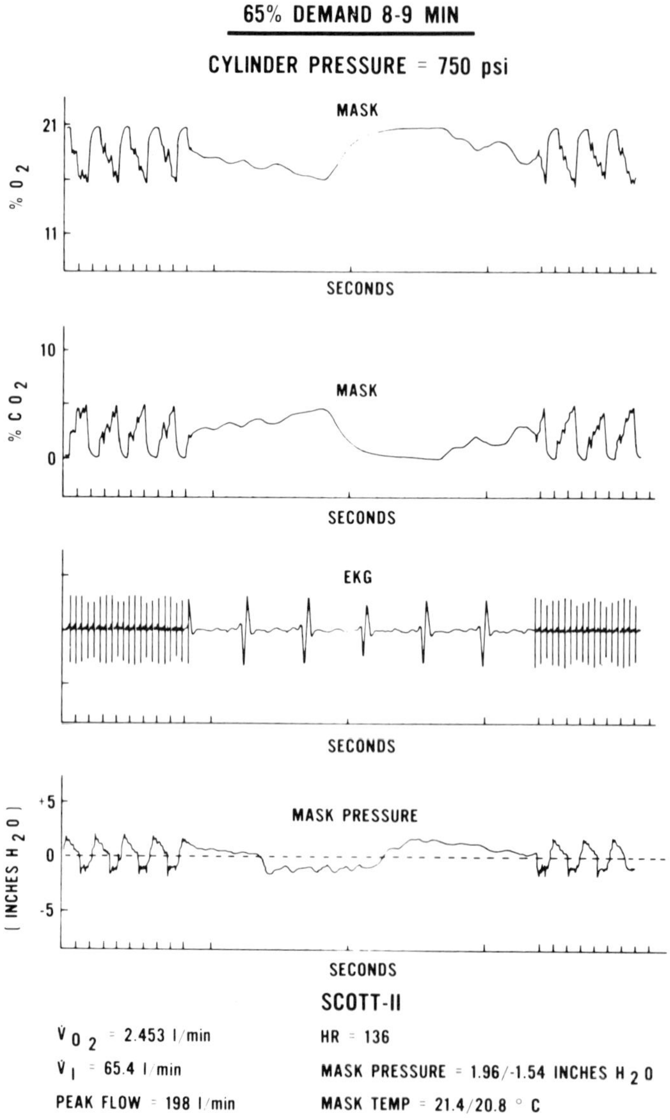

Figure 3. Respiratory responses to treadmill exercise at 65% max $\dot{V}O_2$ while breathing through a demand mode self-contained breathing apparatus.

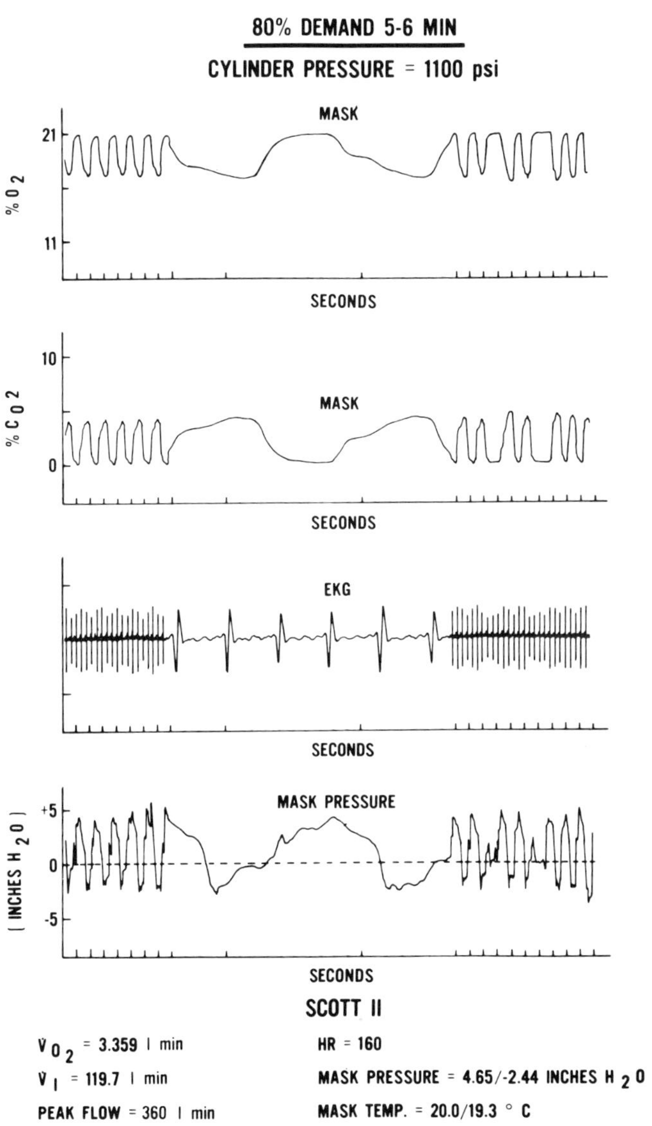

Figure 4. Respiratory responses to treadmill exercise at 80% max $\dot{V}O_2$ while breathing through a demand mode self-contained breathing apparatus.

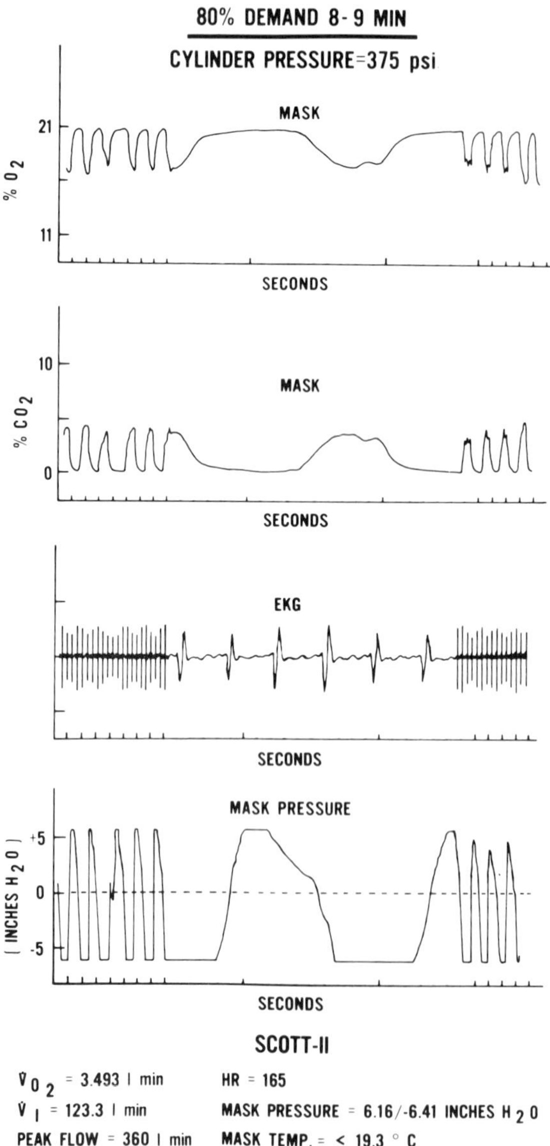

Figure 5. Respiratory responses to treadmill exercise at 80% max $\dot{V}O_2$ while breathing through a demand mode self-contained breathing apparatus with cylinder pressure <500 psi.

1979). (2) Resistance added to inspiration during moderate exercise can be expected to cause discomfort when the pressure drop at the mouth exceeds 17.0 cm H_2O (Bentley et al., 1973). (3) Relatively easy work ($\dot{V}O_2$ of 1.6 liter/min) can be performed without complaint when breathing against an inspiratory resistance of 10 cm H_2O (measured at a flow of 100 liter/min) provided CO_2 in the inspired air does not exceed 3%; when $FICO_2$ exceeds this level, less tolerant individuals may become unacceptably distressed (Love et al., 1979). To the above we can add that our work suggests that a peak pressure swing at the mouth of about 18 cm H_2O represents a near maximal level for tolerance to breathing resistance when man is performing 10 min of work at 80% of max $\dot{V}O_2$.This is in contrast to 17 cm H_2O pressure swing where Bentley et al. (1973) observed the onset of discomfort during 30 min of moderate exercise. We have concluded that during exercise at 80% max $\dot{V}O_2$ a pressure swing at the mouth of 30 cm H_2O imposes an intolerable feeling of suffocation which may only be tolerated for a minute or two in an emergency situation.

References

Air Standardization Co-ordinating Committee. 1979. *The Minimum Physiological Design Requirements for Aircrew Breathing Systems.* Advance Publication 61/3A.

Barnett, T.B. and Rasmussen, B. 1979. Ventilatory and occlusion pressure response to CO_2 and hypoxia with resistive loads. *Acta Physiol. Scand.* 105:23–32.

Bennett, E.D., Jayson, M.I., Rubenstein, D., and Campbell, E.J. 1962. The ability of man to detect added nonelastic loads to breathing. *Clin. Sci.* 23:155–162.

Bentley, R.A., Griffin, O.G., Love, R.G., Muir, D.C., and Sweetland, K.F. 1973. Acceptable levels for breathing resistance of respiratory apparatus. *Arch. Environ. Health* 27:273–280.

Cain, C.C. and Otis, A.B. 1949. Some physiological effects resulting from added resistance to respiration. *J. Aviat. Med.* 20:149–160.

Campbell, E.J. and Howell, J.B. 1963. The sensation of breathlessness. *Brit. Med. Bull.* 19:36–40.

Cerretelli, P., Sikand, R.S., and Farhi, L.E. 1969. Effect of increased airway resistance on ventilation and gas exchange during exercise. *J. Appl. Physiol.* 27:597–600.

Craig, F.N., Blevins, W.V., and Cummings, E.G. 1970. Exhausting work limited by external resistance and inhalation of carbon dioxide. *J. Appl. Physiol* 29:847–851.

Cunningham, D.J. and O'Riordan, J.L. 1957. The effect of a rise in the temperature of the body on the respiratory response to carbon dioxide at rest. *Quart. J. Exptl. Physiol.* 42:329–345.

Ernsting, J. 1981. The genesis and reduction of resistance to breathing in aircraft oxygen delivery systems. *Preprints of Annual Scientific Meeting*, (May) Aerospace Medical Association. pp. 191–192.

Garrard, C.S. and Lane, D.J. 1978. The pattern of stimulated breathing in man during nonelastic expiratory loading. *J. Physiol. (London)* 279:17–29.

Gothe, B. and Cherniack, N.S. 1980. Effects of expiratory loading on respiration in humans. *J. Appl. Physiol.* 49:601–608.

Killian, K.J., Campbell, E.J. and Howell, J.B. 1979. The effect of increased ventilation on resistive load discrimination. *Am. Rev. Respir. Dis.* 120:1233–1238.

Love, R.G., Muir, D.C., Sweetland, K.F., Bentley, R.A., and Griffin, O.G. 1979. Tolerance and ventilatory response to inhaled CO_2 during exercise and with inspiratory resistive loading. *Ann. Occup. Hyg.* 22:45–53.

Myhre, L.G., Holden, R.D., Baumgardner, F.W., and Tucker, D. 1979. *Physiological Limits of Firefighters.* ESL-TR-79-06, Defense Technical Information Center, Alexandria, Virginia, 77 pp.

Otis, A.B., Fenn, W.O., and Rahn, H. 1950. Mechanics of breathing in man. *J. Appl. Physiol.* 2:592–607.

Rebuck, A.S., Betts, M., and Saunders, N.A. 1975. Effect of elastic loading on ventilatory response to hypoxia in conscious man. *J. Appl. Physiol.* 39:548–551.

Rebuck, A.S. and Juniper, E.F. 1975. Effect of resistive loading on ventilatory response to hypoxia. *J. Appl. Physiol.* 38:965–968.

Schaefer, K.E. 1958. Respiratory pattern and respiratory response to CO_2. *J. Appl. Physiol.* 13:1–14.

Silverman, L., Lee, R.C., Lee, G., Drinker, K.R., and Carpenter, T.M. 1943. *Fundamental Factors in the Design of Respiratory Equipment: Inspiratory Air Flow Measurements on Human Subjects With and Without Resistance.* Report No. 1222, Office of Scientific Research and Development, Washington, D.C.

Silverman, L., Lee, G., Yancey, A.R., Amory, L., Barney, L.J., and Lee, R.C. 1945. *Fundamental Factors in the Design of Respiratory Equipment: A Study and an Evaluation of Inspiratory and Expiratory Resistance for Protective Respiratory Equipment.* Report no. 5339, Office of Scientific Research and Development, Washington, D.C.

Silverman, L., Lee, G., Plotkin, T., Sawyers, L.A., and Yancey, A.R. 1951. Air flow measurements on human subjects with and without respiratory resistance at several work rates. *Arch. Indust. Hyg. Occupational Med.* 3:461–478.

Whitelaw, W.A., Derenne, J.-P., and Milic-Emili, J. 1979. Occlusion pressure as a measure of respiratory center output in conscious man. *Respir. Physiol.* 23:181–189.

Wiley, R.L. and Zechman, Jr., F.W. 1966. Perception of added airflow resistance in humans. *Respir. Physiol.* 2:73–87.

Zechman, F., Hall, F.G., and Hull, W.E. 1957. Effects of graded resistance to tracheal air flow in man. *J. Appl. Physiol.* 10:356–362.

J.A. Loeppky and M.L. Riedesel, editors
OXYGEN TRANSPORT TO HUMAN TISSUES

Gravitational Effects on Oxygen Transport

Hilding Bjurstedt

The oxygen transport pathway in the human body consists of two convective transport systems, the lungs and the cardiovascular system, and two diffusing systems, the alveolar-pulmonary capillary and tissue capillary-cell systems. A primary function of these systems is to ensure normal oxygen flow to the tissues of the body. Gravitational forces may limit the oxygen supply to the tissues through interference with both circulatory and respiratory functions. Thus, in the upright healthy individual, normal gravity is strong enough to curtail the cardiac output; if passive standing is maintained, a catastrophic fall in cerebral blood flow will occur sooner or later, interrupting the oxygen flow to the brain. Loss of consciousness therefore ensues even though the oxygen content of the arterial blood may be adequate. On the other hand, gravitational forces may leave cardiac output relatively unaffected as long as the effective force acts transversely to the long axis of the body; in this situation the primary disturbance occurs in the lungs. Proper mixing of blood with the air is prevented, since most of the blood flow goes to dependent lung regions, while most of the ventilation goes to the remaining regions. Thus, pulmonary gas exchange is profoundly disturbed and general asphyxia rapidly ensues.

It is therefore of interest to look at the mechanisms by which gravitational stress may interfere with the flow of oxygen from the ambient air to the body tissues. I would first like to discuss gravitational effects on the pulmonary transfer of oxygen and then some of the transient changes in oxygen flow associated with changes in body position. Finally, I will discuss some of the effects of gravitational stress on man's ability to perform exercise and on the transport of oxygen to working muscles.

Oxygen Transfer in the Lungs

Many of the respiratory and circulatory effects caused by gravitational force may conveniently be studied on the tilt table. Others are subtle or at least difficult to measure, but may be unmasked by exaggerating the force of gravity by the use of a large centrifuge. In the following, I shall use the notation $+G_z$ to refer to gravitational force acting in the head-foot direction as during standing at normal gravity or induced in a centrifuge or in flight maneuvers, tending to displace blood and viscera downwards. For gravitational forces acting transversely to the long axis of the body, the notation $+G_x$ will be used. This is the force that acts on an astronaut lying supine during launch and reentry, tending to push him into his couch.

Because tolerance to increased G stress in the head-foot direction is limited by impaired blood and oxygen flow to the brain, with loss of consciousness rapidly ensuing at +5 to +6 G_z, the possibility that G stress might also seriously affect pulmonary function received little attention until the 1950's. At that time, the use of cuvette oximetry in centrifuge experiments performed on dogs in our laboratory showed that low to moderate $+G_z$ forces applied over several minutes could lead to severe arterial desaturation even though 100% oxygen was breathed and hyperventilation was present (Barr et al., 1959). Barr (1962, 1963) extended these observations to man breathing air and exposed to +4 to +5 G_z for 2 min. In the +5 G_z experiments, the arterial oxygen saturation fell to an average level of 87%. At the beginning of the 1960s, work in many laboratories focused on the effects of $+G_x$ forces on pulmonary function; this interest was prompted by the need for astronauts to be exposed to such forces to achieve orbital velocity and reentry. Wood et al. (1961) were the first to report a marked reduction in the arterial oxygen saturation in man during $+G_x$ acceleration; they recorded a fall to below 85% at +5 G_x.

These early observations of impaired oxygen transfer by the lungs have been confirmed in many subsequent centrifuge studies. There seem to be about equal degrees of desaturation in the $+G_z$ and $+G_x$ situations (Figure 1).

It is well-recognized that gravity is the main factor determining the distribution of both blood and gas within the lungs under physiological conditions. Thus, in the upright lung at lung volumes greater than functional residual capacity, the alveoli in the lower lung are better ventilated than those in the upper lung, and an even greater difference exists in the distribution of blood flow to these regions. As a result of such gravity-dependent ventilation-perfusion inequality, there is an overall loss in PO_2 between mixed alveolar air and arterial blood. In the upright lung, this amounts to about 5 mm Hg and corresponds to a reduction of oxygen transfer by about 2% below that of a lung having even distribution of blood and gas (West, 1962). With increased G forces acting on the lung, the ventilation-perfusion inequality along the force vector is exaggerated. Using experimental values of ventilation/perfusion ratios observed at +3 G_z and combining these with data for the distribution of

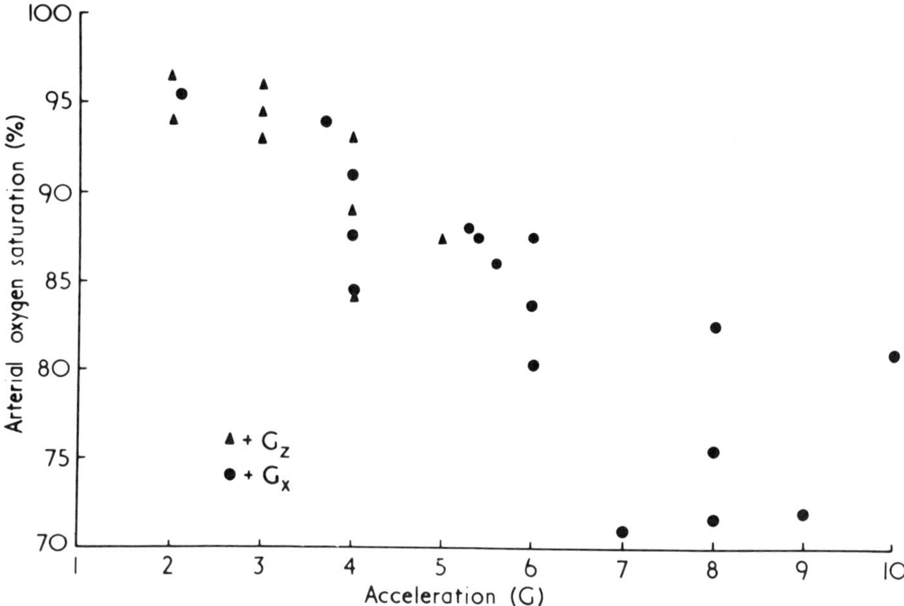

Figure 1. Effects of $+G_z$ and $+G_x$ forces on arterial oxygen saturation in subjects breathing air, as reported from different centrifuge laboratories. Each point represents the average of from 3 to 31 determinations made during exposures lasting not less than 50 sec.

SOURCE: *Modified from Glaister, 1970.*

lung volume, it has been possible to compute functions of a number of horizontal slices of lung tissue lying between the apex and the diaphragm and compare these with functions similarly computed for the upright lung at normal gravity (West, 1962). In this way, it can be shown that for the upright lung a change from normal gravity to $+3G_z$ will cause a fall in arterial PO_2 of less than 5 mm Hg, if attributed solely to exaggerated ventilation-perfusion inequalities (Glaister, 1970). The marked arterial desaturation observed in centrifuge experiments referred to previously can therefore only in part be explained on the basis of a mismatch between ventilation and flow as long as the ventilation/perfusion ratios in dependent regions are assumed to be low but greater than zero.

Instead, the situation must be characterized by considerable shunting of blood past lung units, which receive no ventilation at all. Evidence for the development of large lung regions with zero ventilation during increased G stress first came from field studies in pilots immediately after flight. They showed X-ray shadowing at the lung bases indicative of basal lung collapse, constituting part of the so-called "acceleration atelectasis syndrome." The underlying mechanism is the phenomenon of regional airway closure, which occurs at low lung volumes and leads to trapping of gas in unventilated alveoli and eventually to absorptional atelectasis, a process greatly hastened if 100% oxygen is breathed. During increased gravitational stress, airways close at higher lung volumes than is the case at normal gravity and a region with good ventilation can suddenly be converted to one of zero ventilation as the G level is increased. By use of radioactive xenon techniques on the centrifuge, it has been possible to show that closing volumes may increase up to 40% of vital capacity at $+4\ G_z$, and to even higher values at $+5\ G_x$ (Glaister, 1977).

Acceleration atelectasis may lead to considerable right-to-left shunting and a marked widening of the alveolar-arterial oxygen difference. Figure 2 shows the increase in the "effective alveolar" to arterial oxygen difference resulting from a 2-min exposure to $+5\ G_z$; the magnitude of the shunt could be calculated to average 20% of the cardiac output. Much larger shunts may develop during exposure to G_x forces because of restrictions in lung volume with an increased tendency to airway closure in dependent lung regions. Although breathing 100% oxygen increases the tendency to atelectasis irrespective of the direction of the G force, it initially prevents the arterial oxygen saturation from falling. Even as more and more airways become closed, trapped alveoli containing a

Figure 2. "Effective alveolar"-arterial oxygen differences before and at the end of a 2-min exposure to $+5\ G_z$ with the subjects breathing air. Values are 1-min time averages.

SOURCE: *Barr, 1963.*

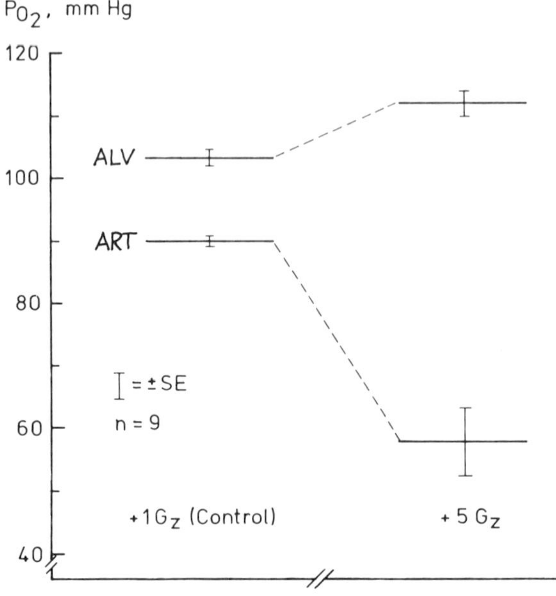

high percentage of oxygen would not act as a shunt until the oxygen became absorbed. Figure 3 shows the delayed desaturation occurring in a subject breathing 100% oxygen at $+5\ G_z$.

From the above considerations, it may be predicted that the gas exchange function of the lung would be more efficient in the weightless condition than it is in our normal force environment. Experiments have utilized parabolic and orbital flight to study the effect of weightlessness on the lung. Various simulation techniques and the method of extrapolating data from various G levels down to zero have been employed. Work in this area has recently been reviewed by Glaister (1977). As might be expected, results in general point to a disappearance of gravity-induced regional inequalities in ventilation/perfusion ratio. All factors tending to produce such inequalities would be at a minimum in the weightless state and, hence, the efficiency of pulmonary transfer of oxygen would be at a maximum.

Transient Changes in Oxygen Flow Associated with Changes in Posture

In a true steady state, oxygen uptake must equal the metabolic consumption but, over short periods of time, oxygen intake at mouth level may differ from the metabolic need. Changes in posture may cause marked transient fluctuations in oxygen uptake, and it is of considerable interest that oxygen uptake may be reduced shortly after subjects are moved to an upright position from supine (Rahn and Ament, 1955). A similar finding has been reported from experiments with brief exposure to moderate $+G_z$ forces in the centrifuge (Glaister, 1963). In both cases, release of the stress is rapidly followed by rather large but transient increases in the oxygen uptake above its preexposure baseline level. Evidently, these changes cannot be understood on the basis of alterations in metabolic rate.

There are at least two mechanisms which could be invoked to explain the surprising feature that the oxygen intake may decrease during the course of G stress in the head-foot direction. The first possibility is that underperfusion of some tissues, especially a severely reduced blood flow through the lower extremities, could lead to anaerobic metabolism with the development of a lactacid oxygen debt which is repaid on release of the G stress. The second possibility is that part of the metabolic oxygen requirement is covered by oxygen stored in the lungs and blood, i.e., by incurring an alactacid oxygen debt.

The nature of the oxygen debt that may develop during several minutes in the upright posture has recently been clarified by work in Luft's laboratory. Passive standing on a tilt table at 60° was employed to minimize the possibility that metabolic oxygen consumption might change appreciably with changes in posture from supine to upright (Loeppky and Luft, 1975). These studies were continued in a subsequent series in which the advantages of simulating

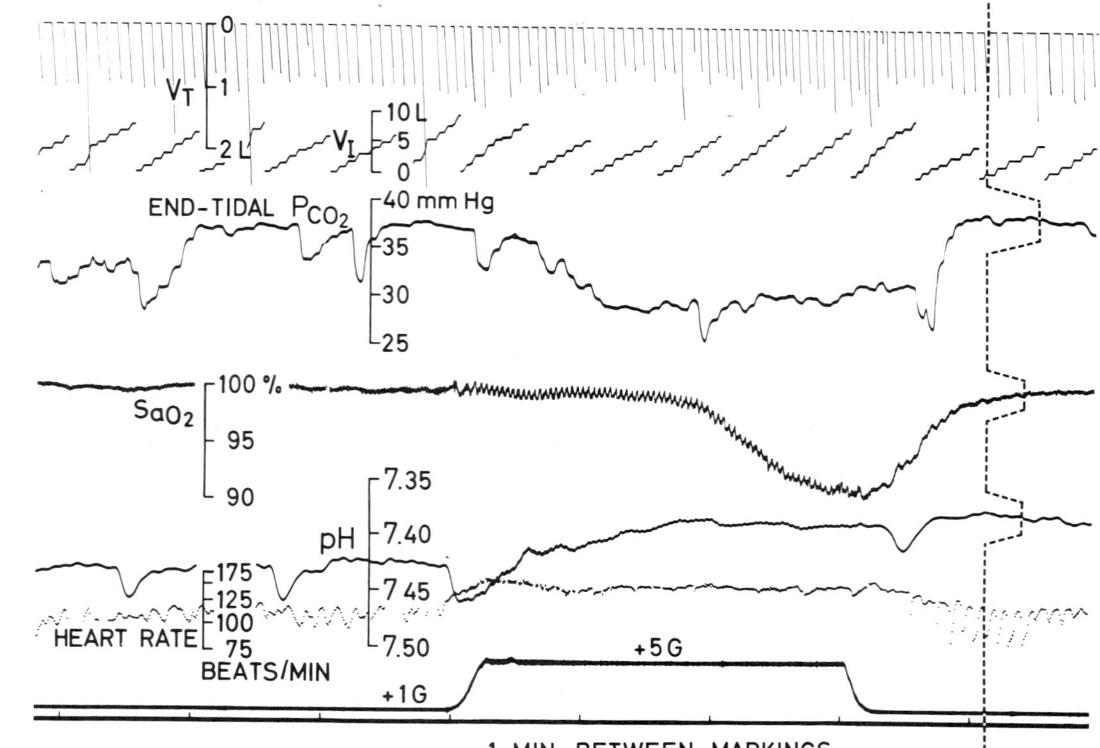

Figure 3. Cardiorespiratory and blood gas responses in a subject exposed to +5 G_z for 3 min breathing 100% oxygen and using an automatically inflated G suit. Note that arterial saturation does not begin to fall until the G stress has acted for 80 to 100 sec.

SOURCE: *Barr et al., 1969.*

orthostasis by applying negative pressure to the lower half of the body (LBNP) were utilized (Loeppky et al., 1978).

In both series of experiments, breath-by-breath measurements of oxygen intake were employed, and the oxygen transfer at the pulmonary capillary membrane was calculated; in this way it was possible to account for fluctuations in oxygen uptake due to posture-dependent changes in functional residual capacity and to calculate the time-course of the oxygen flow across the lung membrane. Assuming metabolic oxygen consumption to remain unchanged, these studies noted that oxygen transfer by the lung membrane dropped when body position changed from supine to standing and remained well below the assumed level of metabolic oxygen consumption for the 10 min that the upright position was maintained. During such a period, the oxygen taken up by the blood in the pulmonary capillaries may be a few hundred ml less than the amount going into the tissues, resulting in a corresponding loss in venous oxygen stores. On reassuming the supine posture, oxygen transfer in the pulmonary capillaries increases sharply as pooled blood with very low oxygen content moves centrally by gravity and passes through the lungs; in this way all the oxygen lost from the blood during standing may be fully repaid within a few minutes. A similar sequence of events was observed in the LBNP experiments.

The results showed, however, that the oxygen deficit developed during orthostasis or LBNP was far greater than the amount calculated from the assumed reduction of the mixed venous oxygen content in these conditions. They also showed that all the oxygen debt incurred in orthostasis and in LBNP is of the alactacid type. To explain the considerable oxygen debt that can be incurred in these conditions, the authors (Loeppky and Luft, 1975; Loeppky et al., 1978) developed a model in which the systemic circulation was represented by two parallel circuits, a "lower" and an "upper" one; the "lower" circuit had a blood flow reduced out of proportion to the decrease in cardiac output, and a venous volume greater than that of the "upper" circuit. By applying this model, the calculated loss in venous oxygen stores that occurs during passive standing and during LBNP could be shown to greatly exceed that obtained in a one-circuit model, and to correspond well to the amount of oxygen actually repaid after release of the stress.

Increased Gravitational Stress and Exercise

Finally, I would like to consider the combined effects of gravitational forces and exercise on oxygen transport. By making measurements in a centrifuge with a cycle ergometer inside the capsule, it is possible to investigate how physiological responses to leg exercise are modified by G stress and vice versa. Experiments in our laboratory (Rosenhamer, 1967) showed that the overall tolerance to $+3\ G_z$ was clearly increased by moderate exercise both subjectively and objectively. These and other experiments (Linnarsson and Rosenhamer, 1968) served to clarify some of the mechanisms through which exercise can markedly reduce certain disturbances caused by increased G stress in resting subjects. An important factor is the action of the leg muscle pump, which boosts venous return and effectively counteracts the G-induced curtailment of the stroke volume. This explains the surprising observation that exercise at high G may lower the heart rate (Nunneley and Shindell, 1975). Both heart rate and arteriovenous oxygen difference increase less with exercise at $+3\ G_z$ than they do at normal gravity; up to and including moderate work loads, the delivery of oxygen to the tissues is largely adequate since the oxygen uptake increases by about the same rate as it does at normal gravity.

With regard to the G-induced disturbances that occur in the pulmonary gas exchange at rest referred to previously, exercise reduces the stress in some ways and augments it in others. Exposure to $+3\ G_z$ at rest increases the ventilatory equivalent, $\dot{V}_E/\dot{V}O_2$, and the dead space ventilation; low levels of exercise improve the efficiency of pulmonary gas exchange (Rosenhamer, 1967; Bjurstedt et al., 1968; Nunneley and Shindell, 1975; Nunneley, 1976). This is in keeping with what is known about the effect of leg exercise in the erect posture at normal gravity; in this situation, gas exchange is improved because G-induced reduction of central blood volume is counteracted and the capillary filling of the lungs, especially in the apexes, is improved.

There are a number of observations which point to the probability of a G-induced limitation to oxygen transport at increasing work load. Thus, Rosenhamer (1967) found that even light exercise at $+3\ G_z$, unlike at normal gravity, widens the alveolar-arterial oxygen difference. As shown in Figure 4, the magnitude of the underlying shunt, expressed as percent of cardiac output, increases with the physiological work load at $+3\ G_z$, whereas the opposite is true during upright exercise at normal gravity. The underlying mechanism is not clear, but a possible explanation is that improved filling of apical capillaries caused by exercise results in a lengthening of the hydrostatic column in the lung, so that the increased G load further increases the capillary pressures at the base of the lung with consequent development of atelectasis. Another indication of a diminishing efficiency in the oxygen transfer is that the ventilation equivalent at a given work load increases with the G level. Also, dead-space ventilation at a given work load increases and the heart rate response is greater.

It seemed of interest to look into the effects of G stress as the performance of the oxygen transport system is pushed to its limit. For this purpose, a series of experiments was carried out in which the work load at $+3\ G_z$ was extended to 900 kpm/min (Bjurstedt et al., 1968). Figure 5 shows the relationship between the oxygen uptake in a group of subjects ($n=8$) with the work load at normal gravity and at $+3\ G_z$; individual data are also included. The higher

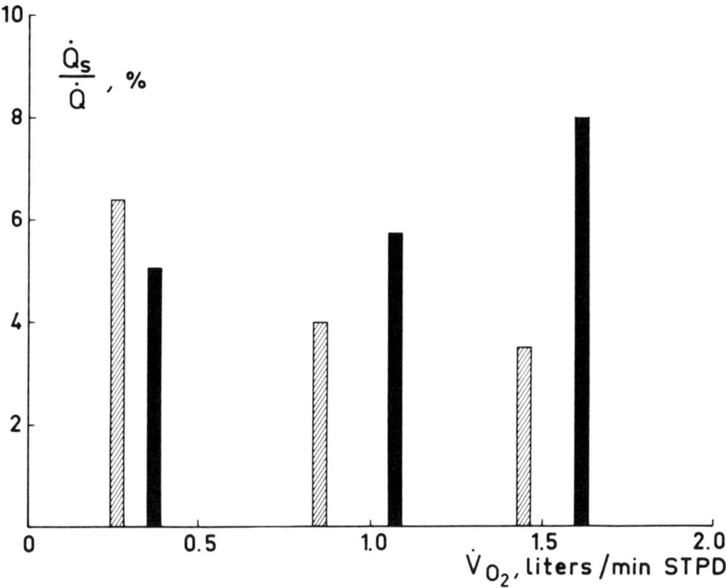

Figure 4. Magnitude of pulmonary shunt in relation to oxygen uptake at $+1$ G_z (shaded columns) and $+3$ G_z (black columns). Left columns refer to resting conditions, middle columns to exercise at 300 kpm/min, and right columns to exercise at 600 kpm/min.

SOURCE: *Rosenhamer, 1967.*

oxygen uptake for the group at $+3$ G_z can be ascribed to G-induced increase of work of postural and respiratory muscles because of increased effective weight of the body and augmented respiration activity. When the work load at $+3$ G_z was increased from 600 to 900 kpm/min, two subjects exhibited a levelling off of oxygen uptake and showed considerably higher arterial lactate values than the rest of the subjects. They also showed a smaller than average increase in oxygen pulse, and the ventilatory equivalent at the highest work load (900 kpm/min) was much higher than average. One subject was unable to complete exercise at 900 kpm/min at $+3$ G_z because of exhaustion. These observations taken together indicate that maximal oxygen uptake is lowered by G-stress and that the primary limitation imposed on the oxygen transport system by such stress occurs in the lungs. With increasing work load, the additional widening of the arteriovenous oxygen difference caused by G stress diminishes (Rosenhamer, 1967). Thus, the G-induced changes in pulmonary gas exchange present a greater handicap to oxygen transport and work capacity than do the changes in the systemic circulation.

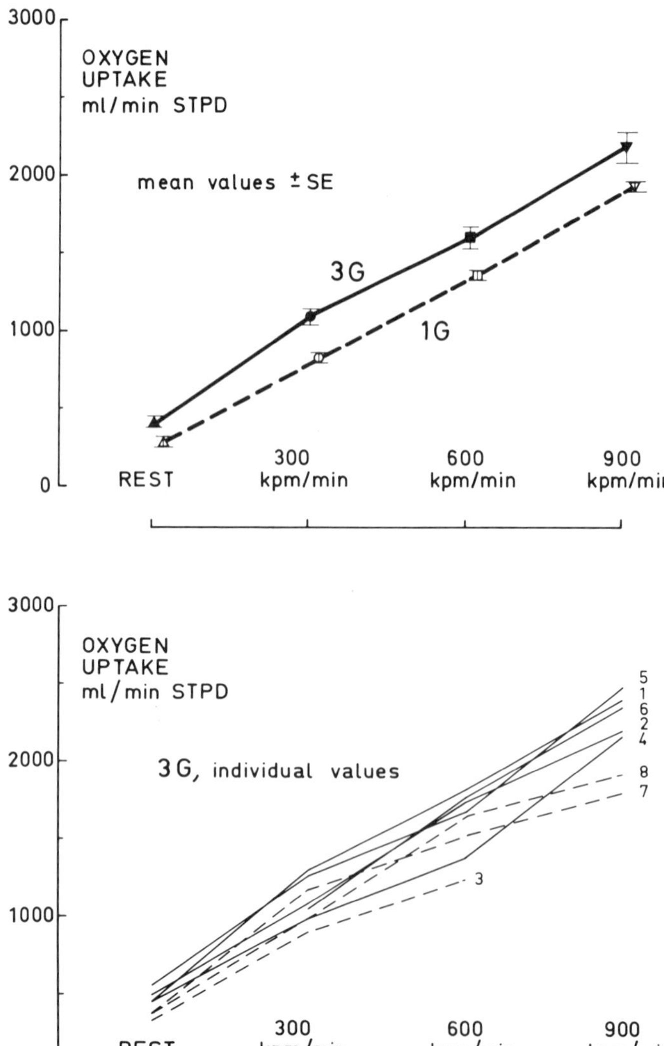

Figure 5. Oxygen uptake vs external work load at +1 and +3 G_z. (Upper graph) Group means for oxygen uptake at rest and during the 6th min of exercise at different work loads (n = 8, except for +3 G_z-exercise at 900 kpm/min where n = 7; vertical bars indicate ±S.E.). (Lower graph) Individual data obtained at +3 G_z. Subjects 3, 7, and 8 showed the highest lactate levels; subject 3 was unable to complete the work at 900 kpm/min.

SOURCE: *Bjurstedt et al., 1968.*

References

Barr, P.-O. 1962. Hypoxemia in man induced by prolonged acceleration. *Acta Physiol. Scand.* 54:128–137.

Barr, P.-O. 1963. Pulmonary gas exchange in man as affected by prolonged gravitational stress. *Acta Physiol. Scand.* 58(Suppl. 207):1–45.

Barr, P.-O., Bjurstedt, H., and Coleridge, J.C. 1959. Blood gas changes in the anesthetized dog during prolonged exposure to positive radial acceleration. *Acta Physiol. Scand.* 47:16–27.

Barr, P.-O., Brismar, J., and Rosenhamer, G. 1969. Pulmonary function and G-stress during inhalation of 100% oxygen. *Acta Physiol. Scand.* 77:7–16.

Bjurstedt, H., Rosenhamer, G., and Wigertz, O. 1968. High-G environment and responses to graded exercise. *J. Appl. Physiol.* 25:713–719.

Glaister, D.H. 1963. *Pulmonary Gas Exchange During Positive Acceleration.* Rep. No. 1212. Flying Personnel Research Committee, M.O.D. (Air Force Dept.), London.

Glaister, D.H. 1970. *The Effects of Gravity and Acceleration on the Lung.* AGARDO-graph No. 133. Advisory Group for Aerospace Research and Development. North Atlantic Treaty Organization, Neuilly-sur-Seine, France.

Glaister, D.H. 1977. Effect of acceleration. In *Regional Differences in the Lung* West, J.B., ed. New York. Academic Press. pp. 323–379.

Linnarsson, D. and Rosenhamer, G. 1968. Exercise and arterial pressure during simulated increase of gravity. *Acta Physiol. Scand.* 74:50–57.

Loeppky, J.A. and Luft, U.C. 1975. Fluctuations in O_2 stores and gas exchange with passive changes in posture. *J. Appl. Physiol.* 39:47–53.

Loeppky, J.A., Venters, M.D., and Luft, U.C. 1978. Blood volume and cardiorespiratory responses to lower body negative pressure. *Aviat. Space Environ. Med.* 49:1297–1307.

Nunneley, S.A. 1976. Gas exchange in man during combined $+G_z$ acceleration and exercise. *J. Appl. Physiol.* 40:491–495.

Nunneley, S.A. and Shindell, D.S. 1975. Cardiopulmonary effects of combined exercise and $+G_z$ acceleration. *Aviat. Space Environ. Med.* 46:878–882.

Rahn, H. and Ament, R. 1955. *The Effects of Posture Upon the Gas Exchange and Alveolar Gas Composition.* WADC-TR-55-357. Wright Air Development Center, Ohio, U.S.A. pp. 327–336.

Rosenhamer, G. 1967. Influence of increased gravitational stress on the adaptation of cardiovascular and pulmonary function to exercise. *Acta Physiol. Scand.* 68(Suppl. 276):1–61.

West, J.B. 1962. Regional differences in gas exchange in the lung of erect man. *J. Appl. Physiol.* 17:893–898.

Wood, E.H., Sutterer, W.F., Marshall, H.W., Lindberg, E.F., and Headley, R.N. 1961. *Effect of Headward and Forward Accelerations on the Cardiovascular System.* Tech. Rep. 60-634, Wright Air Development Division, USAF, Ohio, U.S.A. pp. 1–48.

J.A. Loeppky and M.L. Riedesel, editors
OXYGEN TRANSPORT TO HUMAN TISSUES

Hyperbaria-O_2 Toxicity

Karl E. Schaefer

The normal concentration of oxygen in air is approximately 21%, corresponding to a partial pressure of 0.21 atmosphere absolute (ATA) or 159 mm Hg. In closed systems, such as pressure chambers, air craft, or space craft, the partial pressure of oxygen may increase and result in oxygen toxicity. Oxygen toxicity is likely to be encountered under the following conditions: (1) in underwater swimmers using closed or semiclosed breathing equipment, (2) oxygen tolerance tests used for the selection of diving personnel in the Navy, (3) saturation diving, (4) use of oxygen breathing to shorten decompression times, (5) recompression for therapeutic purposes, and (6) during prolonged resuscitation efforts in cases of respiratory failure.

A rise in oxygen partial pressure may be due to an increase in the percentage of oxygen in ambient air or an elevation of ambient pressure, or a combination of both factors. Increases of partial pressure of oxygen at 1 ATA produce effects on the respiratory and circulatory systems, erythropoiesis and endocrine functions but do not affect the central nervous system (Bean, 1945). Oxygen convulsions that involve the central nervous system, one form of oxygen poisoning, occur only under conditions in which oxygen tensions are in excess of 1 atm (2 ATA).

In threshold values of increased ambient partial pressure of oxygen causing effects on different organ systems, O_2 levels of inspired air are also given in ATA together with alveolar PO_2 values. Dejours et al. (1958) established that the O_2 chemoreceptor drive of respiration (which accounts for 10 to 15% of the resting ventilation) disappears above 170 mm Hg of alveolar O_2 tension; this corresponds to an inspiratory PO_2 of 230 mm Hg which is equivalent to 30% oxygen in the ambient air. Fifty percent O_2 in nitrogen (corresponding to an inspired PO_2 of 360 mm Hg and alveolar PO_2 of 300 mm Hg) appears to be the threshold concentration for elicitation of cardiopulmonary effects. Exposure to this mixture was found to produce a reduction in vital capacity after 24 hr (Comroe et al., 1945) and a transitory slowing of the heart rate (Meda, 1950). Another oxygen threshold exists at an alveolar PO_2 of 300 mm Hg in regard to the combined respiratory sensitivity to CO_2 and O_2. Breath-holding studies under various pressures by Hesser (1962) and Stroud (1959) demonstrated that decreasing the alveolar O_2 tension below 300 mm Hg increases the sensitivity to CO_2.

It is well-established that the inhalation of oxygen concentrations above 65%, corresponding to an oxygen tension higher than 494 mm Hg, has deleterious effects in most warm-blooded animals and leads eventually to death due to pulmonary oxygen toxicity. Oxygen lung toxicity represents an important clinical problem complicating the care of very ill patients (Huber and Drath, 1981).

The toxic effects of oxygen at high pressure (OHP) on the central nervous system were first reported by Paul Bert (1878) who described in detail the incidence of convulsions in various animal species exposed to OHP. Behnke et al. (1936) carried out experiments on human subjects. As a result of these earlier studies, it was generally accepted that 3-hr exposure to 3 ATA and 30 to 40 min to 4 ATA was safe for men at resting conditions.

The development of pulmonary and central nervous system oxygen toxicity depends on partial pressure and the duration of exposure as shown in Figure 1. There is a latent period prior to the onset of toxicity in both the central

Figure 1. Predicted human pulmonary and CNS tolerance to high pressure oxygen.
SOURCE: *Clark and Lambertsen, 1971a.*

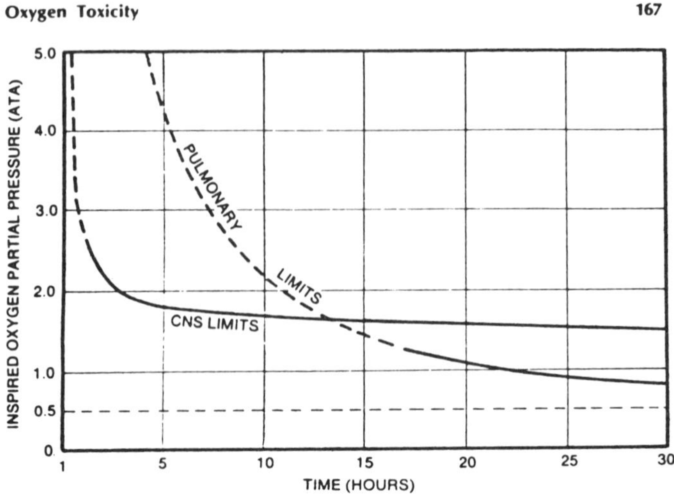

nervous system and the lungs. An inspired PO_2 of 0.5 ATA was selected as a horizontal asymptote indicating pulmonary limits because multiday exposures of men to oxygen pressures ranging from 0.23 to 0.55 ATA did not produce detectable impairment of pulmonary function (Clark and Lambertsen, 1971a). The horizontal asymptote for the central nervous system curve of oxygen toxicity has been placed at 2 ATA because neurological effects rarely occur in men during oxygen breathing at this pressure (Clark and Lambertsen, 1971b). Clark and Fisher (1977) pointed out that the rectangular hyperbola describing quantitatively the time of occurrence of oxygen toxicity in the lungs and the central nervous system (Figure 1) has also been found to apply for oxygen toxicity affecting other functions such as the inactivation of cellular respiration, nerve conduction block, and erythrocyte hemolysis. Practical use of oxygen breathing in underwater swimming has been considered to be limited to 30 ft (Yarbrough et al., 1947) and 25 ft (Donald, 1947). The maximum safe depth for pure oxygen diving is set in the U.S. Navy Diving Manual at 10 m or 33 ft.

Central Nervous System Oxygen Toxicity

Clinical Manifestations

Prodromal signs and symptoms listed in order of their percentage of incidence during underwater exposure include: vertigo, nausea, lip-twitching and other involuntary tremors, convulsions, drowsiness, disorientation, acoustic hallucinations, and paresthesia (Donald, 1947). Symptoms of pulmonary irritation were rarely seen in these experiments because CNS symptoms forced termination before pulmonary symptoms could develop. However in other studies of oxygen toxicity in underwater swimming, in which 14 out of 50 exposures (28%) were terminated due to toxic manifestations, dyspnea was by far the most frequent symptom (Schaefer, 1956). The subjects complaining about dyspnea had a rapid respiratory rate (about 32/min) and reported a resistance to breathing and inspiratory inhibition.

Two cardiovascular findings during exposure to increased partial pressure of oxygen at 1.0 or more atm seem to be well-established: the bradycardia which is of vagal origin (Bean and Rottschafer, 1938; Alella and Meda, 1948; Daly and Bondurant, 1962), and the increase noted in the pulse rate and blood pressure if symptoms of oxygen toxicity develop in man (Benedict and Higgins, 1911; Behnke et al., 1935, 1936; Yarbrough et al., 1947). The reported fixation of pulse rate (Schaefer, 1956, 1965) appears to denote the endpoint of the predominant parasympathetic activity and the approaching release of increased sympathetic activity which is associated with symptoms of oxygen toxicity.

Gillen (1966) reported a higher incidence of oxygen convulsions in experienced divers undergoing the oxygen tolerance test than those previously found in studies of underwater swimmers (Donald, 1947; Yarbrough et al., 1947;

Schaefer, 1956). The conditions during the oxygen tolerance test, which involves a 30-min exposure to pure oxygen breathing at an average of 2.82 ATA, may not be comparable to underwater swimming. It was observed that 11 out of 39 divers had their oxygen symptoms during treatment for decompression sickness or air embolism, which may have lowered the threshold for oxygen poisoning.

Etiology

Neurophysiological studies of oxygen toxicity demonstrated that the seizures appear during or just after a sharp rise in cerebral oxygen tensions as measured with the platinum electrode (Bean, 1961). Normal cerebral blood flow prior to the onset of the first electrical discharges and brain tissue PO_2 levels less than theoretically predicted values were found in rats during hyperbaric oxygenation by Torbati et al. (1978). The same authors very recently reported a 10 to 30% increase in regional metabolic rate for brain glucose uptake before onset of convulsions (Torbati et al., 1981). These findings support the notion that higher regional metabolic rates for oxygen may be responsible for the relatively low elevation in brain PO_2 prior to convulsions and that preconvulsive EEG changes are not due to inhibition of brain energy metabolism.

Investigations of Noell (1955, 1962) on the effect of increased oxygen tension on the visual cell of the rabbit retina demonstrated that oxygen exerts a direct toxic effect which is cumulative. Noell (1962) pointed out that in this cumulative action oxygen poisoning resembles the effects of X-irradiation. This observation supports the theory advanced by Gerschman et al. (1954) that oxygen poisoning and X-irradiation have one common mechanism of action, namely, the formation of free radicals. It has been demonstrated that the lethal effects of X-irradiation are enhanced by high oxygen and reduced by anoxia. Furthermore, agents which give protection against X-irradiation, such as glutathione and cysteine, also afford a protection against oxygen poisoning (Gerschman et al., 1954). It is reasonable to assume that oxidizing free radicals such as HO_2^1, $HO\cdot$, and H_2O_2 would react rapidly and initiate chain reactions.

Under these circumstances, the body does require antioxident defenses against uncontrolled oxidations (Gerschman, 1962). Differences in the available antioxidant defenses might account for the wide range in species and organ susceptibility. The discovery of the superoxide dismutases (McCord and Fridovich, 1969) and the elucidation of their antioxidant function consisting of enzymatic inactivation of superoxide (Fridovich, 1975), contributed greatly in advancing the previously neglected free radical theory of oxygen toxicity. The action of toxic free radicals does not require postulation of an O_2 vasoconstrictor effect on the blood vessels or any specific changes in acid-base parameters. The free radical theory offers therefore an explanation for the occurrence of oxygen toxicity under conditions such as exercise in high PO_2, when changes in circulation and arterial and venous PCO_2 and PO_2 are too small to account for the development of symptoms.

The antioxidant defense mechanisms may become exhausted if too many oxygen free radicals are formed and as a consequence oxidation of essential cellular constituents such as sulfhydryl-containing proteins may occur. A variety of metabolic changes produced under conditions of oxygen toxicity have been described and different investigators have attached major significance to different metabolic changes in the development of oxygen toxicity. Chance and coworkers (1965, 1966) have emphasized the inactivation of the energy-linked reverse electron transport pathway. Wood et al. (1969) have accumulated evidence indicating that changes in brain gamma-aminobutyric acid (GABA) levels are involved in CNS oxygen toxicity. The GABA is known to be a transmitter at central nervous system inhibiting synapses. Hyperoxia has been shown to reduce endogenous output of GABA (Wood et al., 1969), which is thought to cause convulsions by allowing uncontrolled firing of excitatory nerves. This theory has found further support in the findings of Radomsky and Watson (1973) which showed that lithium treatment is effective in inhibiting convulsions and also preventing a decrease in brain GABA which precedes the onset of convulsions in oxygen toxicity.

Rats exposed to 4 ATA 100% O_2 for 3 hr showed preconvulsive inhibition of NaK-ATPase activity during the first hr of exposure, followed by a decrease in cortical (K^+) and an increase in cortical (Na^+) during the second hr. Convulsions occurred during the third hr of exposure (Kovachich et al., 1981). The authors suggest that oxygen convulsions may be caused by this redistribution of electrolytes since accumulation of K^+ in the extracellular fluid may cause depolarization and hyperexcitability.

Exercise (Donald, 1947) and CO_2 inhalation (Marshall and Lambertsen, 1961; Bean and Zee, 1966) have been shown to hasten the onset of oxygen toxicity. Studies of chronic exposure to increased CO_2 levels carried out in rats and guinea pigs demonstrated that the precipitating effect of CO_2 in regard to oxygen toxicity is limited to the acute phase of CO_2 exposure which is associated with a stress effect on the adrenals. During the chronic phase of CO_2 exposure, the stress effect subsides and the onset of oxygen toxicity is delayed (Schaefer, 1974). Animal studies have shown that factors which stimulate metabolism in general cause an enhancement of oxygen toxicity, e.g., epinephrine, norepinephrine, adrenocortical hormones, thyroid hormones, and hyperthermia, while the opposite is true for factors leading to a decrease in metabolism such as hypothyroidism, hypothermia, adrenergic blocking agents, and starvation. Drugs that have been found effective in animal experiments in preventing oxygen toxicity could not be used in man because of existing toxic side effects with the possible exception of disulfiram (Clark and Fisher, 1977).

Most recent studies have demonstrated that aspirin given to rats exposed to 100% O_2 at 6 ATA doubled the time to onset of convulsions (Brady and Bradley, 1981). The proposed mechanism for the action of this anti-inflammatory drug consists of an inhibition of prostaglandins and possibly scavenging of free radicals.

Prevention

It has been emphasized by Edmonds et al. (1976) that the only real practical approach for the prevention of oxygen toxicity is to place limits on the exposure. This is especially important for underwater swimming while breathing oxygen. The Royal British Navy and Royal Australian Navy limit the depth for a resting dive breathing pure oxygen to 9 m and a working dive to 7 m. The U.S. Navy employs a depth-time of exposure table for the same purpose. In therapeutic recompression using oxygen, intermittent periods of air breathing are routinely used which shorten the exposure to high levels of oxygen and thereby reduce the occurrence of oxygen toxicity.

Pulmonary Oxygen Toxicity

Pulmonary oxygen toxicity does not play a role in oxygen diving of relatively short durations lasting minutes or hours. However, in saturation diving, subjects may be exposed to increased oxygen partial pressures for days and weeks. Under these conditions as well as in oxygen recompression therapy, the length of exposure is sufficient to cause pulmonary oxygen toxicity if the ambient oxygen partial pressure is too high.

The limits of oxygen partial pressure to which subjects can safely be exposed for prolonged periods of time have been established in extensive multiday exposures of men. Clark and Lambertsen's earlier prediction (1967) indicated a maximum safe, long-term O_2 pressure of 0.6 ATA. This is in line with the threshold given in the 1962 NASA Life Sciences Data Book (Webb, 1962). Clark and Lambertsen (1971a) later revised the limit and adopted a more conservative figure of 0.5 ATA. Pulmonary functions studied during shallow habitat air dives which lasted up to 30 days with an average resident O_2 partial pressure of 0.51 and 0.57 ATA did not show significant changes which would suggest that the earlier prediction of 0.6 ATA is more nearly correct than the conservative revision (Dougherty et al., 1978).

Fisher et al. (1968) and Clark and Lambertsen (1971b) studied several methods for measuring the rate of development of pulmonary oxygen poisoning in normal men during continuous oxygen breathing at an ambient pressure of 2 ATA. They observed significant changes of the following lung functions at a reversible stage of oxygen poisoning: vital capacity, inspiratory capacity, expiratory reserve volume, inspiratory flow rate, carbon monoxide diffusing capacity, lung compliance, and respiratory rate. Decrease in vital capacity has proved to be a very good indicator of the development of oxygen toxicity in healthy subjects during diving operations.

The rate of development of symptoms has been compared with the decrease in vital capacity during oxygen breathing at 2 ATA (Clark and Lambertsen, 1971b). The sensitivity of vital capacity measurements for monitoring development of pulmonary oxygen toxicity in saturation-excursion diving has recently been demonstrated in an experiment in which subjects were exposed for 8 days to compressed air at 2.53 ATA with daily 9-hr excursions to 4.03 ATA. The mean oxygen tension was 0.61 ATA. One subject showed a progressive fall in daily forced vital capacity (FVC) measurements beginning with the second excursion. Simultaneously, his subjective chest discomfort increased (Dougherty et al., 1978).

In subsequent air saturation-excursion dives (Airsat I, II, and III), observations on vital capacity changes were extended to 31 divers (Dougherty et al., 1981). In Airsat I and II, which involved air saturation at 2.82 ATA and a PO_2 level of 0.57 ATA, air excursions were made to 4.03 and 5.55 ATA. Ten percent of the subjects showed persistent and significant decrements in FVC, but a small early transient drop in FVC occurred in most subjects. In Airsat III, in which subjects were exposed to an air saturation depth of 5 ATA and a PO_2 level of 0.3 ATA, air excursions were made to 7 ATA. Twenty-four hr prior to decompression the subjects were exposed to 5 ATA air, corresponding to PO_2 levels of 0.84 ATA. This resulted in a significant FVC decrement in 30% of the subjects (Eckenhoff et al., 1981).

Pathology

Acute and chronic phases of pulmonary oxygen toxicity have been described. Acute pulmonary oxygen toxicity caused by exposure to oxygen pressures higher than 0.8 ATA, is characterized by atelectasis, interstitial and alveolar edema, hemorrhages, hyaline membrane rupture, and swelling and destruction of type 1 alveolar epithelial cells (Kistler et al., 1966; Clark and Lambertsen, 1971a). The histopathological changes observed in acute pulmonary oxygen toxicity are surprisingly similar to those found in acute pulmonary CO_2 toxicity, except that in the latter the type 2 alveolar epithelial cells are primarily affected (Schaefer et al., 1964; Schaefer, 1965). After 72 hr of exposure to 98.5% oxygen, the thickness of the air-blood barrier was found to be doubled in rats, indicating a severe impairment of gas exchange (Kistler et al., 1966). In chronic pulmonary oxygen toxicity, which occurs during prolonged exposure to pressures between 0.5 and 0.8 ATA, hyperplasia of type 2 alveolar epithelial cells develops along with thickening of alveolar walls and arteriolar hypertrophy. An increased rate of collagen synthesis was found during chronic pulmonary oxygen toxicity, which is probably associated with the observed chronic fibrosis of the lungs (Valimaki et al., 1975).

Etiology

The enzymatic changes observed in pulmonary oxygen toxicity are similar to those found in CNS oxygen toxicity. Moreover, hyperoxia causes metabolic changes in the lungs such as reductions of oxygen uptake and ATP synthesis and the incorporation of radioactive leucine into tissue components by lung homogenates (Gacad and Massaro, 1973; Sanders et al., 1976). A depression of pulmonary serotonin clearance was also found in hyperoxia, suggesting impairment of endothelial cell membrane transport (Block and Fisher, 1977). It appears that these changes in intracellular enzymes and endothelial transport occur in acute pulmonary oxygen toxicity after the antioxidant defense mechanism have been exhausted. This would also explain the markedly higher mortality of older animals exposed to 100% oxygen for prolonged periods of time (Brooksby et al., 1966), since older animals are known to have reduced antioxidant defense mechanisms.

Effects of Hyperoxia on Other Organ Systems

Most of the investigators of oxygen toxicity have focused their attention on the effects of hyperoxia on lungs and brain. However it has been shown that 30-day exposure to 0.33 ATA oxygen, which does not impair pulmonary function in men (Robertson et al., 1964), will produce effects on red cells and endocrine functions (Love et al., 1971; Larkin et al., 1972).

Fisher and Kimzey (1971) have demonstrated that prolonged exposure to increased oxygen levels in spacecraft operations causes abnormal red cell morphology and a decrease in circulating red cell mass. This may be caused by a depression of erythropoiesis induced by the increased oxygen tension, since it is known that the former is closely regulated by the oxygen tension.

The retinal vessels are particularly susceptible to high oxygen pressures. Behnke et al. (1936) were the first investigators to report on subjective visual impairment of subjects at 3 ATA oxygen. Comroe et al. (1945) found occular hypotonia in their studies. Noell (1955, 1962) described in detail the metabolic injuries of the visual cell occurring in the outer nuclear layer during breathing of 100% oxygen. Although Noell (1962) believed that a direct toxic effect of oxygen is the cause of the visual impairment, other evidence showing an oxygen-induced decrease in both retinal and uveal blood flow (Saltzman et al., 1965; Trokel, 1965) suggests that the retinal changes in hyperoxia are caused by an intensive vasoconstriction. Visual acuity changes have also been found in patients following intermittent exposures to 2.5 ATA of oxygen for treatment of osteomyelitis (Hart et al., 1974).

A more recent report on serous otitis media, observed in divers breathing 100% oxygen from semiclosed and closed circuit diving equipment (Strauss et al., 1973), suggested that this syndrome is caused by the absorption of oxygen from the middle ear. Similar observations had been made previously in aviators exposed to high oxygen during flight.

Oxygen Requirements in the Hyperbaric Environment

Hypoventilation and CO_2 retention have been observed frequently at pressures of 4.0 ATA and greater while breathing N_2-O_2 mixtures (Lanphier, 1963; Hesser et al., 1968; Lambertsen et al., 1973; Fagraeus, 1974; Morrison et al., 1976). The limitation of ventilation under pressure has been attributed to the increased respiratory resistance to breathing denser gas mixtures whereby a significant load is put on the respiratory system, the pulmonary circulation and the right heart. The simultaneous study of respiratory functions and electrocardiographic changes in rest and exercise during saturation excursion dives breathing N_2-O_2 mixtures showed that constraints on pulmonary and circulatory functions are correlated with each other. Arrhythmias were only found under conditions in rest and exercise in which the ventilatory response was decreased and CO_2 retention occurred (Wilson et al., 1977; Schaefer et al., 1981).

The constraints on pulmonary and circulatory functions produced by exposure to hyperbaric environments breathing N_2-O_2 mixtures may interfere with oxygen transport and could be the cause of normoxic hypoxia, first reported by Chouteau (1971). He exposed goats to high pressures with normal ambient oxygen pressures of 159 mm Hg and observed symptoms of behavioral disorders and paralysis which could be reversed by increasing the partial pressure of oxygen to 191 mm Hg without changing the absolute pressure.

Similar observations have been reported by Wilson et al. (1977) in a saturation dive in which 3 men were exposed to 7 ATA while breathing a nitrogen-oxygen mixture which contained 0.21 ATA oxygen. Between 1 and 2 hr after pressurization to 7.0 ATA, two of the divers experienced the onset of nausea and shortly afterwards began vomiting. All 3 divers also showed symptoms of vertigo, slurred speech, and cold sensations not usually associated with nitrogen narcosis. Relief of the symptoms occurred following elevation of PIO_2 from 0.21 ATA to 0.30 ATA. Subsequent exercise tests did not cause a return of the symptoms. During the initial period, one of the divers had electrocardiographic changes at rest consisting of a lengthening of the P-R interval from 0.14 sec (control) to 0.21 sec. The P waves became progressively more flattened and disappeared, resulting in a nodal rhythm (Figure 2). Minor S-T elevations,

Figure 2. ECG tracings of a diver during N_2-O_2 dive at 7.0 ATA showing an apparent progressive loss of the P waves. Tracings taken 7 hr after saturation depth (7.0 ATA) was reached show loss of P waves with no retrograde P waves visible.
SOURCE: *Wilson et al., 1977.*

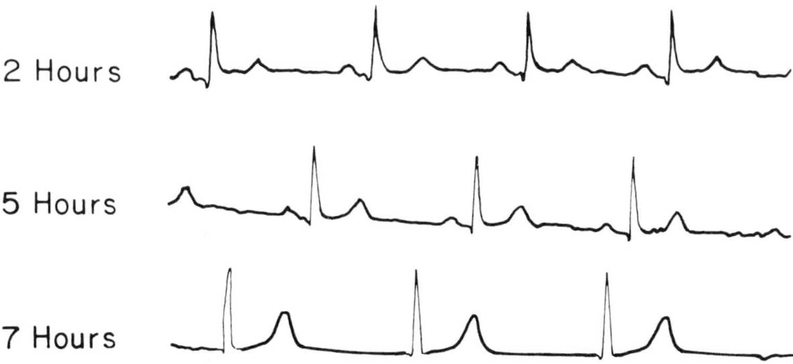

rSR′ complexes in the right precordial lead and diphasic T waves also appeared during this period, indicating a right ventricular conduction delay (Figure 3). After 8 hr of breathing the increased oxygen concentration, the rSR′ complexes and T wave changes had disappeared, and the P waves were more evident. In another diver, premature ventricular contractions had occurred during the initial period of 0.21 ATA oxygen, which disappeared after more oxygen was added (Figure 4).

Although other factors such as an aberrant high pressure nervous syndrome have been considered as causes of the reported symptoms and electrocardiographic changes, tissue hypoxia remains the most likely explanation. This interpretation is supported by recent investigations of Doubt and Evans (1981). They examined excitation-contraction (E-C) variables in intact hearts of cats during normoxic ($PO_2 = 0.35$ ATA) helium dives from 1 to 30 ATA. The E-C delay was measured as the time from onset of ventricular excitation (QRS complex of ECG) to onset of left ventricular pressure (LVP) recorded from the intracavity catheter. The E-C delay increased with depth. Pulsus alternans and alternate variations in beat-to-beat LVP amplitude developed, indicating depressed contractility. Breathing hyperoxic mixtures ($PO_2 = 2$ ATA) at 30 ATA the E-C delay was reduced and the pulsus alternans was abolished

Figure 3. ECG tracings of a diver during N_2-O_2 dive at 7.0 ATA before oxygen concentration was increased. Note flattened appearance of P waves, rSR′ complexes in the right precordial leads and diphasic T waves. Tracings approximately 8 hr after oxygen concentration was increased are on the right. Note disappearance of rSR′ complexes in V1 and diphasic T waves in V2.

SOURCE: *Wilson et al., 1977.*

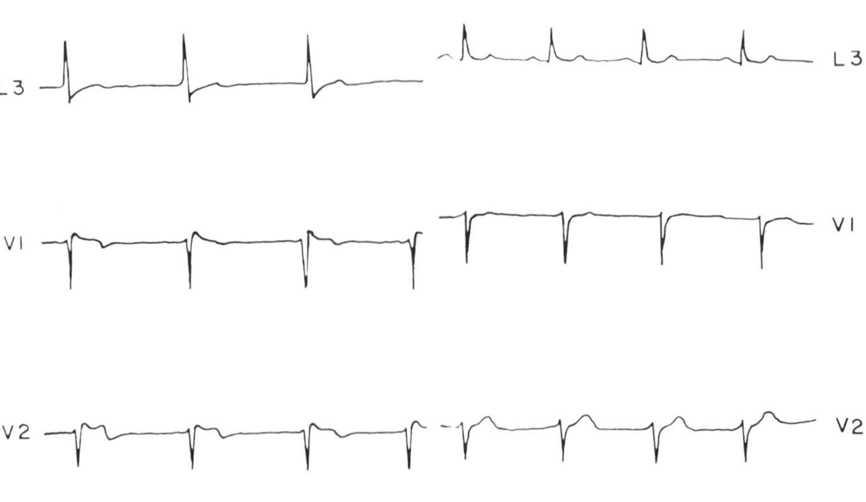

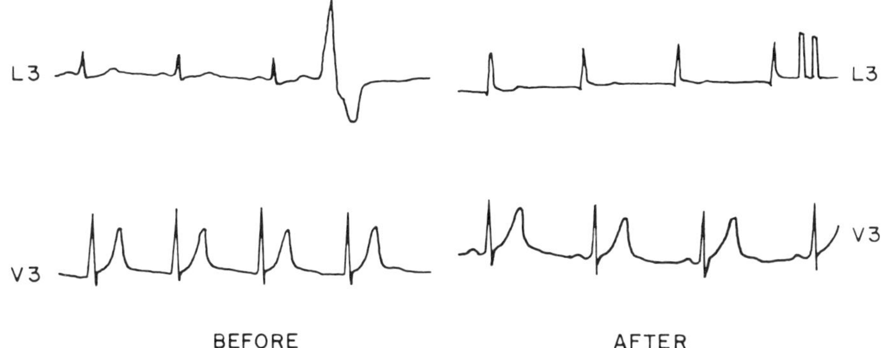

Figure 4. Tracing of a diver during N_2-O_2 dive at 7.0 ATA before oxygen concentration was increased. Note premature ventricular contractions in L3 and the tall T waves in V3. Approximately 8 hr after oxygen concentration was increased, premature ventricular contractions had disappeared, while tall T waves persisted.

SOURCE: *Wilson et al., 1977.*

or lessened. These studies clearly show an ameliorating effect of increased oxygen levels on the performance of the heart.

References

Alella, A. and Meda, E. 1948. Frequenza cardiaca durante la respirazioni di O_2 nell'uomo ed importanza del vago. *Boll. Soc. Ital. Biol. Sper.* 24:581.

Bean, J.W. 1945. Effects of oxygen at increased pressure. *Physiol. Rev.* 25:1–147.

Bean, J.W. 1961. Tris buffer, carbon dioxide, and sympathoadrenal system in reactions to oxygen at high pressure. *Am. J. Physiol.* 201:737–739.

Bean, J.W. and Rottschafer, G. 1938. Reflexogenic and central structures in oxygen poisoning. *J. Physiol. (London).* 94:294–306.

Bean, J.W. and Zee, D. 1966. Influence of anesthesia and carbon dioxide on CNS and pulmonary effects of oxygen at high pressure. *J. Appl. Physiol.* 21:521–526.

Behnke, A.R., Forbes, H.S., and Motley, E.P. 1936. Circulatory and visual effects of oxygen at 3 atmospheres pressure. *Am. J. Physiol.* 114:436–442.

Behnke, A.R., Johnson, F.S., Poppen, J.R., and Motley, E.P. 1935. The effect of oxygen on man at pressures from one to four atmospheres. *Am. J. Physiol.* 110:565–572.

Benedict, F.G. and Higgins, H.L. 1911. Effects on men at rest of breathing oxygen-rich gas mixtures. *Am. J. Physiol.* 28:1–28.

Bert, P. 1878. *La Pression barometrique, recherches de physiologie experimentale.* Paris: Masson. 1168 pp. (English translation: *Barometric Pressure. Researches in Experimental Physiology.* 1943. Hitchcock, M.A. and Hitchcock, F.A., translators. Columbus, Ohio: College Book Co, 1055 pp.

Block, E.R. and Fisher, A.B. 1977. Depression of serotonin clearance by rat lungs during oxygen exposure. *J. Appl. Physiol.* 42:33–38.

Brady, J.I., Jr. and Bradley, M.E. 1981. Effects of nonsteroidal anti-inflammatory drugs on CNS oxygen toxicity. *Undersea Biomed. Res. Suppl.* 8(1):65.

Brooksby, G.A., Dennis, R.L., and Staley, R.W. 1966. Effects of prolonged exposure of rats to increased oxygen pressure. In *Proceedings of the Third International Conference on Hyperbaric Medicine*. Brown, I.W. and Cox, B.G., eds. Washington, D.C.: National Academy Sciences. Publ. 1404: pp. 208–216.

Chance, B., Jamieson, D., and Coles, H. 1965. Energy-linked pyridine nucleotide reduction: inhibitory effects of hyperbaric oxygen *in vitro* and *in vivo*. *Nature* 206:257–263.

Chance, B., Jamieson, D., and Williamson, J.R. 1966. Control of the oxidation-reduction state of reduced pyridine nucleotides *in vivo* and *in vitro* by hyperbaric oxygen. In *Proceedings of the Third International Conference on Hyperbaric Medicine*. Brown, I.W. and Cox, B.G., eds. Washington, D.C.: National Academy of Sciences. Publ. 1404. pp. 15–41.

Chouteau, J. 1971. Respiratory gas exchange in animals during exposure to extreme ambient pressures. In *Proceedings in the Fourth Symposium on Underwater Physiology*. Lambertson, C.J., ed. New York: Academic Press.

Clark, J.M. and Fisher, A.B. 1977. Oxygen toxicity and extension of tolerance in oxygen therapy. In *Hyperbaric Oxygen Therapy*. Davis, J.C. and Hunt, T.K., eds. Bethesda, Maryland: Undersea Medical Society, pp. 61–77.

Clark, J.A. and Lambertsen, C.J., 1967. Pulmonary oxygen tolerance and the rate of development of pulmonary oxygen toxicity in man at two atmospheres inspired oxygen tension. In *Underwater Physiology. Proceedings of the Third Symposium on Underwater Physiology*. Lambertsen, C.J., ed. Baltimore, Maryland: Williams and Wilkins, pp. 439–451.

Clark, J.M. and Lambertsen, C.J. 1971a. Pulmonary oxygen toxicity: a review. *Pharmacol. Rev.* 23:37–133.

Clark, J.M. and Lambertsen, C.J. 1971b. Rate of development of pulmonary oxygen toxicity in man during oxygen breathing at 2.0 ATA. *J. Appl. Physiol.* 30:739–752.

Comroe, J.H., Dripps, R.D., Dumke, P.R., and Demming, M. 1945. Oxygen toxicity: the effect of inhalation of high concentrations of oxygen for 24 hours on normal men at sea level and at a simulated altitude of 18,000 feet. *J.A.M.A.* 128:710–717.

Daly, W. and Bondurant, J.S. 1962. Effects of oxygen breathing on the heart rate, blood pressure, and cardiac index of normal men resting with reactive hyperemia and after atropine. *J. Clin. Invest.* 41:126–132.

Dejours, P., Labrousse, Y., Raynaud, J., Girard, F., and Teillac, A. 1958. Stimulus oxygene de la ventilation au repos et au cours de l'exercise musculaire, a basse altitude (50 m) chez l'homme. *Rev. Fr. Clin. Biol.* 3(2):105–123.

Donald, K.W. 1947. Oxygen poisoning in man. *Brit. M. J.* 1:667–672 and 712. (See also Admiralty Experimental Diving Unit Report No. 16, 1946).

Doubt, T.J. and Evans, D.E. 1981. Excitation-contraction coupling in intact cat hearts during hyperbaric helium-O_2 exposures. *Undersea Biomed. Res. Suppl.* 8(1):67.

Dougherty, J.H., Jr., Frayre, R.L., Miller, C.A., and Schaefer, K.E. 1978. Pulmonary function during shallow habitad air dives (Shad I, II, III). In *Proceedings of the Sixth Symposium on Underwater Physiology*. Schilling, C.W. and Beckett, M.W., eds. Bethesda, Maryland: FASEB, pp. 193–204.

Dougherty, J.H., Jr., Styer, D.J., Eckenhoff, R.G., and Hunter, W.L., Jr., 1981. The effects of hyperbaric and hyperoxic conditions on pulmonary function during prolonged hyperbaric chamber and saturation dives. *Undersea Biomed. Res. Suppl.* 8(1):29.

Eckenhoff, R.G., Hunter, W.L., Jr., Parker, J.W., Dougherty, J.H., Jr., Moeller, G.O., Tappan, D.V., and Jordan, J.C. 1981. Progress of an air saturation dive series; Airsat. *Undersea Biomed. Res. Suppl.* 8(1):39.

Edmonds, C., Lowry, C., and Pennefather, J. 1976. *Diving and Subaquatique Medicine*. Mosman, N.S.W., Australia: diving Medical Center.

Fagraeus, L. 1974. Cardiorespiratory and metabolic functions during exercise in the hyperbaric environment. *Acta Physiol. Scand.* 414(suppl.):1–40.

Fischer, C.L. and Kimzey, S.L. 1971. Effects of oxygen on blood formation and destruction. *Proceedings of the Fourth Symposium on Underwater Physiology*. Lambertson, C.J., ed. New York: Academic Press.

Fisher, A.B., Hyde, R.W., Puy, R.J., Clark, J.M., and Lambertsen, C.J. 1968. Effect of oxygen at 2 atmospheres on the pulmonary mechanics of normal man. *J. Appl. Physiol.* 24:529–536.

Fridovich, I. 1975. Superoxide dismutases. *Ann. Rev. Biochem.* 44:147–159.

Gacad, G. and Massaro, D. 1973. Hyperoxia: influence of lung mechanics and protein synthesis. *J. Clin. Invest.* 52:559–565.

Gerschman, R. 1962. The biological effects of increased oxygen tension. In *Man's Dependence on the Earthly Atmosphere*. Schaefer, K.E., ed. New York: MacMillan, p. 171.

Gerschman, R., Gilbert, D.L., Nye, S.W., Dwyer, P., and Fenn, W.O. 1954. Oxygen poisoning and X-irradiation: a mechanism in common. *Science*. 119:623–626.

Gillen, H.W. 1966. Oxygen convulsions in man. In *Proceedings of the Third International Conference on Hyperbaric Medicine*. Brown, I.W. and Cox, B.G., eds. Washington, D.C.: National Academy of Sciences. Publ. 1404: pp. 217–223.

Hart, G.B., Lee, W.S., Rasmussen, B.D., and O'Reilly, R.R. 1974. Complications of repetitive hyperbaric therapy. In *Proceedings of the Fifth International Hyperbaric Congress, Vol. II*. Trapp, W.G., Banister, E.W., Davison, A.J., and Trapp, P.A., eds. British Columbia: Simon Fraser University, pp. 867–873.

Hesser, C.M. 1962. The role of nitrogen in breath-holding at increased pressures. In *Man's Dependence on the Earthly Atmosphere*. Schaefer, K.E., ed. New York: MacMillan, p. 327.

Hesser, C.M., Fagraeus, L., and Linnarsson, D. 1968. *Cardiorespiratory Responses to Exercise in Hyperbaric Environment.* Report Lab. Aviat. Nav. Med Stockholm, Karolinska Institute.

Huber, G.L. and Drath, D.B. 1981. Pulmonary oxygen toxicity. In *Oxygen in Living Processes: An Interdisciplinary Approach*. Gilbert, D., ed. New York: Springer Verlag, pp. 273–342.

Kistler, G.S., Caldwell, P.R., and Weibel, E.R. 1966. Quantitative electron microscopic studies of murine lung damage after exposure to 98.5% oxygen at ambient pressure: a preliminary report. *Proceedings of the Third International Conference on Hyperbaric Medicine*. Brown, I.W. and Cox, B.G., eds. Washington, D.C.: National Academy of Sciences. Publ. 1404: pp. 169–178.

Kovachich, G.B., Mishra, O.P., and Clark, J.M. 1981. Preconclusive changes in NaK-ATPase activity, K^+ and Na^+ concentrations in the cortex of rats exposed to O_2 at 4.0 ATA. *Undersea Biomed. Res. Suppl.* 8(1):53.

Lambertsen, C.J., Gelfand, R., Lever, M.J., Bodammer, G., Takano, N., Reed, T.A., Dickson, J.G., and Watson, P.T. 1973. Respiration and gas exchange during a 14-day continuous exposure to 5.2% O_2 in N_2 at pressure equivalent to 100 FSW (4 ATA). *Aerospace Med.* 44:844–849.

Lanphier, E.H. 1963. Influence of increased ambient pressure upon alveolar ventilation. In *Proceedings of the Second Symposium on Underwater Physiology*. Lambertsen, C.J. and Greenbaum, L.J., eds. Washington, D.C.: National Academy of Sciences. Publ. 1181: pp. 124–133.

Larkin, E.C., Adams, J.D., Williams, W.T., and Duncan, D.M. 1972. Hematologic responses to hypobaric hyperoxia. *Am. J. Physiol.* 223:431–437.

Love, T.L., Schnure, J.J., Larkin, E.C., Lipman, R.L. and Lecocq, F.R. 1971. Glucose intolerance in man during prolonged exposure to hypobaric-hyperoxic environment. *Diabetes* 20:282–285.

Marshall, J.R. and Lambertsen, C.J. 1961. Interactions of increase PO_2 and PCO_2 effects in producing convulsions and death in mice. *J. Appl. Physiol.* 16:1–7.

McCord, J.M. and Fridovich, I. 1969. Superoxide dismutase. An enzymic function for erythrocuprein (hemocuprein). *J. Biol. Chem.* 224:6049–6055.

Meda, E.I. 1950. Effetti della respirazione di miscele ricche di O_2 sull'apparato cardiovascolare dell'uomo. II. Variazione elettrocardiografiche nell'uomo durante la respirazione di O_2. *Boll. Soc. Ital. Biol. Sper.* 26:931.

Morrison, J.B., Butt, W.S., Florio, J.T., and Mayo, I.C. 1976. Effects of increased O_2-N_2 pressure and breathing apparatus on respiratory function. *Undersea Biomed. Res.* 3(3):217–234.

Noell, W.K. 1955. Visual cell effects of high oxygen pressures. *Fed. Proc.* 14:107.

Noell, W.K. 1962. Effects of high and low oxygen tension on the visual system. In *Environmental Effects on Consciousness*. Schaefer, K.E., ed. New York: MacMillan, p. 3.

Radomsky, M.W. and Watson, W.I. 1973. Effect of lithium on acute oxygen toxicity and associated changes in brain gamma-aminobutyric acid. *Aerospace Med.* 44:387–392.

Robertson, W.G., Hargreaves, J.J., Herlocker, J.E., and Welch, B.E. 1964. Physiologic response to increased oxygen partial pressure. II. Respiratory studies. *Aerospace Med.* 35:618–622.

Saltzman, H.A., Hart, L., Sieker, H.O., and Duffy, E.J. 1965. Retinal vascular response to hyperbaric oxygenation. *J.A.M.A.* 191:290–292.

Sanders, A.P., Gelein, R.S., and Currie, W.D. 1976. The effect of hyperbaric oxygenation on the metabolism of the lung. In *Underwater Physiology V. Proceedings of the Fifth Symposium on Underwater Physiology*. Lambertsen, C.J., ed. Bethesda: FASEB, pp. 483–492.

Schaefer, K.E. 1956. Oxygen toxicity studies in underwater swimming. *J. Appl. Physiol.* 8:524–531.

Schaefer, K.E. 1965. Circulatory adaptation to the requirements of life under more than one atmosphere of pressure. In *Handbook of Physiology, Section* 2, *Circulation, Volume III*. Hamilton, W.F. and Dow, P., eds. Washington, D.C.: American Physiological Society, pp. 1843–1873.

Schaefer, K.E. 1974. Modification of oxygen toxicity by chronic hypercapnia. *Proceedings of the International Union of Physiological Sciences*, New Delhi. 11:350.

Schaefer, K.E., Avery, M.E., and Bensch, K. 1964. Time-course of changes in surface tension and morphology of alveolar epithelial cells in CO_2-induced hyaline membrane disease. *J. Clin. Invest.* 43:2080–2093.

Schaefer, K.E., Dougherty, J.H., Jr., Wilson, J.M., Frayre, R.L., and Knight, D.R. 1981. CO_2 retention and ECG changes in exercise during prolonged hyperbaric N_2-O_2 breathing. *J. Appl. Physiol.*, in press.

Strauss, M.B., Lee, W., and Cantrell, R.W., 1973. Serous otitis media in divers breathing 100% oxygen. *Preprints of Annual Scientific Meeting.* (May 7–10), Aerospace Medical Association.

Stroud, R.C. 1959. Combined ventilatory and breath-holding evaluation of sensitivity to respiratory gases. *J. Appl. Physiol.* 14:353–356.

Torbati, D., Greenberg, J., and Lambertsen, C.J., 1981. Glucose uptake in rat's brain during exposure to hyperbaric oxygenation. *Undersea Biomed. Res. Suppl.* 8(1):52.

Torbati, D., Parolla, D., and Lavy, S. 1978. Blood flow in rat brain during exposure to high oxygen pressure. *Aviat. Space, Environ. Med.* 49:963–967.

Trokel, W. 1965. Effect of respiratory gases upon choroidal hemodynamics. *Arch. Ophthal.* 73:838–842.

Valimaki, M., Juva, K., and Rantanen, J. 1975. Collagen metabolism in rat lungs during chronic intermittent exposure to oxygen. *Aviat. Space Environ. Med.* 46:684–690.

Webb, P., ed. 1962. *NASA Life Sciences Data Book*. Washington, D.C.: National Aeronautics and Space Administration.

Wilson, J.M., Kligfield, P., Adams, G.M., Harvey, C., and Schaefer, K.E. 1977. Human ECG changes during prolonged hyperbaric exposures breathing N_2-O_2 mixtures. *J. Appl. Physiol.* 42:614–633.

Wood, J.D., Watson, W.J., and Murray, G.W. 1969. Correlation between decreases in brain gamma-aminobutyric acid levels and susceptibility to convulsions induced by hyperbaric oxygen. *J. Neurochem.* 16:281–287.

Yarbrough, O.D., Welham, W., Brinton, E.S., and Behnke, A.R. 1947. *Symptoms of Oxygen Poisoning and Limits of Tolerance at Rest and at Work*. Research Report Number 1, U.S. Naval Experimental Diving Unit, Washington, D.C.

J.A. Loeppky and M.L. Riedesel, editors
OXYGEN TRANSPORT TO HUMAN TISSUES

Significance of P_{50} Under Stress

Steven M. Horvath and Ronald L. Jackson

Our original intention was to evaluate the alterations in oxygen affinity when the organism was responding to various stressors. We were somewhat surprised to discover, in evaluating the literature, that in all probability the concept of utilizing P_{50} as a measure of hemoglobin's affinity for oxygen was itself under stress. Traditionally, since it was demonstrated that there were relatively small variations in the shape of the oxygen dissociation curve, a single point from the relatively linear portion of the curve could serve as an indication of Hb affinity. A more marked sigmoidal curve facilitates oxygen conductance by the fact that hemoglobin can act on the steep part of the curve where greater amounts of oxygen can be released with slight changes in the partial pressure of oxygen. However, a single point at half saturation tends to ignore the shape of the curve emphasizing only a possible right or left shift at this midpoint. It is probably more correct to consider that the oxygen dissociation curve has adaptive value because of its shape rather than its shift to the right or left.

Early investigators concerned with determination of hemoglobin-oxygen affinity constructed full or nearly complete oxygen dissociation curves. More recently, several shorter and less time-consuming methods have been developed leading to the concept that a measure of affinity can be obtained by presenting only a single point, i.e., the partial pressure of oxygen at which 50% of the hemoglobin is saturated. The procedures utilized have varied from measuring 1 to 5 points on the steep linear portion of the curve, obtaining a single value approximately estimated to occur as close as possible to the half saturation value and referring such estimates to the standard curves of Dill and Forbes (1941) and Severinghaus (1966). Several potential errors in such representations are clearly evident although most investigators have referred to a standard P_{50} value (sP_{50}) in which pH, PCO_2 and temperature are constant but which in general has ignored the effect of other influences such as 2,3-DPG, etc. on hemoglobin (Horvath et al., 1977).

Variability in P_{50}

Hemoglobin-oxygen affinity is known to be altered in a number of physiological and pathological conditions. However, before evaluating the manner by which alterations in sP_{50} would affect oxygen transport, and so reflect abnormal or stressful conditions, we decided to determine the constancy of its normal value as well as the potential magnitude of intra- and inter-individual variance of this measure. Roughton (1964), in his classic discussion of the transport of oxygen and carbon dioxide by blood, stated "the oxygen dissociation curve of several persons has been determined from time to time over a period of years, and is said to remain approximately constant." Indeed, it appears that one could fully accept this concept, i.e., that the sP_{50} has a value of 26 to 27 Torr since it is repeatedly stated to be such in the literature. We collected and analyzed sP_{50} data from some 100 publications. Surprisingly, the mean value turned out to be 26.4 Torr with a small standard error which is not different from the values obtained from the Dill and Severinghaus standard oxygen dissociation curves. However, when we plotted these data as a mean and included the range of individual values, the constancy of the sP_{50} became somewhat questionable. Figure 1 presents values for standard P_{50} from 11 publications and 2 sets of data from our laboratory. Not all of the literature values could be presented in this graph and we selected representative publications spaced over nearly 40 years in which individual values were given. Although the mean value (26.4 Torr) statistically agrees with previously stated values, it is apparent that an extremely larger inter-individual variation is present which ranges from 22 to 31 Torr. The magnitude of these variations in blood obtained from normal resting individuals is greater than the mean changes reported to occur under a variety of abnormal states or stress situations.

In view of such variability, it was necessary to determine whether intra-individual values were constant or exhibited similar large variations. Giannelli et al. (1977), using a single point procedure to estimate P_{50}, reported that oxyhemoglobin affinity could vary significantly within one individual when determined at intervals separated by several days. In one group, the average reported intra-subject difference was 6.4 Torr. The largest variability in one subject was 8.5 Torr. Shifts of this magnitude would have a significant effect on oxygen delivery to tissues. These large intra-individual variations were apparently not associated with alternations in 2,3-DPG or red cell pH. Although these results were disturbing, several of their procedures could have been responsible for the excessive shifts in P_{50} values.

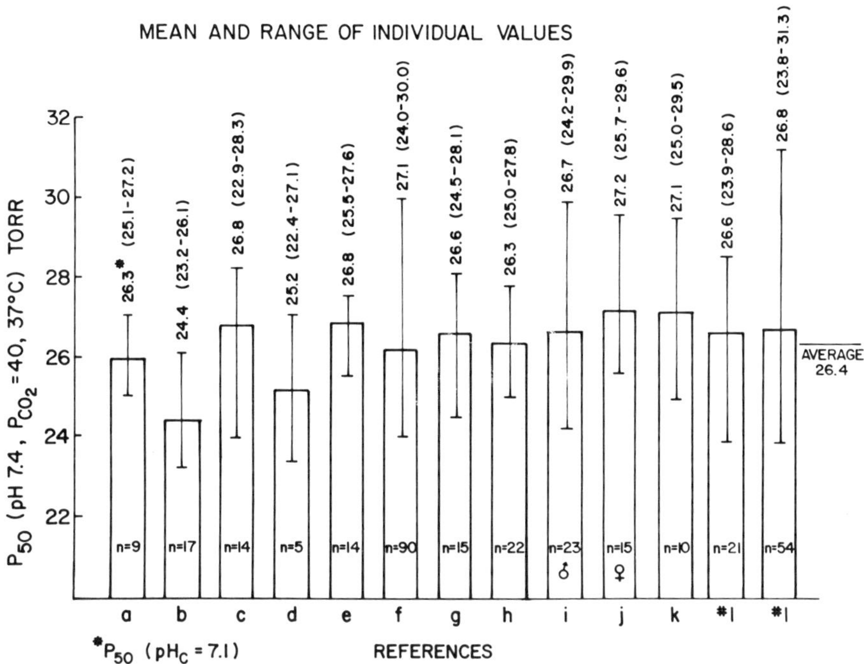

Figure 1. Mean and range of standard P_{50} as reported by 11 investigations [a to k, see Jackson (1981) for references] and 2 studies from our laboratory (#1).

Therefore, we also investigated the within-subject variability of the oxygen dissociation curve of normal, resting individuals. In our 17 subjects (10 men and 7 women), individual sP_{50}s were determined from blood obtained at the same time in the morning on two occasions separated by 48 hr. Blood was collected after a 30-min sitting rest period. Certain precautions to control activity, smoking, food intake, etc. were taken. The initial and 48 hr sP_{50}s for the 17 subjects are shown in Figure 2. There was no statistically significant difference ($P<0.01$) between sP_{50}s determined before and after an interval of 48 hr. The mean $\pm$S.D. of the initial and 48-hr samples were 26.2 ± 1.33 and 26.5 ± 1.32 Torr, respectively, with an average intra-subject difference of 0.72 ± 0.48 Torr. Some differences between the values obtained on these two occasions were observed but the greatest individual variation between days was only 1.5 Torr. Although sP_{50} demonstrated no significant intra-individual variability over 48 hr, it should be noted that there was considerable between-subject variation (range 23.9 to 28.9 Torr) as demonstrated by others (Figure 1). However, not included in the above calculations were two occasions when large intra-subject variation was found. A female subject demonstrated a 2.1 Torr and a male subject showed a 5.2 Torr difference after 48 hr. Upon questioning each individual, we discovered a factor common to both subjects. Each had been involved in a strenuous physical workout; the female, a 10-kilometer run 12 hr earlier and the male a handball match 1 to 2 hr before the sampling. This marked right shift following uncontrolled subject activity could probably account for some of the inter-individual variability illustrated in Figure 1. If reliable comparisons are to be made between control and stressful situations, certain factors such as prior exercise, level of physical fitness, physical training, presence of certain pharmaceuticals and carbon monoxide must be controlled because they will influence the O_2 affinity in blood obtained from resting individuals.

In one subject, oxygen dissociation curves were determined over a 2.5-yr period. The mean $\pm$S.D. for 10 measurements of sP_{50} was 27.5 ± 0.95 Torr (range: 26.8 to 28.5 Torr). However, 4 of the 10 measurements were performed while the subject was breathing 72% oxygen. If only the normoxic, rest data were included ($n=6$) the mean $\pm$S.D. was 27.2 ± 0.33 Torr (range: 26.8 to 27.7 Torr). If only the 4 trials were used when blood was obtained while the subject breathed the hyperoxic air mixture, the mean $\pm$S.D. was 28.0 ± 0.57 Torr (range: 27.2 to 28.5 Torr). Thus, if subjects are selected carefully and conditions are controlled properly, hemoglobin-oxygen affinity appears to be reproducible. However, if conditions are not matched between measurement periods (such as with the intervention of exercise), the sP_{50} can demonstrate wide intra-individual variations.

Exercise and Training

We then proceeded to evaluate alterations in sP_{50} taking into account as fully as possible intra- and inter-subject variability and certain stressor effects. In view of our observations, that prior exercise induced a marked right shift and that exercise, per se, is accompanied by changes in body temperature and some ligands (primarily H^+, CO_2, and 2,3-DPG), maximum exercise should result in significant alterations in oxygen affinity. A limited number of publications were available for this analysis (Table 1). Reported sP_{50}s in resting trained subjects averaged 26.8 Torr with a range from 25.7 to 28.0, while in resting untrained subjects a mean value of 26.2 was found with a range from 23.8 to 27.1 Torr. Highly trained subjects apparently receive no benefit from a shifted curve from their attainment of a high level of physical fitness. Only one study was found in which the same 3 subjects were studied before and after 8 weeks of training (Table 1). In these resting subjects 2,3-DPG increased 7% consequent to training, but sP_{50} showed a mean decrease of 1.2 Torr. The P_{50} in blood obtained after the maximum aerobic test in the untrained state dropped slightly while it increased insignificantly following the same test after training.

From these studies under consideration (Table 1), maximum efforts by untrained subjects resulted in a slight increase in postexercise sP_{50}, but the values ranged from a -0.7 to $+1.6$ Torr. A similar pattern was observed in trained subjects, with a range from 0.0 to $+2.8$ Torr. Therefore, it can only be

Table 1. Influence of Maximal Exercise[b] on sP_{50}.[c]

	Subjects		Standard P_{50}		In vivo P_{50}		Effectors of in vivo shift, Torr			
Ref[a]	n	UT/TR	Rest	Max	Rest	Max	T°	pH	2, 3-DPG	Unknown
l	3	UT	26.9	26.2	27.4	36.3	1.9	5.3	1.0	+0.7
	3	TR(b)[d]	25.7	26.5	25.8	38.9	2.3	6.5	0.0	+4.3
m	6	UT	23.8	24.8	—	—				
	6	TR	25.7	26.7	—	—				
n	10	TR	27.2	30.0	27.0	35.8	0.0	5.5	1.5	+1.5
o	6	UT	26.7	27.7	26.7	38.8	6.6	4.6	1.0	0.0
p	6	UT	25.2	26.7	25.8	—				
	6	TR	27.4	28.9	31.7	—				
q	8	UT	26.5	26.5	—	—				
	10	TR	28.0	28.0	—	—				
r	6	UT	26.4	28.0	—	—				
	10	UT	27.1	28.5	—	—				
s	11	UT	27.0	28.5	27.0	31.1	0.0	2.0	−1.5	+3.1

[a]References from Jackson (1981).

[b]Nonsmokers.

[c]Standard P_{50} $pH_{7.4}$, PCO_2 40 Torr, 37°C.

[d]Same subjects after 8 weeks of training. Max P_{50}: following maximal exercise. UT: Untrained subjects; TR: Trained subjects.

stated that sP_{50} is hardly influenced by the changes in blood parameters resulting from maximum effort. On the other hand, *in vivo* measurements of P_{50} indicate that oxygen affinity is altered. A mean change of +9.4 Torr in 5 studies (Table 1) occurred in both trained and untrained subjects, although data from the one study suggests that training induces a greater right shift with exercise in the *in vivo* oxygen dissociation curve. *In vivo* P_{50} was significantly increased with exercise to a greater extent (+13.1 Torr) in the trained than in the untrained state (+8.9 Torr). This right shift in the trained subject was greater than could be predicted from the effects of temperature, 2,3-DPG, and pH effects. Although the available data is meager and to some degree variable, it does suggest that *in vivo* P_{50} may provide more useful information than sP_{50}. It is also of some importance that consideration be given to determination of the other factors influencing *in vivo* values, since it is apparent that the known factors do not account for all the shifts observed (Table 1).

Altitude

It is commonly accepted that newcomers to and permanent residents at high altitude have a decreased hemoglobin-oxygen affinity. This right shift of the

Figure 2. Reproducibility of sP_{50} in resting subjects measured at two intervals separated by 48 hr.

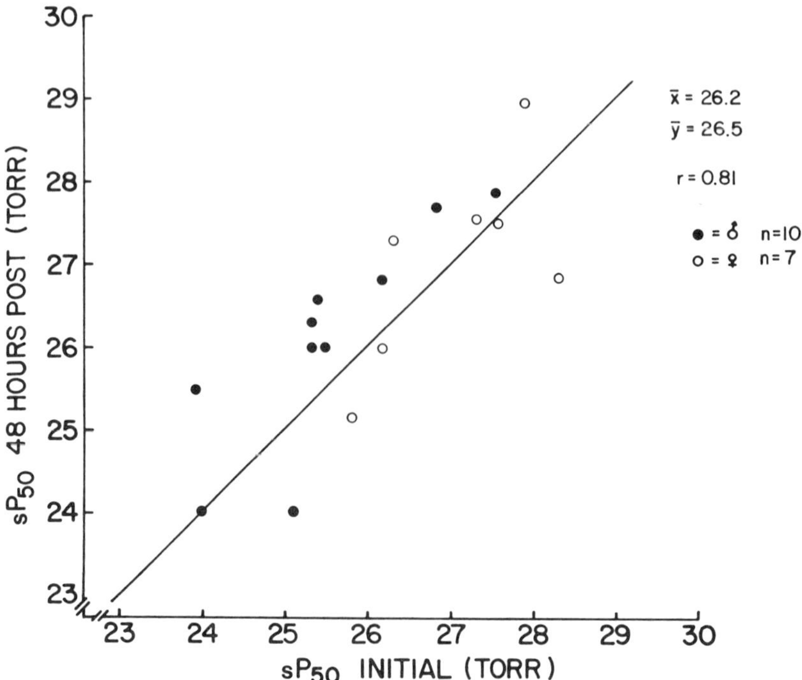

oxyhemoglobin dissociation curve, noted as an increase in P_{50}, is supposedly of adaptative value since facilitation of oxygen unloading would occur at the tissue level. However, not all investigators have concurred; in fact, some data suggest that the shift is nonexistent or even to the left. At altitude, the physiological levels of P_{50} are mainly the result of counteracting effects, i.e., the increase in 2,3-DPG (right) and the decrease in arterial PCO_2 (left). Unfortunately, these two separate and diverse effects have not been adequately considered in most studies made on man at altitude. In Figure 3 are presented available data obtained on natives to various altitudes. The trend line is a composite of the information obtained by Keys et al. (1936) and Torrance et al. (1970/71). Most investigators have only reported mean values or mean values ±S.E. but a few provided individual data so that ranges can be presented. In some instances, the range is of such magnitude that questions as to the validity of assuming a right shift must be raised. More to the point is the rather large and unexpected variations reported by different investigators in P_{50} of natives living at equivalent altitudes. Whether this reflects the variability observed among individuals even at sea level or is a consequence of different techniques and inability to obtain adequate data on all the factors which could modify the curve remains open for further investigations. One ligand which has been expressly related to a right shift in these natives has been 2,3-DPG but even this effect may be questioned, since significant increases in 2,3-DPG have only been reported to occur in natives living at altitudes in excess of 4300 m.

Figure 3. P_{50} in residents (natives) of various altitudes. Blocks represent mean values. Ranges are also given when individual values were available.

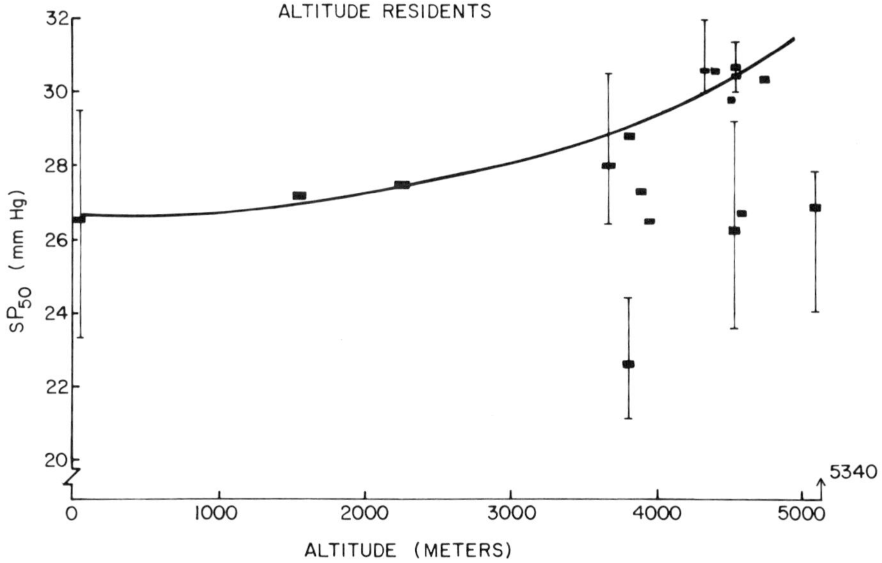

The values for P_{50} of sojourners to various altitudes exhibits a similar degree of confusion. Although in general it appears that P_{50} is increased, the magnitude of these increases do not correlate either with the altitude attained or the duration of stay at the respective altitude (Figure 4). For example, the right shift at 4500 m varied from 0.8 to 4.4 Torr in 4 studies made on subjects in residence for less than 4 days. In subjects resident for longer periods in two studies at this same altitude, the reported right shifts were 2.2 and 4.5 Torr. Increases in 2,3-DPG are inadequate to account for the right shifts reported. The organic phosphate levels remained relatively constant from 1550 to 4330 m and only increased significantly at 4500 m. It is of some interest that the response of sojourners appears to be exaggerated, i.e., a larger shift when compared to native residents except at altitudes in excess of 4000 m (Torrance et al. 1970/71). Adequate explanations for this divergent response is not available at this time but presents an interesting area for future research.

Another research opportunity exists in that all studies to date have utilized men as subjects, neglecting the possible influence of sex differences. In a preliminary study in our laboratory on 6 men and 3 women exposed for 40 hr to a final altitude of 4300 m, the men had a minimal right shift (0.2 Torr)

Figure 4. P_{50} in sojourners ascending to specific altitudes. The left side of the figure presents data on individuals during their first four days at the respective altitude while the right side of the figure presents data obtained on individuals who had been at altitude for more than 4 days. Numbers of subjects in each study are shown.

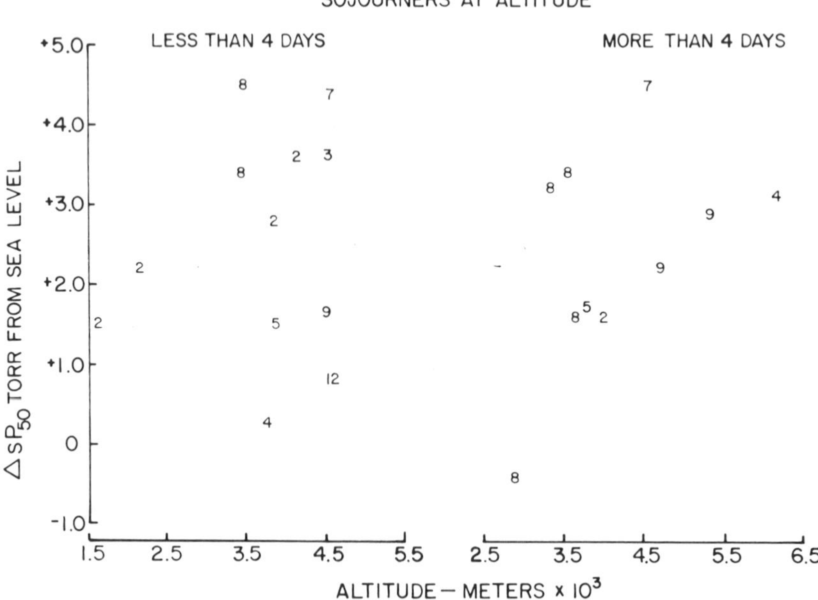

despite a 22% increase in 2,3-DPG and the women exhibited a right shift of 2 to 3.2 Torr with a mean increase of 6% in 2,3-DPG. The woman having the largest shift had a 5% decrease in her 2,3-DPG level.

Luft (1972) has suggested on theoretical grounds that the shape of the Hb-O_2 dissociation curve is such that a right shift may be of some benefit at altitudes below 3500 m, but not at higher altitudes. The hyperventilation present at these higher altitudes is a much more effective means of assisting the oxygen transport mechanism than is the shift in the mid-portion of the dissociation curve. Many animals successfully adapted to high altitudes do not have 2,3-DPG or elevated total hemoglobin and some have a left-shifted curve. Hebbel et al. (1978) have also raised questions as to the value of a right-shifted curve. Their "human llamas" (individuals with high oxygen affinity hemoglobins) who had a sP_{50} of 17.1 Torr at sea level showed a marked improvement in their maximum aerobic capacity on ascent to 3100 m in contrast to the anticipated decrease in aerobic capacity which was observed in their siblings with normal hemoglobins (sP_{50} of 27 Torr). The apparently normal human response to altitude, a decrease in Hb oxygen affinity, may be maladaptive. Those investigators who have not reported alterations in P_{50} consequent to altitude exposure may have been studying individuals with a different kind of altitude adaptation. It is clear that further and more intensive studies are required to clarify the significance of P_{50} at altitude. Probably more information on oxygen transport could be obtained if the entire Hb-O_2 dissociation curve was determined rather than relating to a fixed and immutable single point.

Disease

Many diseases are characterized by a reduction in arterial oxygen saturation (hypoxemia) or by alterations in many of the factors that affect hemoglobin's affinity for oxygen. Hasselbalch (1917), in attempting to disprove an early suggestion that the position of the oxyhemoglobin dissociation curve was constant, found to his dismay that it was indeed so in normal individuals. However, Hasselbalch was not one to give up easily and he turned his investigations toward the study of patients who had been hospitalized for a variety of reasons, including pernicious anemia, uremia, gout, and diabetic coma. Although 3 of the 8 patients examined displayed normal curves, the remainder had curves strikingly different from those of the normal subjects. Since Hasselbalch's virtually unknown research, many other disease entities have been studied. Table 2 presents information from various sources up to the present. Right- and left-shifted curves have been reported with suggestions that compensatory mechanisms had occurred, thus allowing for a more efficient transport of oxygen. Agreement as to the direction of curve shifts is far from universal. In fact, some investigators have reported normal curves for individuals with disorders indicated by others to result in large shifts in P_{50}. As Astrup

Table 2. Some Reported Changes in sP_{50} (pH 7.4, PCO_2 40 Torr, 37°) in Pathological and Physiological States.

Decreased sP_{50} (left shift)	Increased sP_{50} (right shift)
Acute alkolosis	Acute acidosis
Increased carboxyhemoglobin	Anemia
Hypothyroidism	Hyperthyroidism
Hypophosphatemia	Hyperphosphatemia
Hexokinase deficiency	Pyruvate kinase deficiency
Cyanate ingestion	High altitude
Hemodialysis	Chronic lung disease
Chronic antacid use	Chronic heart disease
Increased fetal hemoglobin	Angina pectoris
Transfusion of stored blood	Low cardiac output
Hyperbaric exposure	Uremic anemia
Anesthesia	Acute maximal exercise
Diabetes	Steroids
Septic shock	Hemoglobinopathies
Hemoglobinopathies	

(1969) stated, "we have been able to confirm some of the published abnormal P_{50} values, but we do not get the uniform pattern of which the literature gives the impression." He cites a number of examples, including myxedema, anemia, liver cirrhosis, and uremic acidosis, where P_{50}s varied from normal to abnormal. His statement is as appropriate today as it was in 1969.

Although we have not presented in any detail the altered hemoglobin-oxygen affinities in diseased individuals, it is apparent that much more information is needed to clarify P_{50} changes in disease. It is even more important to determine the biochemistry of the regulatory processes involved. The role of various factors on Hb-O_2 affinity have not been adequately determined. More attention also needs to be given to the effects that the presence of carbon monoxide, the age of the erythrocytes, the age of the individual, etc. have on hemoglobin's affinity for oxygen. It is apparent that even in disease, the use of sP_{50} to define the state of the individual is under stress.

Summary

We were unable, due to space restraints, to consider all of the published material on P_{50}. We found the same confused state regarding changes in P_{50} in all of the areas we examined. It is apparent that the present tendency to assume that sP_{50} effectively reflects measurements of alterations in $Hb-O_2$ affinity is open to question. The uncritical and unqualified utilization of this index can lead to serious misunderstandings regarding the ability of Hb to transport oxygen. We need to reevaluate the significance of this one-point value.

ACKNOWLEDGMENT
This work was supported in part by the Air Force Office of Scientific Research, Air Force Systems Command, under Grant AFOSR 78-3534.

References

Astrup, P. 1969. Oxygen dissociation curves in some diseases. *Forsvarsmedicin* 5:199–204.

Dill, D.B. and Forbes, W.H. 1941. Respiratory and metabolic effects of hypothermia. *Amer. J. Physiol.* 132:685–697.

Giannelli, S., Lambright, B.R., and Marin, M.Z. 1977. Spontaneous variability of the hemoglobin affinity for oxygen. *Crit. Care Med.* 5:150–153.

Hasselbalch, K.A. 1917. Wasserstoffzahl und Sauerstoffbindung des Blutes. *Biochem. Z.* 82:282–288.

Hebbel, R.P., Eaton, J.W., Kronenberg, R.S., Zanjani, E.D., Moore, L.G., and Berger, E.M. 1978. Human llamas: adaptation to altitude in subjects with high hemoglobin oxygen affinity. *J. Clin. Invest.* 62:593–600.

Horvath, S.M., Malenfant, A., Rossi, F., and Rossi-Bernardi, L. 1977. The oxygen affinity of concentrated human hemoglobin solutions and human blood. *Amer. J. Hematol.* 2:343–354.

Jackson, R.L. 1981. *Oxygen Transport During Exercise.* Ph.D. Thesis. University of California, Santa Barbara.

Keys, A., Hall, F.G., and Barron, E.S.G. (1936). Position of oxygen dissociation curve of human blood at high altitude. *Amer. J. Physiol.* 115:292–307.

Luft, U.C. 1972. Principals of adaptation to altitude. In *Physiological Adaptations: Desert and Mountain.* Yousef, M.K., Horvath, S.M., and Bullard, R.W., eds. New York: Academic Press. pp. 143–156.

Roughton, F.J. 1964. Transport of oxygen and carbon dioxide. In *Handbook of Physiology. Section 3. Respiration, Vol. 1.* Fenn, W.O. and Rahn, H., eds. Washington D.C.: American Physiological Society. p. 778.

Severinghaus, J.W. 1966. Blood gas calculator. *J. Appl. Physiol.* 21:1108–1116.

Torrance, J.D., Lenfant, C., Cruz, J., and Marticorena, E. 1970/71. Oxygen transport mechanisms in residents at high altitudes. *Respir. Physiol.* 11:1–15.

SECTION VI:

Clinical Problems in Oxygen Transport

J.A. Loeppky and M.L. Riedesel, editors
OXYGEN TRANSPORT TO HUMAN TISSUES

Detection of Early Airways Dysfunction

Ronald J. Knudson

Introduction

In this symposium on oxygen transport, it is appropriate to consider the airways upon which gas transport ultimately depends. Obstruction of airways is a leading cause of hypoxemia and chronic obstructive airways disease a major cause of disability and death. As a result, there is a practical interest in the etiology, natural history, and early detection of this ubiquitous disease. From this interest, a series of hypotheses has evolved which, though unproved, have assumed an aura of truth. As an introduction to the subject of the detection of early disease, a brief review of these hypotheses is appropriate, recognizing that this list may be incomplete.

First, it has been assumed that chronic potentially disabling chronic obstructive lung disease begins early in life. This has found support in the observation of functional changes in young people exposed to excessive air pollution or who smoke cigarettes and the finding of emphysematous changes in lungs of young people dying of nonrespiratory causes.

Secondly, it is assumed that the disease, beginning early in life, is gradually progressive and only after time does the disease become clinically apparent in the fourth or fifth decade of life. Patients with significant chronic airways obstruction show a slightly increased rate of decline of forced expiratory volume in one second (FEV_1) which may be twice the normal rate of decline of 25 to 30 ml per year. For functional impairment to result, it is reasoned, this rate of decline must have been present for many years.

Thirdly, cigarette smoking was considered to be the primary cause of chronic airways obstructive disease because most patients had been smokers. We now realize, however, that only a small proportion of smokers develop significant obstructive disease and other risk factors have been identified. Disabling obstructive lung disease appears to be the product of the convergence of innate host susceptibility and extrinsic contributing risk factors.

Fourthly, the earliest changes which ultimately lead to chronic airways obstruction are thought to occur in peripheral airways smaller than 2 mm in diameter. There is morphologic evidence that changes do occur in these peripheral structures (Hogg et al., 1968; Macklem et al., 1971; Niewoehner et al., 1974; Cosio et al., 1977), some of which are reversible. From these observations, arose the concept of "small airways disease" and certain physiological tests were proposed to detect these abnormalities.

The end result of this sequence of hypotheses was the proposal that tests could be employed which would detect peripheral airways dysfunction and this would allow us to detect those individuals in whom the early processes were at work which would lead, if left unchecked, to clinically significant and ultimately disabling chronic obstructive lung disease. At this point, appropriate intervention could alter or reverse an otherwise inexorable disease process. In short, we could detect early airways obstructive disease before the development of overt obstruction was revealed by slowing of forced expiration.

To be readily applicable for screening of persons who do not perceive themselves as ill, tests must be relatively simple to administer requiring a minimum of time and causing minimal discomfort. Since 1972, we have been engaged in a longitudinal epidemiological study of respiratory health in a random, stratified, cluster sample of the white, non-Mexican-American population of Tucson, Arizona (Lebowitz et al., 1975). The population sample was based on all members of approximately 1650 households. At regular intervals, health information was obtained using self-administered questionnaires and lung function tests performed. In this population study, we had the opportunity to administer two of these tests purported to detect early disease, and to consider the theoretical bases for these tests.

Closure of Small Airways

Theoretical Basis

The analysis of the concentration of inert gas during full expiration from total lung capacity (TLC) has been proposed as a method of detecting the small airways dysfunction considered to be a manifestation of early developing obstructive airways disease. Fowler (1949) analyzed expired nitrogen following inspiration of 100% oxygen, introducing a test which reveals certain pulmonary abnormalities (Comroe and Fowler, 1951). This test was further refined, using either a bolus of a foreign gas such as xenon, argon, or helium introduced at the beginning of inspiration from residual volume (RV) or analyzing expired N_2 following a full inspiration of nitrogen free gas. The now familiar sequence of changes of expired inert gas concentration define what has come to be known as the closing volume test (Figure 1). After an initial rise in concentration constituting phases I and II, a gradually increasing concentration (phase III) is observed, normally followed by a terminal rise in concentration (phase IV). The terminal rise was considered to be the result of closure of small airways in dependent portions of the lung and the volume at which this occurred was termed the closing volume (Holland et al., 1968). Closure of small terminal airways had been demonstrated histologically (Hughes et al., 1970) and physiologically (Burger and Macklem, 1968; Engel et al., 1975). It was assumed that the measurement of closing volume, therefore, would be a sensitive test of small airways dysfunction in that diseased airways might close prematurely and phase IV occur at a higher than normal volume.

There are basic differences in principle between the bolus and resident nitrogen methods of measuring closing volume (Travis et al., 1973). The distribution of a bolus of foreign gas inhaled from RV and, hence, the volume at which phase IV occurs during subsequent expiration is determined by the sequence of opening and subsequent closure of airways at low lung volume. The nitrogen method, on the other hand, also depends on the regional differences in volume change during inspiration to TLC. Our own data (Knudson et al., 1977) and those of others (Farebrother et al., 1973; Stanescu et al., 1977) show that there are systematic differences between the two techniques.

When the test was applied to populations potentially at risk, it was the nitrogen slope of phase III, expressed as % N_2/liter, which proved to be the single measurement most sensitive in revealing an abnormality (Buist and Ross, 1973; Buist et al., 1973; Knudson and Lebowitz, 1977; Oxhøj et al.,

Figure 1. The plot of expired inert gas concentration against lung volume during slow expiration. If inspiration began with a bolus of foreign gas, that gas is sampled. If 100% oxygen was inspired, nitrogen is sampled.

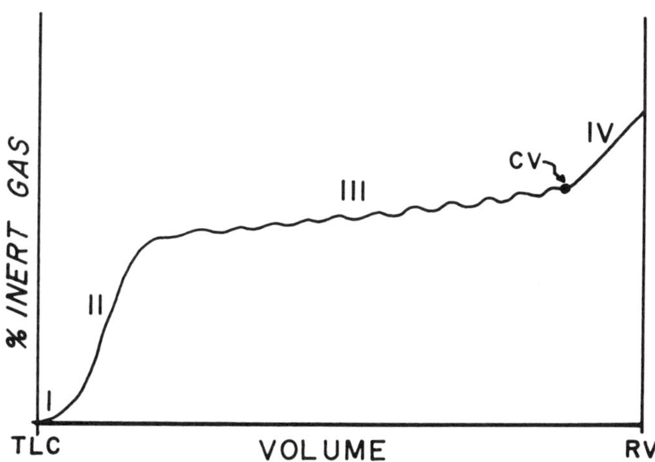

1977). An increased slope identified a larger proportion of subjects considered to be other than normal than any other measurement derived from the single breath nitrogen test. What is the meaning of an abnormality in the single breath test? Will an abnormality be followed by changes which define the presence of airways obstructive disease and will it therefore detect early disease?

Application of Test

To explore these questions, we compared single breath N_2 data with maximum expiratory flow-volume parameters in 725 subjects, 25 to 54 yr of age, from our random population sample. For each measurement, we developed regression equations based on that segment of the population sample which met predefined criteria for "normal," i.e., subjects who were free of any cardiorespiratory symptoms or disease and had never smoked cigarettes. The normal limit was then defined as the percent predicted value which encompassed 95% of "normal" subjects, the "normal 95th percentile." Using this definition by which 5% of normal subjects would be considered abnormal, we then compared the sensitivity of measurements by determining the proportion of remaining population subgroups considered to be abnormal by a given test parameter. In particular, we compared the nitrogen slope of phase III, the most sensitive measurement from the single breath test, with the maximum expiratory flow after 75% of the vital capacity had been expired ($\dot{V}max_{75}$), the flow-volume measurement found to be the most sensitive in revealing abnormality (Knudson et al., 1976a, b). Whereas 17.9% of the subjects were judged abnormal by the slope of phase III and 24% were abnormal by $\dot{V}max_{75}$, in only 9.5% were *both* abnormal. Among asymptomatic subjects who regularly smoked cigarettes (n = 116), 9.5% had an abnormal slope of phase III while 21.5% had an abnormal $\dot{V}max_{75}$ with only 4.3% having both abnormalities. This lack of concordance was even observed among the 114 subjects who reported having physician-confirmed asthma, chronic bronchitis, or emphysema. In this group, 17.3% had an abnormal slope, 23.4% an abnormal $\dot{V}max_{75}$, and 8.2% had both test abnormalities. It did not appear, therefore, that the single breath test, thought to be more sensitive, was of necessity abnormal when there was evidence of obstruction revealed by expiratory slowing.

The question remained whether an abnormality revealed by the single breath test might yet have prognostic significance. We compared the slope of phase III with FEV_1, both expressed as percent of predicted, for 458 subjects who failed to meet our criteria for being free of any past or present cardiorespiratory problem. Of 97 subjects who had a normal FEV_1 but an abnormal slope of phase III, 86 had FEV_1 values which, though in the normal range, were below 100% of predicted. Did the abnormal slope therefore predict decline in FEV_1? Four and a half years later, we had accumulated longitudinal FEV_1 data and could not demonstrate that an abnormal slope of phase III was a predictor of accelerated decrease in FEV_1.

It could be argued that this period of follow-up was not long enough to demonstrate the significance of the single breath abnormality. On the other hand, the single breath test may reveal an abnormality which is not necessarily a precursor of chronic obstructive lung disease. It may indicate a peripheral airway dysfunction which is transient or readily reversible or at least not of great clinical significance.

Critique

The original explanation for the sequence of changes in nitrogen concentration during expiration was based on gravity dependent interregional inhomogeneity and sequential airway closure. Studies performed under varying gravitational conditions have demonstrated how gravity can affect the slope of phase III (Michels and West, 1978). However, other studies on open chested dogs, (Engel et al., 1974) demonstrated that a nitrogen slope can occur in the absence of a gravity gradient and can be modified by breath-holding. Several factors, therefore, may influence the nitrogen slope. The test maneuver is done slowly and intraregional stratified inhomogeneity may affect the slopes with intraregional gas mixing contributing to the upward slope. Moreover, during the time of the slow expiration, the differences in rate of oxygen uptake and CO_2 elimination within a given region will affect the total N_2 concentration in the region (Van Liew and Avieli, 1981; Cormier and Bélanger, 1981). Differences in active gas exchange have been cited as the cause of an increased nitrogen slope following exercise. Neither the precise mechanisms operating during the single breath test nor the significance of an abnormality are clear. The utility of the test in population screening is still unclear. In a sense, the test appears to provide an answer in search of a question. The caveat enunciated by Comroe and Fowler (1951) is still pertinent. When they first described their new test, they pointed out that "the test does not diagnose specific types of pulmonary disease, but directs attention to a definite abnormality which can be explored more fully by other methods."

Density Dependence of Maximum Expiratory Flow

Theoretical Basis

Density dependence of maximum expiratory flow ($\dot{V}max$) has also been employed as another test purported to reveal small airways dysfunction based on the principal that flow is partly a function of the physical properties of the gas expired (Schilder et al., 1963; Barnett, 1967). Despas et al. (1972) compared maximum expiratory flow-volume (MEFV) curves in asthmatics who breathed air and then a mixture of 80% helium and 20% oxygen (HeO_2). A failure to increase $\dot{V}max$ after breathing HeO_2, they suggested, was indicative of obstruction in peripheral airways smaller than 2 to 3 mm. Dosman et al. (1975) proposed that this phenomenon identified early small airways dysfunction in smokers whose MEFV curves breathing air were still normal. As a result,

MEFV curves with air and HeO_2 were considered to be potentially useful in detection of early airways obstruction.

The theoretical basis for this test was derived from the concept that $\dot{V}max$ at a given lung volume was determined by lung elastic recoil pressure [Pst(L)] at that lung volume and the resistance of airways upstream of the points at which lateral airway pressure was equal to pleural pressure, the equal pressure points (EPP). In the mid-vital capacity when EPP are located in central airways, the upstream segment is, in effect, a summed conduit. The cross-sectional area of the conduit decreases from terminal airways toward central airways and resistive pressure losses can be largely accounted for by convective acceleration. Flow would then be highly density dependent. If, however, EPP were located in more peripheral airways, flow in the upstream airways would be predominantly laminar and independent of gas density (Figure 2). If obstruction was present in small peripheral airways and their resistance therefore

Figure 2. Schematic of airway cross-section by airway generation showing distribution of the several flow patterns. If EPP are normally located, flow is determined primarily by convective acceleration. In the presence of peripheral airway narrowing, EPP are more peripherally located and flow in the upstream segment is thought to be primarily laminar.

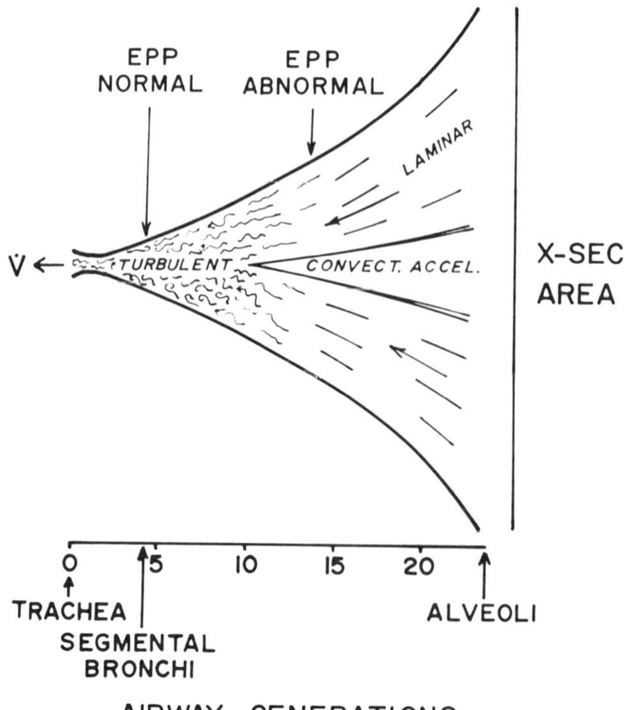

greater, then in order to preserve normal $\dot{V}max$ breathing air, the EPP would be located more peripherally than normal, a phenomenon which might be revealed by the failure to increase $\dot{V}max$ by breathing the less dense HeO_2 mixture. Testing for density dependence of $\dot{V}max$, it was thought, would reveal this peripheral airway abnormality. This, of course, requires that the subject perform a series of forced vital capacity (FVC) maneuvers breathing air and then HeO_2 and that the vital capacities are similar for the comparisons of flow to be made.

Application of Test

During a recent survey of the Tucson study population, such studies were done. Each subject performed at least 3 FVC maneuvers breathing air and then, after 3 vital capacities breathing HeO_2, performed 3 additional FVC maneuvers while still breathing the HeO_2. Testing was administered by trained nurse-interviewers using a dry rolling seal spirometer (Cardiopulmonary Instruments Model 220) with MEFV curves recorded on a rapid responding X-Y recorder (Hewlett Packard 7041M). For 1162 of the 1584 subjects so tested, the best air and best HeO_2 vital capacities agreed to within 5% and only these data were used for subsequent analysis. Helium response was measured by superimposing the air and HeO_2 curves, matching at TLC and, using the outer envelope of each set of curves, expressing density dependence as the ratio of the $\dot{V}max$ breathing HeO_2 to that breathing air ($\dot{V}_H/\dot{V}_A$) at 50 and 75% of the best air vital capacity (VC). The point of convergence of the two curves, the volume of isoflow ($V_{iso}\dot{V}$) was expressed as the ratio of the expired volume at which that occurred to the vital capacity (Hutcheon et al., 1974) and is shown in Figure 3.

There were 290 subjects who met the criteria for being totally free of past or present cardiorespiratory symptoms or disease and who never smoked cigarettes. Values for $\dot{V}_H/\dot{V}_A$ at 50% VC showed considerable variability and even of this normal subgroup, 78 had values equal to or less than 1.0 and would be considered total nonresponders. Because there appeared to be opposite effects of age in young and older subjects, data were analyzed separately for subjects aged 19 to 24 yr and those over the age of 25 years. Results are shown in Table 1. There was a significant increase in $\dot{V}_H/\dot{V}_A$ with age in the young and a significant decline with age in those over age 25 years. In addition, the mean $\dot{V}_H/\dot{V}_A$ was significantly greater in males than females. The coefficient of variation (100×mean/S.D.) was of considerable magnitude for all measurements and in general was greatest for the $V_{iso\dot{V}}/VC$. Inasmuch as the $\dot{V}_H/\dot{V}_A$ at 50% VC showed the smallest coefficient of variation, subsequent analyses focused on this measurement of density dependence.

An abnormal forced expiratory volume in the first second of expiration, FEV_1, is generally recognized as the single measurement which identifies overt airways obstruction. Accordingly, we compared the FEV_1 breathing air with $\dot{V}_H/\dot{V}_A$ at 50% VC. To define an abnormality in density dependence, we

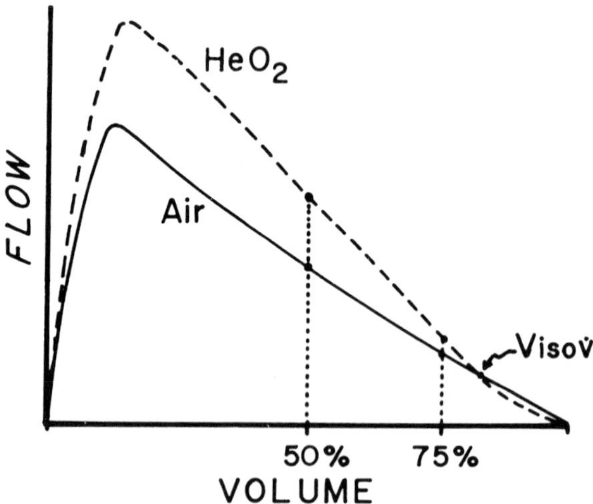

Figure 3. Comparison of normal air and HeO_2 maximum expiratory flow-volume curves. The increase in flow after 50 and 75% of the vital capacity has been expired is expressed as the ratio of the two flows, $\dot{V}_H/\dot{V}_A$. The isoflow volume ($V_{iso\dot{V}}$) is the volume point at which the curves converge and flows are identical.

adopted the criteria used by Meadows et al. (1980) whereby a $\dot{V}_H\dot{V}_A$ of less than 1.20 would be considered abnormal and such subjects considered "nonresponders." Our "normal 95th percentile" in defining an abnormal FEV_1 is a value below 72.4% predicted. Only one of our normal control subjects had an abnormal FEV_1 and that person had an abnormal $\dot{V}_H/\dot{V}_A$. However, 17% of the normal group would be considered nonresponders, all but one of whom had values for FEV_1 within the normal range.

Of 207 subjects who met the same "normal" criteria for being asymptomatic but who smoked cigarettes, only 4 had an abnormal FEV_1 and, of these, only 2 were nonresponders. Only 24% would be considered nonresponders and 47 of these 49 people had a normal FEV_1. There were no significant differences in the mean $\dot{V}_H/\dot{V}_A$ at 50% between smokers and nonsmokers when the two groups of equally asymptomatic males or females were compared. Thus we could not reproduce the results of Dosman et al. (1975) who found that decreased density dependence distinguished smokers from nonsmokers.

Of the remaining 656 subjects who failed to meet the criteria for having been free of symptoms or disease, 25.9% were nonresponders, 6.1% had an abnormal FEV_1 and both abnormalities appeared in 3.7%. Of these subjects, 69 reported having physician confirmed asthma, chronic bronchitis, or emphysema. Of this group, 23.2% had an abnormal FEV_1 but 37.5% of those with an abnormal FEV_1 had normal density dependence. Of these 69 people with confirmed disease, 39.1% were nonresponders and 14.4% had both an abnormal FEV_1 and $\dot{V}_H/\dot{V}_A$.

Table 1. Density Dependence Measurements from Asymptomatic Nonsmokers; Age Regressions by Sex.

Parameter	n	Slope coefficient	Constant	P value[a]	Mean	SD	Coefficient of variation
Males ≥ 25 years	76						
$\dot{V}_H/\dot{V}_A$ 50%VC		−.00296	1.56904	.01352	1.430	.219	15%
$\dot{V}_H/\dot{V}_A$ 75%VC		−.00395	1.48134	.00471	1.296	.250	19%
$V_{iso\dot{V}}/VC$		−.00493	1.06007	.00001	.829	.181	21%
Females ≥ 25 years	120						
$\dot{V}_H/\dot{V}_A$ 50%VC		−.00173	1.44615	.09318 (NS)	1.349	.239	17%
$\dot{V}_H/\dot{V}_A$ 75%VC		−.00447	1.42847	.00149	1.179	.277	23%
$V_{iso\dot{V}}/VC$		−.00478	.97298	.00014	.706	.244	35%
Males < 24 years	51						
$\dot{V}_H/\dot{V}_A$ 50%VC		.02508	.96206	.00010	1.439	.141	10%
$\dot{V}_H/\dot{V}_A$ 75%VC		.02072	.89460	.03132	1.288	.221	17%
$V_{iso\ \dot{V}}/VC$		.00829	.71520	.02962	.873	.087	10%
Females < 24 years	43						
$\dot{V}_H\dot{V}_A$ 50%VC		.01951	.94217	.02502	1.315	.179	14%
$\dot{V}_H\dot{V}_A$ 75%VC		−.00011	1.19270	.49662 (NS)	1.191	.221	19%
$V_{iso\dot{V}}/VC$		.01125	.58150	.15220 (NS)	.797	.193	24%

[a]P value for slope of age regression.

Age regression equation: Parameter = Slope coefficient X age (yr) + constant.

The use of density dependence as a screening test presents several problems. We applied the test in a field survey situation, unlike Dosman et al. (1975) who performed their tests under controlled laboratory conditions using a body plethysmograph. Moreover, ours was a randomly selected population sample. The test has been shown to exhibit poor reproducibility (Bevan et al., 1980; Bonsignore et al., 1980). To minimize this source of error, we used the outer envelope of the MEFV curves but the coefficients of variation still showed considerable intersubject variability compared to the results of Dosman et al. (1975). Having defined our population subgroups based on answers to a self-administered health questionnaire, we found a significant number of nonresponders in a population which met the criteria for being normal. At the other end of the spectrum, we found that density dependence or lack thereof did not identify subjects with physician confirmed respiratory disease. There is poor correspondence between FEV_1 and $\dot{V}_H/\dot{V}_A$. Of the 45 persons in the total population sample who had an abnormal FEV_1, 40% would be considered normal responders to HeO_2. This is quite similar to the results reported by Meadows et al. (1980) who found that half of their patients with airways obstruction had normal density dependence. We find ourselves in agreement with Lam et al. (1981) who concluded that the helium flow-volume curve has little utility in population screening.

When comparing two MEFV curves obtained when breathing two gases, one is faced with several sources of variability. The air MEFV curve itself shows intersubject variability (Green et al., 1974; Knudson et al., 1976b). Green et al. (1974) sought to explain this variability by the phenomenon of dysanapsis, a difference in development and relative size of airways and lung parenchyma. Those differences might be expected to introduce an additional source of variability in HeO_2 MEFV curves. The magnitude of the density dependent convective accelerative resistance would depend on the size of central airways relative to the summed cross-sectional area of peripheral airways. Castile et al. (1980) postulated that, if two individuals with lungs of equal size were compared, the one with smaller central airways would have lower $\dot{V}max$ with air, but a greater increase in $\dot{V}max$ breathing HeO_2 than the one with larger central airways because of the greater convective accelerative resistance in the individual with smaller airways.

Chest roentgenograms in posterior-anterior and lateral views had been obtained on 733 of the subjects tested. From these roentgenograms, TLC had been computed and, based on measurements of tracheal diameter in both projections, tracheal cross-sectional area had been calculated. The ratio of tracheal cross-section to TLC was taken as an estimate of the magnitude of convergence of the summed cross-sectional airway from alveoli to trachea. In theory, a larger ratio would mean that central airways are larger in relation to volume and one might predict that flow, corrected for size, would be greater breathing air but the magnitude of density dependence, expressed as $\dot{V}_H/\dot{V}_A$ would be less. When mean cross-section/TLC ratios were compared by sex, females had significantly greater ratios than males. In view of the fact that females had lower mean $\dot{V}_H/\dot{V}_A$ values than males, this made the original hypothesis attractive. However, when $\dot{V}_H/\dot{V}_A$ was compared to cross-section/TLC for all 399 adults over age 25 yr, though there was a trend toward an inverse relationship, it did not even approach significance. Thus we could not confirm the hypothesis that the relative size of central airways had a clear relationship to density dependence.

Critique

These attempts to apply the test of density dependence and the disappointing results lead one to reexamine the original concepts upon which the test was based. That original concept involved certain simplifying assumptions regarding the location of the EPP and airway geometry. It also assumed that the patterns of flow were the same for both gases and that classic laws of fluid mechanics could be applied.

The mathematical description of a given flow regime is the expression of the relationship between pressure losses and flow when airway geometry, gas density and gas viscosity are taken into consideration. The descriptions of classic pressure-flow relations are summarized in Table 2. In each of these equations, a geometric constant appears. If we assume that the driving pressure is Pst(L) and it is the same for HeO_2 and air, and if we also assume that the flow regimes and airway geometry are the same for air and HeO_2, then we can set the ratio of geometric constants equal to 1.0 and predict the $\dot{V}_H/\dot{V}_A$ in terms of the ratio of air/HeO_2 density and viscosity functions for the possible flow regimes. These predictions are also listed in Table 2.

In summary, according to the Poiseuille equation, when flow is laminar and the velocity profile parabolic, flow is independent of gas density and will vary with viscosity and the predicted $\dot{V}_H/\dot{V}_A$ is 0.95. When flow is disturbed by boundary layer growth in a branched system, density and viscosity contribute equally in determining flow (Pedley et al., 1970a, b, 1971) and $\dot{V}_H/\dot{V}_A$ would be 1.35. Density dependent inertial pressure losses constitute a major portion of the pressure losses when flow is turbulent and the predicted $\dot{V}_H/\dot{V}_A$ would be 1.50. Because the total cross-sectional area diminishes from peripheral to central airways, convective accelerative resistance should be a major determi-

Table 2. Predictions Based on Classic Flow-Pressure Descriptions.

Type of flow resistance	Equation	Predicted $\dot{V}_H/\dot{V}_A$
Poiseuille laminar	$P = K_1\,\mu\dot{V}$	0.95
Boundary layer growth	$P = K_2\,\mu^{0.5}\,\rho^{0.5}\,\dot{V}^{1.50}$	1.35
Turbulent	$P = K_3\,\mu^{0.25}\,\rho^{0.75}\,\dot{V}^{1.75}$	1.50
Convective acceleration	$P = K_4\,\rho\dot{V}^2$	1.62

ρ = density; μ = viscosity; K_n = geometric constant.

nant of flow and pressure losses would be totally inertial and $\dot{V}_H/\dot{V}_A$ would then achieve a maximum of 1.62.

However, under conditions of maximum expiratory flow, all of these flow patterns exist simultaneously as a continuum, density and viscosity contributing in varying degrees to pressure losses in the various airway generations. Because no single pressure-flow relationship can describe the entire tracheobronchial tree, Wood et al. (1976) proposed a unified equation (see Table 2) incorporating the variable effects of density and viscosity:

$$P = K\mu^{2-a}\rho^{a-1}\dot{V}^{a} \tag{30.1}$$

where a can vary from 1 to 2, depending on the flow regime. The value of a, therefore, varies in proportion to Reynolds number (Re) the dimensionless expression:

$$Re = du\rho/\mu \tag{30.2}$$

where d is tube diameter and u is flow velocity. For a given flow through a tube of a given diameter, Re will vary with the ratio ρ/μ and therefore the flow regime, and a, will also vary accordingly. Thus, it is not the case that flow regimes and patterns of pressure losses would be identical when breathing air and HeO_2. Some subjects in our study and in the studies of others (Despas et al., 1972; Dosman et al., 1975; Castile et al. 1980) were able to achieve $\dot{V}_H/\dot{V}_A$ values in excess of the maximum predicted value of 1.62. This suggests that there are fundamental differences in responses to the two gases and that even the assumption of identical airway geometry may also be questioned. Indeed, the data of Mink and coworkers (Mink et al., 1979; Mink and Wood, 1980) have shown that EPP may not be in the same location breathing air and HeO_2.

Similar predictions may be examined based on the wave speed theory of flow limitation. According to this concept, maximum expiratory flow is determined when the local flow velocity at some critical point in the airways equals the tube wave speed (Griffiths, 1975; Shapiro, 1977; Elliott and Dawson, 1977; Dawson and Elliott, 1977, 1980; Mead, 1980). The critical velocity at that choke point is determined by the balance between gas density and the change in airway cross-sectional area (dA) for a given change in airway transmural pressure (dPtm). Flow at a wave speed ($\dot{V}$ws) is then expressed:

$$\dot{V}ws = \left(\frac{1}{\rho}\right)^{0.5}\left(\frac{dPtm}{dA}\right)^{0.5}A^{1.5} \tag{30.3}$$

From this relationship, it follows that flow would be greater if the density of the gas was lower, the airway stiffer, or the cross-sectional area greater.

If all conditions were the same breathing air and breathing HeO_2, that is, if the choke points were in the same location and dPtm/dA and A were also the same, then $\dot{V}$max would simply vary with gas density and $\dot{V}_H/\dot{V}_A$ would be 1.62. Mink and coworkers (Mink et al., 1979; Mink and Wood, 1980) observed that the choke points breathing HeO_2 were upstream of where they were breathing air and conditions are indeed different breathing the two gases, as they would have to be if $\dot{V}_H/\dot{V}_A$ was less than the predicted value of 1.62. It is quite possible, and indeed likely, that compared to the location when breathing air, the choke points when breathing HeO_2 may be further upstream in airways which are more compliant. It is not even clearly inevitable that choke points occur downstream of EPP throughout expiration.

That the conditions which determine maximum expiratory flow for HeO_2 and air differ seems inescapable. The choke points and EPP are very likely in different locations, the flow patterns and Reynolds numbers differ, and the airway geometry and pertinent airway elastic properties also differ for the two gases. As a result of these complex and still poorly understood factors, the use of density dependence as a test specific for peripheral airways dysfunction does not seem well founded.

Summary

The precise anatomic or structural changes in airways which produce abnormalities in these tests are not completely defined. If they do indeed reveal peripheral airways dysfunction, the long-term significance of such dysfunction or its relationship to chronic obstructive airways disease is also poorly understood. The original hypotheses which led investigators to attempt to utilize these tests in screening for detection of early obstructive disease may not have been well-founded and the original rationale for the tests themselves may have been too simplistic. Nevertheless, the utilization of the tests, while not achieving the intended goals, has been useful. The results may not have provided the answers hoped for but they have raised new questions. Therein may lie the value of this inquiry.

ACKNOWLEDGMENT

This work was supported by Specialized Center of Research Grant HL 14136 from the National Heart, Lung, and Blood Institute.

References

Barnett, T.B. 1967. Effects of helium and oxygen mixtures on pulmonary mechanics during airway constriction. *J. Appl. Physiol.* 22:707–713.

Bevan, C., Collins, C., and Legg, S.J. 1980. Reproducibility of the volume of isoflow in small airway function. *Proc. Physiol. Soc.* 19P.

Bonsignore, G., Bellia, V., Ferrara, G., Mirabella, A., Rizzo, A., and Sciarabba, G. 1980. Reproducibility of maximum flows in air and HeO_2 and of $\Delta\dot{V}max_{50}$ in the assessment of the site of airflow limitation. *Europ. J. Respir. Dis.* 61 (Suppl.106):29–34.

Buist, A.S. and Ross, B.B. 1973. Quantitative analysis of the alveolar plateau in the diagnosis of early airway obstruction. *Am. Rev. Respir. Dis.* 108:1078–1087.

Buist, A.S., Van Fleet, D.L., and Ross, B.B. 1973. A comparison of conventional spirometric tests and the test of closing volume in an emphysema screening center. *Am. Rev. Respir. Dis.* 107:735–743.

Burger, E.J. and Macklem, P.T. 1968. Airway closure: demonstration by breathing 100% O_2 at low lung volumes and by N_2 washout. *J. Appl. Physiol.* 25:139–148.

Castile, R.G., Hyatt, R.E., and Rodarte, J.R. 1980. Determinants of maximal expiratory flow and density dependence in normal humans. *J. Appl. Physiol.* 49:897–904.

Comroe, J.H., Jr. and Fowler, W.S. 1951. Lung function studies. Detection of uneven alveolar ventilation during a single breath of oxygen. *Am. J. Med.* 10:408–413.

Cormier, Y.F. and Bélanger, J. 1981. The influence of active gas exchange on the slope of phase III at rest and after exercise. *Am. Rev. Respir. Dis.* 123:213–216.

Cosio, M., Ghezzo, H., Hogg, J.C., Corbin, R., Loveland, M., Dosman, J., and Macklem, P.T. 1977. The relations between structural changes in small airways and pulmonary-function tests. *N. Engl. J. Med.* 298:1277–1281.

Dawson, S.C. and Elliott, E.A. 1977. Wave-speed limitation on expiratory flow—a unifying concept. *J. Appl. Physiol.* 43:498–515.

Dawson, S.C. and Elliott, E.A. 1980. Use of the choke point in the prediction of flow limitation in elastic tubes. *Fed. Proc.* 39:2765–2770.

Despas, P.J., Leroux, M., and Macklem, P.T. 1972. Site of airway obstruction in asthma as determined by measuring maximal expiratory flow breathing air and a helium-oxygen mixture. *J. Clin. Invest.* 51:3235–3243.

Dosman, J., Bode, F., Urbanetti, J., Martin, R., and Macklem, P.T. 1975. The use of a helium-oxygen mixture during maximum expiratory flow to demonstrate obstruction in small airways in smokers. *J. Clin. Invest.* 55:1090–1099.

Elliott, E.A. and Dawson, S.C. 1977. Test of wave-speed theory of flow limitation in elastic tubes. *J. Appl. Physiol.* 43:516–522.

Engel, L.A., Grassino, A., and Anthonisen, N.R. 1975. Demonstration of airway closure in man. *J. Appl. Physiol.* 38:1117–1125.

Engel, L.A., Utz, G., Wood, L.D.H., and Macklem, P.T. 1974. Ventilation distribution in anatomical lung units. *J. Appl. Physiol.* 37:194–200.

Farebrother, M.J., Paredez Martinez, R.P., Soejima, R., and McHardy, G.J. 1973. The point of onset of "airway closure" measured with argon and nitrogen: a comparison of results obtained by two methods. *Clin. Sci. (London)* 44:181–184.

Fowler, W.S. 1949. Lung function studies. Uneven pulmonary ventilation in normal subjects and in patients with pulmonary disease. *J. Appl. Physiol.* 2:283–299.

Green, M., Mead, J., and Turner, J.M. 1974. Variability of maximum expiratory flow-volume curves. *J. Appl. Physiol.* 37:67–74.

Griffiths, D.J. 1975. Negative-resistance effects in flow through collapsible tubes. *Med. Biol. Eng.* 13:785–802.

Hogg, J.C., Macklem, P.T., and Thurlbeck, W.M. 1968. Site and nature of airway obstruction in chronic obstructive lung disease. *N. Engl. J. Med.* 278:1355–1360.

Holland, J., Milic-Emili, J., Macklem, P.T., and Bates, D.V. 1968. Regional distribution of pulmonary ventilation and perfusion in elderly subjects. *J. Clin. Invest.* 47:81–92.

Hughes, J.M., Rosenzweig, D.Y., and Kivitz, P.B. 1970. Site of airway closure in excised dog lungs: histologic demonstration. *J. Appl. Physiol.* 29:340–344.

Hutcheon, M., Griffin, P., Levison, H., and Zamel, N. 1974. Volume of isoflow. A new test in detection of mild abnormalities of lung mechanics. *Am. Rev. Respir. Dis.* 110:458–465.

Knudson, R.J., Burrows, B., and Lebowitz, M.D. 1976a. The maximum expiratory flow-volume curve: its use in the detection of ventilatory abnormalities in a population study. *Am. Rev. Respir. Dis.* 114:871–879.

Knudson, R.J. and Lebowitz, M.D. 1977. Comparison of flow-volume and closing volume variables in a random population. *Am. Rev. Respir. Dis.* 116:1039–1045.

Knudson, R.J., Lebowitz, M.D., Burton, A.P., and Knudson, D.E. 1977. The closing volume test: evaluation of nitrogen and bolus methods in a random population. *Am. Rev. Respir. Dis.* 115:423–434.

Knudson, R.J., Slatin, R.C., Lebowitz, M.D., and Burrows, B. 1976b. The maximal expiratory flow-volume curve: normal standards, variability, and effects of age. *Am. Rev. Respir. Dis.* 113:587–600.

Lam, S., Abboud, R.T., Chan-Yeung, M., and Tan, F. 1981. Use of maximal expiratory flow-volume curve with air and helium-oxygen in the detection of ventilatory abnormalities in population surveys. *Am. Rev. Respir. Dis.* 123:234–237.

Lebowitz, M.D., Knudson, R.J., and Burrows, B. 1975. Tucson epidemiological study of obstructive lung diseases. I. Methodology and prevalence of disease. *Am. J. Epidemiol.* 102:137–152.

Macklem, P.T., Thurlbeck, W.M., and Fraser, R.G. 1971. Chronic obstructive disease of small airways. *Ann. Intern. Med.* 74:167–177.

Mead, J. 1980. Expiratory flow limitation: a physiologist's point of view. *Fed. Proc.* 39:2771–2775.

Meadows, J.A., III, Rodarte, J.R., and Hyatt, R.E. 1980. Density dependence of maximal expiratory flow in chronic obstructive pulmonary disease. *Am. Rev. Respir. Dis.* 121:47–53.

Michels, D.B. and West, J.B. 1978. Distribution of pulmonary ventilation and perfusion during short periods of weightlessness. *J. Appl. Physiol.* 45:987–998.

Mink, S., Ziesmann, M., and Wood, L.D.H. 1979. Mechanisms of increased maximum expiratory flow during HeO_2 breathing in dogs. *J. Appl. Physiol.* 47:490–502.

Mink, S.N. and Wood, L.D.H. 1980. How does HeO_2 increase maximum expiratory flow in human lungs? *J. Clin. Invest.* 66:720–729.

Niewoehner, D.E., Kleinerman, J., and Rice, D.B. 1974. Pathologic changes in the peripheral airways of young cigarette smokers. *N. Engl. J. Med.* 291:755–758.

Oxhøj, H., Bake, B., and Wilhelmusen, J. 1977. Ability of spirometry, flow-volume curves, and the nitrogen closing volume test to detect smokers. A population study. *Scand. J. Respir. Dis.* 58:80–96.

Pedley, T.J., Schroter, R.C., and Sudlow, M.F. 1970a. Energy losses and pressure drop in models of human airways. *Respir. Physiol.* 9:371–386.

Pedley, T.J., Schroter, R.C., and Sudlow, M.F. 1970b. The prediction of pressure drop and variation of resistance within the human bronchial airways. *Respir. Physiol.* 9:387–405.

Pedley, T.J., Schroter, R.C., and Sudlow, M.F. 1971. Flow and pressure drop in systems of repeatedly branching tubes. *J. Fluid Mech.* 46:365–383.

Schilder, D.P., Roberts, A., and Fry, D.L. 1963. Effect of gas density and viscosity on the maximal expiratory flow-volume relationship. *J. Clin. Invest.* 42:1705–1713.

Shapiro, A.H. 1977. Steady flow in collapsible tubes. *J. Biomech. Eng.* 99:126–147.

Stănescu, D., Veriter, C., and Brasseur, L. 1977. Difference between the He bolus and N_2 technique for measuring closing volume. *J. Appl. Physiol.* 42:859–864.

Travis, D.M., Green, M., and Don, H. 1973. Simultaneous comparison of helium and nitrogen expiratory "closing volumes." *J. Appl. Physiol.* 34:304–398.

Van Liew, H.D. and Arieli, R. 1981. Exchanges of oxygen and carbon dioxide alter inert gas pattern in single breath tests. *J. Appl. Physiol.* 50:487–492.

Wood, L.D.H., Engel, L.A., Griffin, P., Despas, P., and Macklem, P.T. 1976. Effect of gas physical properties and flow on lower pulmonary resistance. *J. Appl. Physiol.* 41:234–244.

J.A. Loeppky and M.L. Riedesel, editors
OXYGEN TRANSPORT TO HUMAN TISSUES

Oxygen Therapy

John C. Mithoefer

The history of the use of oxygen in clinical medicine is one of the examples in physiology and medicine where an important discovery was made but could not be put to effective use until a thorough understanding of physiological mechanisms had been established upon which to base its application. Following Priestly's discovery of "dephlogisticated air" in 1774, oxygen was used in an empirical and often irresponsible way to treat a variety of illnesses and its medical use soon fell into disrepute. Nearly 150 years passed before J.S. Haldane, with his brilliant background in respiratory physiology, treated some soldiers who had been poisoned by phosgene gas and noted that oxygen administration improved their cyanosis and general clinical condition (Haldane, 1927). This event, in 1915, marked the beginning of modern oxygen therapy. Haldane went on to develop methods for the administration of oxygen and he recognized its toxic effect when administered for more than a limited period of time in pure form, and he predicted its general use in clinical medicine. Oxygen was next used in the treatment of pneumonia and it was then soon applied to the management of cardiac disease and other disorders characterized by hypoxia. During this period, probably the most important contributor to the field of oxygen therapy was the late Dr. Alvin Barach who, among many other contributions, developed the first cooled oxygen tent and other devices for administering the gas and recognized the potential danger of oxygen administration in producing respiratory acidosis in certain patients with emphysema (Barach, 1925). Largely as a result of his work, oxygen became widely accepted in clinical medicine but its use remained rather imprecise because there were no practical ways of measuring the concentration that was being administered or the response that was being achieved in the blood. This began to change after the development of practical blood gas electrodes in the late 1950s (Severinghaus and Bradley, 1958) and in 1960 E.M.J. Campbell introduced an important reorientation towards the subject of oxygen administration (Campbell, 1967). A cautious attitude had developed towards the use of oxygen in the management of chronic obstructive pulmonary disease, after it was recognized that it could have a deleterious effect by producing ventilatory depression and respiratory acidosis. Campbell showed that by administering small doses of oxygen to patients in jeopardy of ventilatory depression, the arterial oxygen saturation could be moved onto the relatively flat portion of the oxyhemoglobin dissociation curve where further increase in partial pressure would produce little further gain in saturation and that this could usually be done without causing clinically significant hypercapnia. He devised disposable Venturi masks which allowed the delivery of a precise inspired oxygen concentration and stressed the importance of considering the use of oxygen in terms of a dose-response relationship. The dose is established by the particular Venturi mask which is chosen; they are available to administer concentrations of 24, 28, 35, and 40% oxygen. The response was taken to be the effect that a given inspired concentration of oxygen has on the arterial PO_2. In addition to the use of Venturi masks, low flow oxygen by nasal cannulae, which had been introduced by Barach, continued to be used effectively in patients who were in danger of ventilatory depression because, in the minds of many, the actual dose being given did not matter so much since its response in the arterial blood could be measured. The major disadvantage of low flow oxygen administration is that for a given rate of flow the inspired concentration is dependent upon the tidal volume and the frequency and the pattern of ventilation (Mithoefer, 1980). For patients who did not require a low dose of oxygen, it became generally accepted that nasal cannulae or catheters could be used to deliver oxygen at inspired concentrations up to 40% with flows up to 6 liter/min. Tight fitting oxygen masks were found to be capable of producing inspired concentrations of approximately 60% if the rate of flow was 8 liter/min and, if a reservoir bag was added to the mask, nearly 100% oxygen administration could be achieved. It became recognized that 100% oxygen can be used safely for at least 24 hr in patients who are not in danger of ventilatory depression but beyond this period of time there is rapid deterioration of gas exchange and pulmonary function. It became accepted that the highest inspired concentration of oxygen which will have no deleterious effects after prolonged use is about 40%. Regardless of the method of administration, it is usually desirable to monitor the effect of oxygen and to follow the course of the underlying disease by blood gas analysis. If adequate oxygenation cannot be achieved at a safe inspired concentration, then positive end-expiratory pressure should be applied, usually in association with the use of mechanical ventilation. Low dose oxygen is indicated only in patients who are in danger of ventilatory depression, as in obstructive disease associated with hypercapnia. The appropriate dose can be chosen by the use of a predictive diagram if the arterial

PO_2 is known during air breathing or any other inspired concentration up to and including 40% oxygen (Mithoefer et al., 1971).

In 1974, it was shown that although the arterial PO_2 is a useful index of the gas exchange function of the lung, in many circumstances its value can misrepresent the state of tissue oxygenation (Mithoefer et al., 1974). It was suggested that the mixed venous PO_2 is a more reliable index of oxygenation at the tissue level and this concept was applied to oxygen therapy. In that same year, S.M. Tenney showed, by mathematical analysis, that the pressure of oxygen in the venous blood which drains a tissue represents the driving pressure of oxygen for that area of the tissue most in jeopardy from hypoxia and that the venous blood, under most conditions, is approximately equal to the mean tissue oxygen pressure (Tenney, 1974).

Even before Tenney's analysis was published, a number of investigators had assumed that the partial pressure of oxygen in mixed venous blood was a useful index of total body tissue oxygenation (Lutch and Murray, 1972; Mithoefer et al., 1974). Obviously, since the oxygen consumption and blood flow differs among various organs, mixed venous PO_2 will always be higher than the blood which drains some organs and lower than that coming from others. Nevertheless, the mixed venous PO_2 has turned out to be a useful index of tissue oxygenation in clinical medicine. An important exception occurs when arteriovenous shunting is present, as in septic shock. Mixed venous PO_2 can then seriously misrepresent the state of tissue oxygenation and be normal or high in the face of severe tissue hypoxia and metabolic acidosis (Miller et al., 1979).

In 1974, the effect of oxygen administration on both arterial and mixed venous blood was reported in patients with chronic obstructive pulmonary disease (Mithoefer et al., 1974). It was found that the patients could be classified into two major groups, normocapnic and hypercapnic (A and B) and that each of these could be subdivided into those with normal mixed venous PO_2 (I) and those with mixed venous hypoxia (II). The response of oxygen administration will be considered for each of these 4 groups.

Group IA: Normocapnia and normal mixed venous PO_2. The results of oxygen administration in this group are shown in Figure 1. The percent inspired oxygen concentration is on the abscissa, the mixed venous PO_2 on the ordinate. Although these patients had moderate to severe abnormalities in mechanical dysfunction as shown by standard tests of pulmonary function, gas exchange in the lung was not seriously deranged (mean arterial PO_2: 70 mm Hg) and mixed venous oxygenation was normal at rest, breathing air. With oxygen administration arterial PO_2 rose to very high levels while the mixed venous PO_2 hardly changed, up through an inspired concentration of 40%. This response is similar to that which is seen in normal subjects and is the result of the fact that the arterial blood is high up on the flat portion of the oxyhemoglobin dissociation curve while the mixed venous PO_2 is on the steep slope.

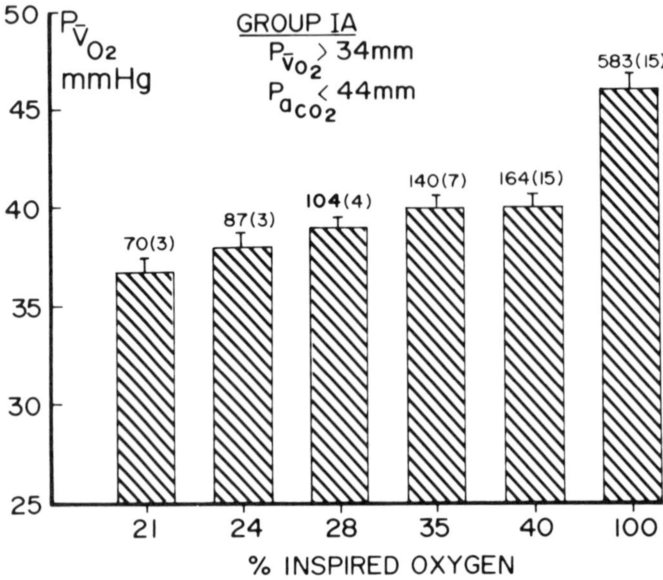

Figure 1. The effect of inspired oxygen concentrations on mixed venous and arterial PO_2 in Group IA, 6 normocapnic patients with normal mixed venous PO_2. Vertical lines above the bars indicate standard error of the mean for mixed venous PO_2. Numbers above each bar represent the arterial PO_2 with standard error of the mean in parentheses.

SOURCE: *Mithoefer et al., 1974.*

Oxygen administration results in large gains of partial pressure in the arterial blood but small increases in saturation. Since the cardiac output usually did not change significantly, the small gain in saturation was transferred to the mixed venous blood with very little resultant increase in pressure because of the steep slope of the curve at that point. Since mixed venous PO_2 is not significantly increased by low inspired oxygen concentrations in these patients, they should not be given an inspired concentration of less than 40% if for some reason they require supplementary oxygen. Low dose oxygen is inappropriate in this group. These patients can be identified as having a normal mixed venous PO_2 by analysis of the arterial blood. In this group, the arterial PCO_2 is normal or low (below 45 mm Hg) and the arterial PO_2 is above approximately 64 mm Hg.

Group IIA: Normocapnia and reduced mixed venous PO_2. This group is an example of how the arterial PO_2 can misrepresent the state of mixed venous and tissue oxygenation. In the past, indications for oxygen administration were based upon the level of arterial PO_2; the critical value at which to administer oxygen varied among authors from 40 to 60 mm Hg. In this group (Figure 2),

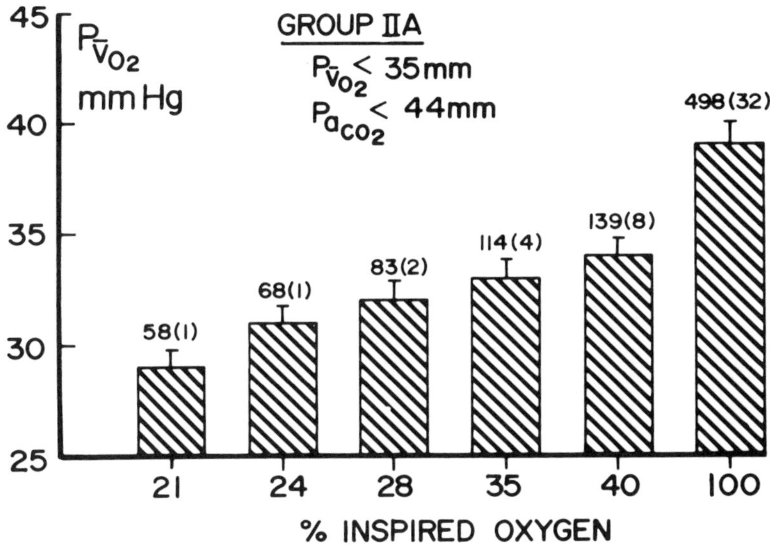

Figure 2. The effect of inspired oxygen concentrations on mixed venous and arterial PO_2 in Group IIA, 12 normocapnic patients with reduced mixed venous PO_2. Vertical lines above the bars indicate standard error of the mean for mixed venous PO_2. Numbers above each bar represent the arterial PO_2 with standard error of the mean in parentheses.

SOURCE: *Mithoefer et al., 1974.*

during air breathing the arterial PO_2 was 58 mm Hg yet there was significant mixed venous hypoxia, the mean value being below 30 mm Hg. Increments of supplementary oxygen produced a brisk rise in arterial PO_2 up to 139 mm Hg with a 40% inspired concentration but the mixed venous PO_2 rose very little, not reaching the lower limit of normal even with 40%. The large increase with 100% oxygen was the result of the addition of dissolved oxygen to the blood. The mechanisms responsible for the sluggish rise in mixed venous PO_2 are similar to those described in the discussion of Group IA. In Group IIA, mixed venous hypoxia is not the result of pulmonary insufficiency alone, but a consequence of inadequate delivery of oxygen to the tissues because of a low cardiac output or hemoglobin concentration or both. In the management of these patients, efforts should be directed toward the restoration of a more normal oxygen delivery system in order to convert them to Group IA. While this is being done, there is no justification for administering less than 40% oxygen since these patients are not in danger of ventilatory depression from oxygen administration. This group can be identified by analysis of the arterial blood where the PCO_2 will be normal or low and the arterial PO_2 less than 65 mm Hg, the lower the arterial PO_2 during air breathing at rest, the lower will be the mixed venous PO_2. Mixed venous hypoxia can be predicted from the arterial blood, though right heart catheterization may be indicated in some patients. If these patients cannot be converted to Group IA by an improvement in their cardiac output and by establishing an optimal level of hemoglobin concentration, then they are candidates for continuous long-term oxygen administration.

Group IB: Hypercapnia and normal mixed venous PO_2. These patients have a very severe abnormality of pulmonary gas exchange with large venous admixtures but they have compensated for this by maintaining a high cardiac output and developing compensatory polycythemia, most have chronic cor pulmonale and are in danger of ventilatory depression from oxygen administration. Because the arterial PO_2 (50 mm Hg) is on the steep portion of the oxyhemoglobin dissociation curve, even small increases in arterial PO_2 result in significant gains in saturation and hence, the mixed venous PO_2 rises briskly in response to oxygen (Mithoefer et al., 1974). From the standpoint of tissue oxygenation, these patients are ideal candidates for low dose oxygen therapy and most of them must be considered for long term continuous oxygen administration. Patients in Group IB (Figure 3) can be identified by analysis of the arterial blood which shows chronic hypercapnia (PCO_2 greater than 44 mm Hg) and an arterial PO_2 of approximately 50 mm Hg or greater.

Figure 3. The effect of inspired oxygen concentrations on mixed venous and arterial PO_2 in Group IB, 3 hypercapnic patients with normal and mixed venous PO_2. Numbers above each bar represent the arterial PO_2.

SOURCE: *Mithoefer et al., 1974.*

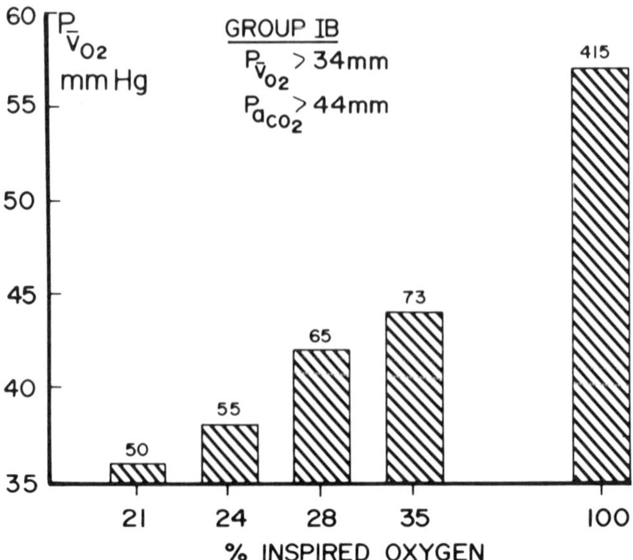

Group IIB: Hypercapnia and reduced mixed venous PO_2. These patients also have very severe abnormalities of pulmonary gas exchange with chronic hypercapnia, but they have not made adequate compensations for this; usually the cardiac output and hemoglobin concentration are both inadequate. They have severe mixed venous hypoxia at rest breathing air but this responds well to small increments of supplementary oxygen (Figure 4). In these patients, as in Group IIA, the mixed venous and tissue hypoxia are not the result simply of pulmonary insufficiency but the combined effect of many or all of the disturbances of oxygen delivery. In the management of these patients, efforts should be made to improve cardiac output and restore hemoglobin concentration to an optimal level, while improving pulmonary gas exchange. They are in danger of ventilatory depression from oxygen administration but usually respond in a satisfactory manner to low doses of oxygen. These patients can often be restored to a more satisfactory level of function by converting them to Group IB through an improvement in cardiac output and hemoglobin concentration. In any case, many of them are candidates for long-term continuous oxygen administration. These patients can be identified by analysis of the

Figure 4. The effect of inspired oxygen concentrations on mixed venous and arterial PO_2 in Group IIB, 12 hypercapnic patients with reduced mixed venous PO_2. Vertical lines above the bars indicate standard error of the mean for mixed venous PO_2. Numbers above each bar represent arterial PO_2 with standard error of the mean in parentheses.

SOURCE: *Mithoefer et al., 1974.*

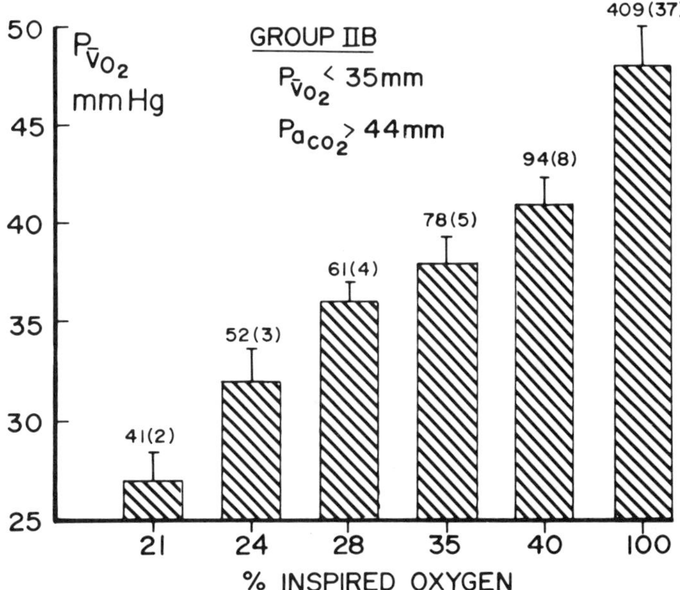

arterial blood where the PCO_2 will be greater than 44 mm Hg and the arterial PO_2 less than 50 mm Hg. Mixed venous hypoxia can be predicted without resorting to right heart catheterization.

In summary, low dose oxygen should be reserved for patients who are in jeopardy of ventilatory depression and respiratory acidosis as a result of the administration of high concentrations of oxygen. In all other situations, when oxygen administration is required for the correction of hypoxia, the most desirable prolonged dose is 40% and even this concentration may not correct mixed venous and tissue hypoxia even though it produces a large rise in arterial PO_2. When mixed venous and tissue hypoxia have been recognized, either by the interpretation of an arterial blood gas analysis or the direct measurement of mixed venous PO_2, it is important to realize that tissue hypoxia is not the result of pulmonary disease alone but is a consequence of failure in oxygen delivery usually as a result of a low cardiac output or hemoglobin concentration or both.

Oxygen administration in the home is appropriate in selected patients with chronic obstructive pulmonary disease or other forms of pulmonary or cardiac insufficiency in which chronic hypoxia is disabling (Block et al., 1977). The method of administration is usually by low flow oxygen through nasal cannulae; the source of the oxygen can be a conventional high pressure oxygen cylinder, a low pressure liquid oxygen source or molecular sieves which concentrate oxygen from the ambient air. In chronic obstructive pulmonary disease, domiciliary oxygen should be administered to selected patients in Group IIA, IB, and IIB. Some ventilatory depression may occur in patients with chronic CO_2 retention but the increased hypercapnia that may develop is usually well tolerated since significant acidemia is usually prevented by renal compensation. A cooperative study was recently reported on 203 patients with chronic obstructive pulmonary disease which compared 24-hr with 12-hr domiciliary oxygen administration (Nocturnal Oxygen Therapy Trial, 1980). It showed that over a mean duration of 19.3 months, those patients who received supplementary oxygen for only 12 hr (including sleep) had nearly twice the mortality rate of those receiving it for 24 hr. The reduction in mortality was particularly striking in patients with hypercapnia, nocturnal hypoxia, severe abnormalities in pulmonary function tests, cerebral dysfunction, normal pulmonary artery pressure, and a relatively well-preserved capacity for work. In addition to appearing to prolong life, continuous oxygen therapy can improve many of the manifestations of chronic hypoxia such as pulmonary hypertension and polycythemia and it often relieves symptoms and improves neuropsychological function and the quality of life. Furthermore, it has been shown that continuous oxygen administration can decrease the number of days of hospitalization as well as the number of outpatient visits for patients with chronic obstructive pulmonary disease and that this can more than make up for the cost of long-term oxygen therapy (Oxygen Therapy Committee, 1977).

References

Barach, A.L. 1925. The therapeutic use of oxygen in acute respiratory disturbances. *Med. Clin. North Am.* 9:471–487.

Block, A.J., Burrows, B., Kanner, R.E., Lilker, E.S., Mithoefer, J.C., and Petty, T.L. 1977. Oxygen administration in the home. *Am. Rev. Respir. Dis.* 115:897–899.

Campbell, E.J.M. 1967. The J. Burns Amberson Lecture: the management of acute respiratory failure in chronic bronchitis and emphysema. *Am. Rev. Respir. Dis.* 96:626–639.

Haldane, J.S. 1927. *Respiration.* New Haven: Yale University Press.

Lutch, J.S. and Murray, J. 1972. Continuous positive-pressure ventilation: effects on systemic oxygen transport and tissue oxygenation. *Ann. Intern. Med.* 76:193–202.

Miller, M.J., Cook, W.R., and Mithoefer, J.C. 1979. Limitation of the use of mixed venous PO_2 as an indicator of tissue hypoxia. *Clin. Res.* 27:401A.

Mithoefer, J.C. 1980. Oxygen therapy. In *Pulmonary Diseases and Disorders Vol. 2.* Fishman, A.P., ed. New York: McGraw-Hill, Co. pp. 1581–1586.

Mithoefer, J.C., Holford, F.D., and Keighley, J.F. 1974. The effect of oxygen administration on mixed venous oxygenation in chronic obstructive pulmonary disease. *Chest* 66:122–132.

Mithoefer, J.C., Keighley, J.F., and Karetzky, M.S. 1971. Correspondence. *Ann. Intern. Med.* 75:326.

Nocturnal Oxygen Therapy Trial Group. 1980. Continuous or nocturnal oxygen therapy in hypoxemic chronic obstructive lung disease. *Ann. Intern. Med.* 93:391–398.

Oxygen Therapy Committee. 1977. Oxygen administration in the home. *Am. Rev. Respir. Dis.* 115:897–899.

Severinghaus, J.W. and Bradley, A.F. 1958. Electrodes for blood PCO_2 and PO_2 determination. *J. Appl. Physiol.* 13:515–520.

Tenney, S.M. 1974. A theoretical analysis of the relationship between venous blood and mean tissue oxygen pressures. *Respir. Physiol.* 20:283–296.

J.A. Loeppky and M.L. Riedesel, editors
OXYGEN TRANSPORT TO HUMAN TISSUES

Assisted Ventilation

Roger C. Bone

Introduction

When mechanical ventilation is indicated in the management of patients with respiratory failure, two major goals are desirable. First, to maintain an alveolar ventilation appropriate for the metabolic requirements of the patient, and second, to correct arterial hypoxemia and maximize oxygen transport. This presentation describes the methods of establishing an efficient ventilatory pattern during mechanical ventilation and how to manage arterial hypoxemia and improve oxygen transport. It also focuses on various bedside techniques for assessing abnormalities in the patient's ventilatory and circulatory status.

The goal is to maintain an alveolar ventilation appropriate to the needs of each individual patient and not necessarily attempt to establish normal blood gas levels. Establishing a $PaCO_2$ level that results in a near normal pH is an appropriate goal in initial management. For example, if chronic carbon dioxide elevation with compensatory bicarbonate retention was present prior to illness, decreasing $PaCO_2$ to normal levels will cause alkalosis. Alkalosis from too great a reduction in $PaCO_2$ carries a risk of cardiac arrhythmias, seizures, or both, and may subsequently make it more difficult to wean the patient from the ventilator (Bone, 1980b).

Mechanical Ventilators

Mechanical ventilators are described by the way in which they terminate inspiratory flow. Volume-cycled machines stop inspiration when a preset volume is delivered. Pressure-cycled machines stop inspiration when a preset pressure is reached. Other types of ventilators exist, but are not in common use. These include time-cycled and flow-cycled machines.

Although more expensive, volume-cycled ventilators are often preferred for ventilatory support of acutely ill patients because the tidal volume delivered by them remains fairly constant despite varying airway resistance and varying lung or chest wall compliance. However, if there is a leak in the system, the patient will not receive the entire prescribed volume. With a pressure-cycled ventilator, tidal volume and alveolar ventilation will vary with changes in lung or chest wall compliance and airway resistance.

The patient's primary disease will have a major bearing on the ventilator used and the settings selected when initiating management. For example, a patient with normal lungs suffering drug overdose is managed differently from a patient with chronic obstructive lung disease. For most patients, the following steps are taken in initiating ventilation. First, the tidal volume is usually set at 10 to 15 ml/kg and at a rate of 8 to 12 breaths/min. For the patient with chronic obstructive lung disease, a tidal volume of about 10 ml/kg is usually selected to reduce the risk of pulmonary barotrauma and hyperinflation (Bone, 1980b). Hyperventilation in these patients will often decrease cardiac output and decrease total oxygen delivery.

Volume Ventilator

With a volume ventilator, the machine delivers the prescribed volume unless the pressure limit is exceeded. Once the tidal volume is selected, one should set the pressure limit 5 to 10 cm H_2O above the pressure required to deliver that tidal volume. An alarm normally sounds when the pressure limit is reached, indicating that the patient has not received the volume selected.

Pressure Ventilator

With a pressure-cycled ventilator, an end-inspiratory pressure is set rather than a tidal volume. Therefore, the tidal volume must be measured separately to determine what volume is delivered with a given pressure. Since tidal volume will vary with changes in lung and chest wall compliance or secretions in the airways, the tidal volume should be monitored constantly or else the patient's ventilation may fall to an inadequate level. This is one important disadvantage of pressure-cycled ventilators. In addition, the pressure and flow generating capabilities of typical pressure ventilators may be inadequate for patients with stiff lungs, such as patients with the adult respiratory distress syndrome or for patients with high ventilatory requirements.

Tidal Volumes

Patients ventilated with small tidal volumes, less than 8 ml/kg, should probably receive periodic hyperinflations or sighs to prevent microatelectasis. The sigh volume is usually set at 1.5 to 2 times the tidal volume, delivered at 5 to 10-min intervals. Patients with large tidal volumes, in the range of 10 or more ml/kg, probably will not require periodic sighs.

Flow Rate

Both volume- and pressure-cycled ventilators provide variable inspiratory flow rates. The flow rate selected should allow the expiratory time to exceed the inspiratory time. This provides for full exhalation of the tidal volume and avoids compromise of the cardiac output by allowing adequate time for venous return. It is usually considered best to let the patient have approximately twice as much time for exhalation as for inhalation. With severe air flow obstruction, expiratory time may need to be even longer to allow lung emptying and avoid progressive increases in end-expiratory lung volume and hyperinflation of pulmonary segments, which could result in alveolar rupture and decreased oxygen transport by decreasing preload.

Respiratory Rate

Settings of respiratory rate also are found on both types of ventilators. This is the rate at which the patient is ventilated if he makes no respiratory effort. The observed rate for the patient who triggers the machine may be higher than the set rate because of self-induced inspirations. A respiratory rate should be set for these patients as a protective measure. The rate set can be somewhat lower than the triggered rate.

Sensitivity

The sensitivity setting on mechanical ventilators allows the patient to trigger an inspiration. Reducing the sensitivity will require greater patient effort to initiate a breath. If the setting is too insensitive, the patient will be unable to initiate a breath at any pressure. If the setting is too sensitive, many machines will self-cycle, resulting in hyperventilation of the patient. Hyperventilation often causes a reduction in cardiac output by decreasing the $PaCO_2$.

Intermittent Mandatory Ventilator

Most ventilators now provide for intermittent mandatory ventilation (IMV) as described by Downs et al. (1974). The IMV allows the patient to spontaneously breathe a humidified gas mixture through the circuit at will while also receiving intermittent positive pressure lung inflations at a predetermined rate and tidal volume. The IMV can be accomplished by modification of the inspiratory circuit of any ventilator.

Oxygen Concentration

Most volume-cycled ventilators allow the inspired oxygen concentration to be set at any point from 21 to 100%. The lowest setting which results in adequate oxygenation should be used to avoid oxygen toxicity. Pressure-cycled ventilators generally have two settings: 100% oxygen and "air mix." The "air mix" setting delivers a concentration of 40 to 90% oxygen, depending on the impedance to air flow. With stiffer lungs or greater airway resistance, a higher concentration of oxygen is delivered. This problem can be avoided if the gas for a pressure-cycled ventilator is delivered through an oxygen-air blender.

The appropriate initial oxygen concentration depends upon the clinical circumstances. Unless previous information assures one that a lower setting will be adequate, 100% oxygen should be delivered initially. This is a time when many things can go wrong, such as ventilator malfunction, improper placement of the endotracheal tube, or inefficient alveolar ventilation from the selected tidal volume and rate.

Humidifiers

Gas delivered by an endotracheal tube bypasses the upper respiratory mucosa and must be warmed and humidified. All ventilators should have a heated humidifier. Most newer ventilators have a sensor to monitor the temperature of the humidified inspired gas.

Monitoring Spirometer

A monitoring spirometer should be added to any ventilator which does not have one. When expired tidal volumes are measured, the volume includes two components: first, the volume delivered to the patient's lungs, and second, the volume used to expand the distensible tubing of the ventilator. The volume change in the tubing must be subtracted from the total volume collected in the spirometer to accurately measure the volume delivered to the patient's lungs. This volume correction usually is in the range of 3 to 5 ml/cm H_2O of peak pressure for adult ventilator circuits (Bone, 1981).

Arterial Blood Gases

Following the initial set-up, a measurement of arterial blood gases is mandatory. Blood gas evaluation is the only way to assess the adequacy of oxygenation and ventilation. The sample should be taken approximately 30 min after the initial setting is made. The adequacy of oxygenation is assessed from the PaO_2 value. A PaO_2 of about 60 mm Hg is acceptable. The adequacy of alveolar ventilation is determined from the amount of CO_2 in the arterial blood. The desired $PaCO_2$ value will depend on the patient's pH.

Alveolar Ventilation

If the patient's ventilation is fully controlled by the machine, achieving the desired $PaCO_2$ and alveolar ventilation are relatively easy. Once the $PaCO_2$ has been measured, changes can be made in the tidal volume or respiratory frequency to achieve the desired $PaCO_2$. Alveolar ventilation is inversely related to the $PaCO_2$ value. To lower the $PaCO_2$, the alveolar ventilation must be increased and vice versa. The required change in ventilation can be easily calculated. Even if the extent of dead space in the ventilatory system is not known, it makes up a fairly constant portion of the tidal volume. Thus, changes in total ventilation will cause proportionate changes in the alveolar ventilation and in the $PaCO_2$. One can calculate a new respiratory rate using the following equation:

$$\text{Desired respiratory rate} = \text{Previous rate} \times \frac{\text{Previous } PaCO_2}{\text{Desired } PaCO_2} \quad (32.1)$$

For example, if 12 breaths/min result in a $PaCO_2$ of 80 mm Hg and the desired $PaCO_2$ is 60 mm Hg, then the new setting should be 16 respirations/min.

Occasionally, patients who trigger the ventilator will spontaneously over-ventilate. In these cases, a simple decrease in the set respiratory rate or tidal volume will not suffice. There are three alternatives to correct this hyperventilation when serious alkalosis results. One alternative is sedation so that the patient no longer triggers the ventilator. Another is to place the patient on IMV and reduce the set rate appropriately. A third choice is to add mechanical dead space to the system, but with this method many patients will increase their triggering rate and maintain the alkalosis.

Arterial Oxygenation

To establish and maintain adequate arterial oxygen saturation requires a PaO_2 of about 60 mm Hg. The lowest possible inspired oxygen concentration should be used to meet this goal. Using an oxygen concentration of greater than 50% for prolonged periods can result in oxygen toxicity. If a PaO_2 of over 50 mm Hg is not achieved with 50% oxygen or less, positive end-expiratory pressure (PEEP) may be cautiously added to the system. This capability is found on most volume ventilators and allows a variable pressure to be maintained in the airway at end-exhalation (Ashbaugh et al., 1967). The PEEP increases the end-expiratory lung volume or functional residual capacity.

While oxygen is carried in bulk combined with hemoglobin, delivery to tissue depends on its partial pressure in the blood which is a reflection of oxygen available to be delivered from hemoglobin. A fall in the PaO_2 without a change in $PaCO_2$ suggests that blood oxygenation is deteriorating despite constant alveolar ventilation. In the acutely ill patient, this is usually due to ventilation-perfusion imbalance or intrapulmonary shunting. An important feature of shunting is that hypoxemia cannot be abolished by giving 100% oxygen, because shunted blood totally bypasses ventilated alveoli. A shunt usually does not result in a raised $PaCO_2$ in arterial blood because the chemoreceptors sense any elevation in $PaCO_2$ and respond by increasing ventilation.

The alveolar oxygen tension can be estimated from the following abbreviated formula which is often used for clinical purposes:

$$PAO_2 = PIO_2 - \frac{PaCO_2}{R} \quad (32.2)$$

The PIO_2 is equal to barometric pressure (P_B) minus water vapor pressure (47 mm Hg at body temperature) multiplied by the inspired oxygen fraction, (FIO_2). The respiratory quotient (R) is approximately 0.8 in the steady state resting condition. It is assumed to be 0.8 in respiratory failure although this is not always the case.

The correction for R varies depending on FIO_2 as can be seen from the nonsimplified alveolar equation:

$$PAO_2 = FIO_2(P_B - 47) - PACO_2\left(FIO_2 + \frac{1 - FIO_2}{R}\right) \qquad (32.3)$$

Although this equation appears more formidable, if $PaCO_2$ is used rather than $PACO_2$ (they are assumed equal) and 100% oxygen is inhaled, the equation shows that PAO_2 is simply the difference between inspired PO_2 and $PaCO_2$. It is highly important that the actual FIO_2 is known precisely to avoid errors in the calculated PAO_2.

The arterial oxygen tension divided by the alveolar oxygen tension is called the a/A ratio. This ratio is relatively stable with varying FIO_2 unlike the classic alveolar-arterial (A-a) gradient. Thus, it is a useful index of changes in lung function when a patient's oxygen concentration is changed. The normal a/A ratio is 0.75 or greater. The ratio can also be used to predict the new PaO_2 that will result from a change in inspired oxygen concentration (Gilbert and Keighley, 1974).

Ventilation-Perfusion Status

The three compartment lung model of Riley and Cournand (Figure 1) is a convenient way to express gas exchange in the patient requiring mechanical ventilation since physiological dead space and physiological shunt can be readily measured in the patient requiring mechanical ventilation as described below.

Physiological Dead Space

Some patients have an elevated $PaCO_2$ despite a seemingly normal ventilation or require a high total ventilation to maintain a normal $PaCO_2$. The relation-

Figure 1. The three compartment lung model of Riley and Cournand.
SOURCE: *Bone, 1980a.*

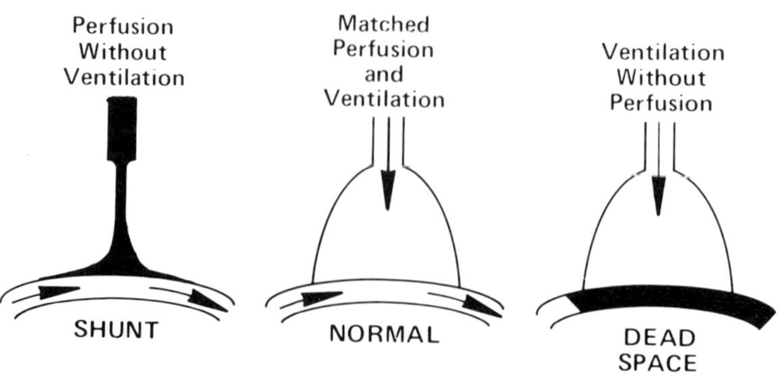

ship between CO_2 production and alveolar ventilation shows that this can occur either if the patient's CO_2 production is high or if a large portion of the total ventilation is wasted in physiological dead space. Physiological dead space represents wasted ventilation because it is the portion of the tidal volume which does not participate in gas exchange. Dead space consists of non-perfused or poorly perfused alveoli (alveolar dead space) in addition to the volume of the conducting airways (anatomical dead space) and that added by ventilator tubing connections.

The CO_2 production and wasted ventilation can be evaluated by making a 3-min collection of expired gas and a simultaneous measurement of arterial PCO_2. The CO_2 production/min is calculated from the expired volume and expired CO_2 concentration. The wasted ventilation, as a proportion of dead space to total ventilation (V_D/V_T) is calculated from the arterial PCO_2 and the carbon dioxide tension in the mixed expired gas ($P\overline{E}CO_2$) from the modified Bohr equation for $PaCO_2$ as follows:

$$\frac{V_D}{V_T} = \frac{PaCO_2 - P\overline{E}CO_2}{PaCO_2} \qquad (32.4)$$

Physiological dead space is increased in respiratory failure due to obstructive lung disease and adult respiratory distress syndrome. Dead space also is increased when pulmonary perfusion is reduced in patients with pulmonary emboli, and those whose lungs are overinflated during positive pressure ventilation (Bone et al., 1981). An estimation of physiological dead space in adult respiratory distress syndrome has shown it to have a striking relationship to survival (Figure 2).

Physiological Shunt

Another useful index of ventilation-perfusion inequity is the physiological shunt (also called venous admixture, or wasted blood flow). The shunt equation can be used in the following form:

$$\dot{Q}s/\dot{Q}t = \frac{CiO_2 - CaO_2}{CiO_2 - C\bar{v}O_2} \qquad (32.5)$$

Where $\dot{Q}s$ refers to blood flow through the shunt and $\dot{Q}t$ to total lung blood flow, while CiO_2, CaO_2, and $C\bar{v}O_2$ refer to the oxygen content of ideal end-pulmonary capillary, arterial, and mixed venous blood, respectively. The normal value of $\dot{Q}s/\dot{Q}t$ is less than 5%. If this shunt fraction is determined on other than 100% oxygen, hypoxemia due to V/Q inequity may result in an overestimation. When the shunt is measured while breathing 100% oxygen, an overestimation may still result if inadequate time is given to completely wash out poorly ventilated alveoli. The PO_2 electrodes may also underestimate the true PO_2 at high PO_2s when compared to blood tonometered with 100% O_2. The magnitude of the physiological shunt is directly related to cardiac output. Increasing cardiac output by volume expansion or by pharmacological means

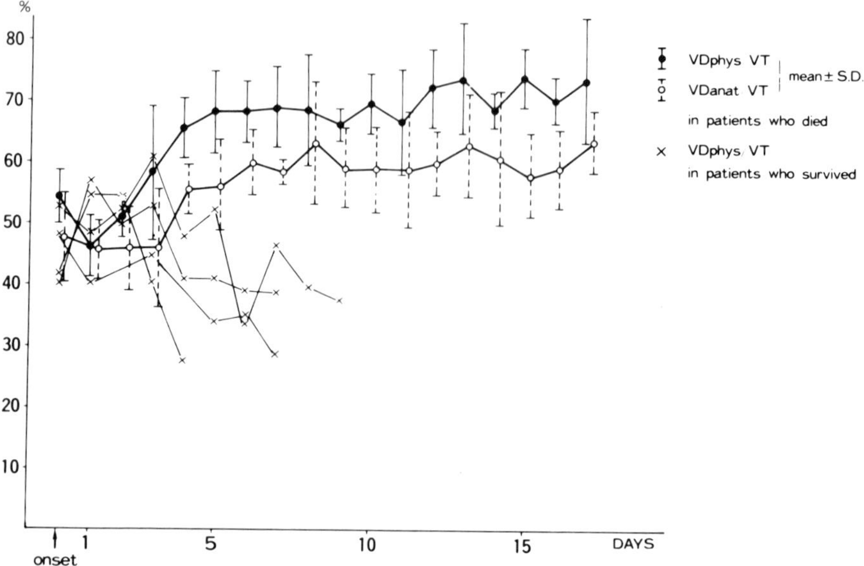

Figure 2. Physiological and anatomical dead space from patients with the adult respiratory distress syndrome.

SOURCE: *Shimada et al., 1979.*

increases the shunt fraction in septic shock (Jardin et al., 1979). Thus, the magnitude of the shunt should always be interpreted in relationship to cardiac output. Often in the critically ill patient, arteriovenous oxygen difference is estimated rather than measured. This often leads to considerable inaccuracy in the estimation of the physiological shunt.

Oxygen Delivery

In the patient with severe respiratory failure, improvement in tissue oxygenation is the goal. Positive end-expiratory pressure is often given to increase the arterial oxygen content. Since oxygen delivery is the product of cardiac output and arterial oxygen content, the cardiac output or some index of changes of cardiac output should be followed as PEEP is changed. Success in using PEEP must be measured by improvement in PaO_2 and also be demonstrating that adequate oxygen delivery is being achieved. This can be a problem with lung injury that is not equal in each lung (Carlon et al., 1978). Several studies have shown that even when PaO_2 increases, significant reduction in cardiac output can result from PEEP. If PEEP results in a decreased cardiac output, the patient may be hypovolemic and cardiac filling pressure may be less than adequate during PEEP. In this case, intravascular volume repletion is indicated. Alternatively, the patient may have primary cardiac dysfunction and require inotropic agents. Positive end-expiratory pressure is used most commonly for patients with adult respiratory distress syndrome. In some situations, PaO_2 is not improved and may even be worsened by PEEP if blood flow is diverted from normal to abnormal lung tissue.

The mixed venous oxygen tension ($P\bar{v}O_2$) is a useful monitor of oxygen delivery. If $P\bar{v}O_2$ decreases as PEEP is increased, a reduction in oxygen delivery to the tissues probably has occurred. When the $P\bar{v}O_2$ is used to measure changes in circulatory function, PaO_2 and hemoglobin concentration must also be considered. Infusion of large amounts of saline or colloid can change the hematocrit. Thus, the PaO_2 and hematocrit should be assessed along with the $P\bar{v}O_2$. The $P\bar{v}O_2$ has gained popularity as an index of tissue oxygenation, a trend facilitated by the relative ease with which $P\bar{v}O_2$ measurements can be made from the pulmonary artery catheter. Tenney has discussed the theoretical relationship between $P\bar{v}O_2$ and tissue oxygen tension, pointing out that $P\bar{v}O_2$ in most situations is a good approximation of tissue oxygen tension (Tenny, 1974). At best, the $P\bar{v}O_2$ is a weighted mean of tissue oxygenation because of variable flow rates and extraction in different organs. Blood drawn from a central venous catheter is not truly mixed and pulmonary artery catheter is necessary. A $P\bar{v}O_2$ of less than 30 mm Hg is a sign of severe tissue hypoxia. We usually obtain a $P\bar{v}O_2$ whenever a PaO_2 sample is drawn with a Swan-Ganz catheter in place. We have recently shown that $P\bar{v}O_2$ is an accurate measure of tissue oxygen in hemorrhagic and hypoxic shock, but is falsely high with endotoxin shock because of arteriovenous shunting peripherally (Hiller and Bone, 1978). Also, Cain and Chapler (1978) have shown that the $P\bar{v}O_2$ at which lactate appeared was different in patients with anemia and hypoxic hypoxia. Danek et al. (1980) have recently shown that $P\bar{v}O_2$ may not be quite as useful as previously assumed to estimate oxygen delivery during a PEEP trial. When the patient is in a basal state with a constant oxygen consumption, cardiac output is inversely related to the arteriovenous oxygen content difference as shown by the Fick equation:

$$\frac{O_2 \text{ consumption}}{\text{cardiac output}} = CaO_2 - C\bar{v}O_2 \qquad (32.6)$$

With the simultaneous measurement of PaO_2, $P\bar{v}O_2$, and hemoglobin, $CaO_2 - C\bar{v}O_2$ can be calculated. In the absence of a pulmonary artery catheter, PEEP should be employed *only* if blood pressure, urine, and CNS status are monitored to ensure that adequate tissue perfusion is being achieved.

A clinical example of maximizing oxygen delivery is shown below. A 24-yr-old female with the adult respiratory distress syndrome secondary to thrombotic thrombocytopenic purpura is treated with PEEP. One can calculate the optimum level of PEEP to use by the results shown in Table 1. The

Table 1. Hemodynamic Profile of a Patient with Adult Respiratory Distress Syndrome Being Treated With Various Levels of PEEP.

	Unit	5 cm H_2O PEEP	10 cm H_2O PEEP	15 cm H_2O PEEP
Blood pressure	mm Hg	140/80	130/82	112/82
Pulse	Min^{-1}	100	90	103
Wedge pressure	mm Hg	10	13	15
Pulmonary artery pressure	mm Hg	45/22	37/17	51/15
Cardiac output	liter/min	5.9	5.8	4
Blood gases				
pH		7.30	7.39	7.32
$PaCO_2$	mm Hg	28	38	32
PaO_2	mm Hg	50	80	55
Sat	percent	85	95	82
Hemoglobin	g	12	12	12
Urine	ml/hr	50	50	30
Oxygen delivery	ml/min	845	933	554

optimum level of PEEP is 10 cm H_2O because it is associated with the best tissue oxygen delivery (933 ml O_2/min). The calculation for 10 cm PEEP is as follows:

$$\text{Tissue delivery of oxygen} = \text{cardiac output} \times CaO_2$$

$$CaO_2 = [\text{Hgb}(g/100\ ml) \times 1.39(ml/g) \times \text{Sat}/100] + (0.003 \times PaO_2) \quad (32.7)$$

$$= [12 \times 1.39 \times 0.95] + 0.24 = 15.8 + 0.24 = 16.1\ ml/100\ ml$$

$$\text{Cardiac output} \times CaO_2 = 5800\ ml/min \times 16.1\ ml/100\ ml = 933\ ml/min.$$

In summary, information gathered from the circulatory system should be added to that gathered from general examinations and respiratory measures. From all these observations, tests, and measurements, it is possible to provide optimal ventilatory care to the patient. Attention to advances in the ability to monitor cardiopulmonary function should continue to improve the care of patients who require mechanical ventilation.

ACKNOWLEDGMENTS

This work was supported by NIH Academic Career Award 1K07 HL00518-01 and the Arkansas Lung Association.

References

Ashbaugh, D.G., Bigelow, D.B., Petty, T.L., and Levine, B.E. 1967. Acute respiratory distress in adults. *Lancet* 2:319–323.

Bone, R.C. 1980a. Treatment of severe hypoxemia due to the adult respiratory distress syndrome. *Arch. Intern. Med.* 140:85–89.

Bone, R.C. 1980b. Treatment of respiratory failure due to advanced chronic obstructive lung disease. *Arch. Intern. Med.* 140:1018–1021.

Bone, R.C. 1981. Monitoring respiratory function in the patient with the adult respiratory distress syndrome. In *Seminars in Respiratory Medicine Vol. 2. Adult Respiratory Distress Syndrome.* Hudson, L., ed. New York: B.C. Decker. pp. 140–150.

Cain, S.M. and Chapler, C.K. 1978. O_2 extraction by hind limb versus whole dog during anemic hypoxia. *J. Appl. Physiol.* 45:966–970.

Carlon, G.C., Ray, C., Klein, R., Goldiner, P.L., and Miodownik, S. 1978. Criteria for selective positive end-expiratory pressure and independent synchronized ventilation of each lung. *Chest* 74:501–507.

Danek, S.J., Lynch, J.P., Weg, J.G., and Dantzker, D.R. 1980. The dependence of oxygen uptake on oxygen delivery in the adult respiratory distress syndrome. *Am. Rev. Respir. Dis.* 122:387–395.

Downs, J.B., Perkins, H.M., and Modell, J.H. 1974. Intermittent mandatory ventilation. *Arch. Surg.* 109:519–523.

Gilbert F. and Keighley, J.F. 1974. The arterial/alveolar oxygen tension ratio: an index of gas exchange applicable to varying inspired oxygen concentrations. *Am. Rev. Respir. Dis.* 109:142–145.

Hiller, C. and Bone, R. 1978. Assessment of correlation between tissue oxygen and mixed venous oxygen during hemorrhage and hypoxemia. *Clin. Res.* 26:448A.

Jardin, F., Eveleigh, M.C., Gurdjain, F., DeLille, F., and Margairaz, A. 1979. Venous admixture in human septic shock. *Circulation* 60:155–160.

Shimada, Y., Yoshiya, I., Tanaka, K., Sone, S., and Sakurai, M. 1979. Evaluation of the progress and prognosis of adult respiratory distress syndrome: simple respiratory physiologic measurement. *Chest* 76:180–186.

Tenney, S.M. 1974. A theoretical analysis of the relationship between venous blood and mean tissue oxygen pressures. *Respir. Physiol.* 20:283–296.

SECTION VII:

Abstracts of Participants

Body Composition and Aging: A Longitudinal Study Spanning Four Decades

Albert R. Behnke, Jr. and L.G. Myhre

ABSTRACT

Population studies suggest that in the adult male body fat increases with advancing age. Increases in body fat allegedly replace metabolically active cells lost by normal degeneration during the aging process. However, the validity of extrapolating data from such cross-sectional population studies to the individual aging man remains subject to question. Body composition data reported here were collected at irregular intervals from one male subject throughout more than four decades of adult life. Body fat and lean body mass (LBM) were derived from body density which was determined by underwater weighing or by body volume measures calculated from either water or helium displacement. Total body potassium (TBK) was measured by a 4-π whole body liquid scintillation counter, and total body water (TBW) was determined by either antipyrine, tritiated water, or ethanol methods. The close relationship between LBM and TBW was little affected by wide fluctuations in body weight throughout adult life. LBM declined at a relatively steady rate averaging about 3.6% per decade from age 30 through 70; thereafter, the rate of loss increased markedly to a level averaging about 9% per decade. Data for TBK suggest a similar rate of decline up through age 55 and decreasing even more sharply than did LBM after age 70. These data seem to confirm the reported decreases in lean tissue with aging. However, after age 70 the rate of loss of TBK exceeds that for LBM, indicating that during the advanced years of adult life the degenerative loss of active lean tissue is in part replaced by other tissue which is both low in fat and in potassium.

Changes in Ventral Medullary ECF pH During Correction of Metabolic Acidosis

Donald G. Davies and W.F. Nolan

ABSTRACT

Changes in arterial blood acid-base balance and medullary ECF pH were measured in 5 chloralose-urethane-anesthetized, gallamine-paralyzed, artificially ventilated New Zealand white rabbits during acute metabolic alkalosis induced by the i.v. infusion of 0.2 M $NaHCO_3$ over 30 min. Ventral medullary ECF pH was measured with micro-pH electrodes (1–2 μ tip diameter) positioned in the ventral medulla. The following results were obtained:

Time (min)	pHa	$PaCO_2$	$[HCO_3]a$	ECF pH
0	7.258 (0.018)	2.69 (0.7)	11.7 (0.8)	7.060 (0.089)
30	7.454[a] (0.045)	26.4 (0.7)	18.4[a] (2.0)	7.226[a] (0.061)

Values are mean ± S.E.
[a]Significant at the 0.01 level.

We conclude that metabolic changes in blood acid-base balance are rapidly reflected in ventral medullary ECF. This mechanism could alter minute ventilation in peripheral chemodenervated animals. (Supported by NIH Grant HL 25984.)

Measurement of Human Fetal Aortic Blood Flow Using Doppler Ultrasound

Marlowe E. Eldridge

ABSTRACT

Currently the only noninvasive method of assessing fetal well-being is fetal heart rate (FHR) monitoring. Clinical studies correlating ominous FHR patterns to pregnancy outcome show a high incidence of false positive tests (70%). In addition, ominous FHR patterns correlate poorly with fetal acidosis. Studies of hemodynamic responses to hypoxia in fetal sheep suggest that fetal descending aortic flow may be a better predictor of fetal hypoxia. Recent developments in combining real-time imaging ultrasound with pulse Doppler ultrasound have made it possible to noninvasively study human fetal circulatory dynamics. This study used a 5 MHz real-time two-dimensional echo/pulse Doppler duplex scanner (DS) to measure noninvasively and quantitatively abdominal aortic blood flow ($\dot{Q}_A$) in 14 normal human fetuses. The fetuses were studied at 4-week intervals from 14 weeks gestational age (GA) to parturition. GA and fetal weight (FW) were estimated from biparietal and transverse abdominal diameters. Aortic velocity ($\bar{v}$) was calculated from the Doppler shifted frequency and the Doppler incidence angle (determined from the cursor/vessel intercept on the DS monitor). Aortic diameter (D) was measured directly from the DS image. Means ($\pm$S.D.) for $\bar{v}$ and D were 27 ± 11 cm/sec and 0.41 ± 0.12 cm, respectively. Both $\bar{v}$ and D increased with GA. $\dot{Q}_A$ (cm^3/min), computed as $\bar{v} \times \pi D^2/4$ (cm^2)$\times 60$ (sec/min), showed a nonlinear increase from 83 ± 19 (cm^3/min) at 20 weeks GA to 527 ± 54 (cm^3/min) at 38 weeks. A reduction in $\dot{Q}_A$ was often seen after 38 weeks. The general shape of the curve is similar to a fetal weight curve. $\dot{Q}_A$/FW was 185 ± 38 cm^3/kg/min and showed little change with GA. This preliminary study shows that the DS system may be used to characterize human fetal aortic blood flow *in utero*. Since the method is noninvasive, it may be used repeatedly throughout gestation to determine and follow fetal circulatory status and placental perfusion. Furthermore, the technique seems ideally suited for assessing fetal well-being in high-risk pregnancies and during complicated labor.

An O_2 Transport Model With Diffusion Impairment and Anatomical Shunt

Wesley M. Granger and D.A. Miller

ABSTRACT

A theoretical study of the O_2 transport system has been generated that includes both pulmonary diffusion and an anatomical shunt. Wagner and West (1972. *J. Appl. Physiol.* 33:62) previously examined the effects of diffusion; however, for computational facility, they assumed that the mixed venous PO_2 remained constant at 40 mm Hg. This assumption would be violated in a real system since a variety of parameters could lower the arterial PO_2 (PaO_2) and consequently the mixed venous PO_2 (PvO_2). The model has been programmed using MIMIC simulation language. An iterative procedure changes the mixed venous O_2 content until it satisfies the arteriovenous O_2 content difference as determined by O_2 consumption and cardiac output (Qt). Part of the impetus for this study was the unpredictable changes in PaO_2 in dogs with oleic acid induced pulmonary edema (Lynch et al. 1979. *J. Appl. Physiol.* 46:315). In these dogs with impaired gas exchange, PaO_2 generally increased with increased cardiac output but frequently the opposite result was observed. This result apparently was not due to ventilation-perfusion abnormality since V/Q measurements indicated that the gas exchange units consisted either of normal or shunt units. The V/Q of the normal units was not influenced by changes in cardiac output. Because of this apparent minimal influence of V/Q, we chose to study the effects of changing cardiac output in the presence of diffusion impairment and anatomical shunt. The analysis consisted of observing the effects of changing cardiac output on PaO_2, PvO_2, and shunt fraction (Fs). The effects of increasing Qt from 2.5 to 20 liter/min were studied in three situations: (1) an anatomical shunt only, (2) diffusion impairment only, and (3) with both conditions. The diffusion impairment showed a decrease in PaO_2 and increases in PvO_2 and Fs as cardiac output was increased. An anatomical shunt showed an increase in PaO_2 and PvO_2 as Qt increased, while Fs remained constant. The combined analysis with both conditions showed that under some parameter conditions PaO_2 increases in the low Qt range and then decreases in the high Qt range. In this combined condition, Fs and PvO_2 increased with Qt over its whole range. During the course of the study, it was also found that increasing the hemoglobin concentration had similar effects as did cardiac output. The theoretical effects of changing Qt on PaO_2, PvO_2, and Fs in this model can explain the experimental findings in oleic acid induced pulmonary edema.

Maximum Expiratory Flow-Volume (MEFV) Curves in the Diagnosis of Exercise-Induced Bronchospasm (EIB)

Francois Haas and A. Haas

ABSTRACT

Diagnosis of EIB is frequently predicted on change in either peak expiratory flow rate (PEFR) or forced expiratory volume at 1 sec (FEV_1), parameters that are overly dependent on patient cooperation and effort. In order to assess the most reliably sensitive parameter(s) for detecting EIB, we investigated the effects of treadmill running on PEFR, FEV_1, forced vital capacity (FVC), the ratio FEV_1/FVC, forced expiratory flow at 25 and 50% VC (FEF_{25}, FEF_{50}), and forced expiratory flow between 25% and 75% VC (FEF_{25-75}) in 101 volunteers. EIB, as assessed by a reproducible postexercise drop of 5% in one or more of these MEFV parameters, was observed in 60 subjects. All 60 showed a significant reversal in this reduction after bronchodilator. Reductions in FEF_{50} and FEF_{25-75} were the most reliably sensitive discriminators of EIB in this sample, accurately identifying 60 and 58%, respectively, of the EIB group. Despite a general trend for those subjects with the more impaired preexercise MEFV curves to have more severe EIB, we could not use these resting curves to predict the actual degree of EIB. Of the 60 subjects with diagnosed EIB susceptibility, 45 had a history of current or childhood asthma, 10 had complained of postexertional coughing, and 5 had denied any respiratory problems or sensations. Three subects who had complained of post exertional shortness of breath and coughing, however, had no appreciable change in the MEFV parameters on any of 3 separate test occasions. However, these individuals, who represented 5% of the EIB susceptible group, consistently demonstrated marked airflow reduction in the terminal 15% of their MEFV curves. We conclude that, for any given patient, EIB cannot be accurately diagnosed from a single airflow parameter and that the complete MEFV curve should be analyzed for change to fully assess susceptibility to EIB.

Effects of Naloxone on Oxygen Transport During Exercise

Philip P. Hamilton, G. Surbey, and G. M. Andrew

ABSTRACT

Recent studies have verified the presence of both highly specific opiate receptors in the CNS of vertebrates and endogenous opiate-like substances in man (including $\alpha, \beta, \gamma, \delta$ endorphin) with analgesic activity indistinguishable from that of morphine. On the basis of endorphin administration or alternatively by injection of naloxone (an opiate receptor antagonist), several roles of the opiate-receptor endorphin system have been suggested, including neuromodulator and endocrine regulation, inhibitory neurotransmitters, pain perception and analgesia, and possibly the mechanism of acupuncture analgesia. An interesting concept is the role of endogenous opiates in modulation of the pain associated with intense physical exercise. Highly competitive athletes frequently experience pain in training sessions. Does this chronic exposure to painful stimuli increase the secretion of endogenous opiates and increase an individual's pain tolerance, thereby allowing a competitive advantage? A recent study has reported a marked (5-fold) increase in serum β endorphin in elite male athletes during maximal exercise. The researchers suggested that this increase may be related to pain control. The present double-blind study was designed to observe the effects of administration of naloxone on maximal exercise performance. Five highly trained middle distance runners were studied on four occasions, during maximal exercise on a graded treadmill. The first two testing sessions were used to determine each subject's maximal oxygen uptake. During the third and fourth tests, either naloxone (0.04 mg/Kg) or a normal saline placebo of equivalent volume was administered intravenously preexercise. Preliminary analysis of results for placebo and naloxone suggest a trend toward marginal reduction with naloxone in work performance, aerobic capacity and related ventilatory functions. Only in respect to heart rate were consistent significant differences observed. It is tentatively concluded that inhibition of the opiate receptor mechanism, if this was in fact achieved by the dose of naloxone presently employed, does not markedly affect progressive maximal exercise performance. (Supported by grants from Health and Welfare, Canada and Queen's University Advisory Research Committee.)

Fast Chemosensory Mechanisms in the Lung?

Neal B. Kindig

ABSTRACT

There is evidence that fast chemosensitive mechanisms respond to local CO_2 disturbances in the lung (Wasserman, Luft, and Filley) before peripheral or central chemoreceptors have time to act. Such reception must respond to directional CO_2 flux and is more likely related to differential changes between blood and alveolar gas, blood and endothelial cells, or different components of blood than to absolute levels of alveolar or blood gases alone. The normal hematocrit of blood in the circulation is about 0.45 while it is less than 0.3 in the capillary bed where mean red blood cell (RBC) velocity must, therefore, exceed mean plasma velocity by a factor of two. Either the plasma must wash back over advancing RBCs, or collateral channels must contain plasma with few RBCs. In gas exchange areas, RBCs are in close contact with capillary walls (0.18 microns, Weibel) and are separated longitudinally by plasma plugs. Carbonic anhydrase (CA) is profusely available in RBCs and probably on the surface of endothelial cells, while its availability in plasma is less certain. Endothelial cells have intimate contact with both alveolar gas and RBCs during capillary transit. Thus conditions exist for endothelial cell PCO_2 and HCO_3^- to remain in equilibrium with alveolar gas throughout the respiratory cycle. The venous CO_2 in entering RBCs equilibrates less rapidly with alveolar gas, but before the completion of capillary transit. Plasma equilibration is even less rapid, but is aided by the CA in RBCs via ionic shifts. Initial changes of pH in well-buffered RBCs may be faster and of greater magnitude than in poorly buffered plasma. End-capillary disequilibrium is in dispute. Directional bicarbonate flux from plasma to RBCs to endothelial cells is enhanced by raised venous PCO_2 and is retarded or reversed by raised alveolar PCO_2 at the end of inspiration. The corresponding endothelial membrane potential may provide a distributed mechanism for converting CO_2 flux into physiological signals for rapid adjustment to the CO_2 environment.

Human Neuromuscular Diseases: Models for Studying Oxygen Transport to Skeletal Muscle

Steven F. Lewis, R.G. Haller, J.D. Cook, and C.G. Blomqvist

ABSTRACT

In dynamic exercise, the slope ($\Delta\dot{Q}/\Delta\dot{V}O_2$) of the linear relation between cardiac output ($\dot{Q}$) and oxygen uptake ($\dot{V}O_2$) is virtually constant ($\simeq 5.5$) regardless of age, sex, body weight, max $\dot{V}O_2$, active muscle mass, and relative load. The precise regulatory mechanisms are unknown but probably include afferent impulses from the motor cortex and from metabolic receptors in skeletal muscle. Previous studies indicate that certain rare disorders of skeletal muscle with abnormal carbohydrate metabolism, e.g., McArdle's syndrome, produce a mismatch between oxygen transport and utilization. We identified 4 patients with a hyperkinetic circulation specific to exercise, i.e., normal $\dot{Q}$ and arteriovenous O_2 difference ($a-\dot{v}O_2D$) at rest but excessive $\Delta\dot{Q}/\Delta\dot{V}O_2$ and low a-vO_2D in exercise. Diagnoses and maximal exercise responses ($\bar{X} \pm$ S.E.) in these patients and in normal controls, paranormals (muscle pains without demonstrable disease), a patient with myasthenia gravis and patients with dystrophic myopathies but normal circulation are shown in the table.

Hemoglobin and hematocrit were normal in all subjects. A diet rich in medium-chain fatty acids normalized the response in the patient with carnitine deficiency. Our data indicate that both abnormal lipid and carbohydrate muscle metabolism may cause a hyperkinetic response. The normal $\Delta\dot{Q}/\Delta\dot{V}O_2$ in patients with dystrophic myopathy, myasthenia gravis, and in the paranormal group provides evidence against central or nonspecific peripheral factors such as pain, weakness, and atrophy as contributors to the hyperkinetic response. Normalization associated with a change in substrate is consistent with a critical role of the metabolic muscle receptors. Further studies in patients with metabolic muscle disease may provide important information on the regulatory mechanisms that normally maintain a tight coupling between systemic oxygen transport and demand.

	Age (yr)	N	HR (bpm)	$\dot{Q}$ (ml/kg/min)	$\dot{V}O_2$ (ml/kg/min)	$\Delta\dot{Q}/\Delta\dot{V}O_2$	$a\text{-}vO_2D$ (ml%)
McArdle's disease	22	2	180	166	16.6	9.4	9.8
Carnitine deficiency	28	1	185	260	16.2	16.0	6.3
Ragged-red fibers	10	1	161	288	21.4	11.8	7.4
Normals	29 ± 1	5	192 ± 4	257 ± 16	41.4 ± 1.6	4.8 ± 0.3	16.3 ± 0.6
Paranormals	29 ± 5	6	169 ± 8	210 ± 22	28.5 ± 1.8	5.5 ± 0.2	13.8 ± 0.6
Myasthenia gravis	18	1	152	161	20.8	6.2	12.9
Dystrophic myopathies	23 ± 4	4	173 ± 10	170 ± 14	23.2 ± 2.8	5.1 ± 0.8	13.6 ± 1.1

Infant Birth Weight at High Altitude is Related to Maternal Arterial Oxygenation

Lorna G. Moore, S.S. Rounds, D. Jahnigen, R.F. Grover, and J.T. Reeves

ABSTRACT

Infant birth weight decreases at high altitude as a result of fetal growth retardation (McCullough et al. 1977. *Arch. Environ. Health* 32:36), but not all babies are born small. We hypothesized that characteristics of the mother render some babies susceptible to growth retardation at high altitude and that, in particular, maternal characteristics which lowered arterial oxygen content would contribute to smaller size full-term births. To test this hypothesis, we measured arterial oxygenation serially during pregnancy and again postpartum in 44 residents of Leadville, Colorado (elev. 3100 m). Three maternal characteristics (ventilation, hemoglobin concentration, and smoking habits) were related to the birth weight of the offspring. Mothers of smaller babies (<2900 g, n=10) compared to mothers of larger babies (>3500 g, n=11) were characterized by relative hypoventilation (a difference of 2 to 3 liter/min BTPS in resting ventilation during pregnancy and postpartum), no change or a decrease in ventilation and arterial O_2 saturation during pregnancy and a 2.3 g% decrease in hemoglobin concentration during pregnancy, which combined to lower arterial O_2 content in the third trimester. Third trimester values of maternal ventilation and arterial O_2 content were related to infant birth weight (r=0.41, P=<.01 and r=0.40, P<.01, respectively) among all the women studied. Maternal smoking at 3100 m was associated with a 2 to 3-fold greater reduction in infant birth weight (546 g) than reported from sea level. Thus, maternal arterial oxygenation during pregnancy may be important for predicting fetal growth retardation. (Supported by March of Dimes 6-169, American and Colorado Heart Associations 80-837 and NIH HL-14985.)

Blood Gas Equilibrium of CO_2 in Lungs

Johannes Piiper

ABSTRACT

Since 1968, experimental data have been reported from several laboratories indicating that in rebreathing equilibrium PCO_2 in arterial blood is below PCO_2 in lung gas. Furthermore, Jennings and Chen (1975. *J. Appl. Physiol.* 38:382) found arterial PCO_2 to be below mixed-expired PCO_2 in awake dogs breathing 5–10% CO_2 in steady state. In our laboratory, however, we were unable to reproduce these paradoxical PCO_2 differences. (1) Neither in isolated dog lung lobes nor in anesthetized dogs were significant gas-blood PCO_2 differences found in rebreathing equilibrium (Scheid et al. 1972. *J. Appl. Physiol.* 33:582); (2) in anesthetized dogs in hypercapnia (breathing 5–10% CO_2) PCO_2 in arterial blood was close to alveolar PCO_2, and always higher than mixed-expired PCO_2 (Scheid et al. 1979. *J. Appl. Physiol.* 47:1074); (3) recently, in joint experiments with Dr. D. Jennings, this result was confirmed in unanesthetized dogs in hypercapnia (unpublished). Thus the results from our laboratory are in agreement with the conventional view that the physiological equilibrium condition for CO_2 in lungs is that of equal PCO_2 in blood and gas. The reported paradoxical, negative blood gas PCO_2 differences probably constitute artifacts.

Inhibition of Glycolysis Increases Sensitivity of Rat Lungs to Hypoxic Vasoconstriction

Hilary S. Stanbrook and I.F. McMurtry

ABSTRACT

It has been suggested that depression of oxidative phosphorylation is the underlying action of hypoxia in the mechanism of hypoxic pulmonary vasoconstriction. If so, then inhibition in the lung of a compensatory rise in rate of glycolysis might increase pressor sensitivity to hypoxia. We studied dose-response curves to airway hypoxia in isolated, blood-perfused rat lungs equilibrated with either 3 mM iodoacetate or 50 mM 2-deoxyglucose, inhibitors of glycolysis, and found greater pressor responses at higher PO_2s as compared to control preparations. Dose-response curves to angiotensin II and KCl were not similarly affected. Inhibition of glycolysis was shown by reduced rates of perfusate lactate accumulation. To exclude possible effects of blood cells or of decreased prostaglandin synthesis, similar studies were performed in rat lungs perfused with a physiological salt solution containing 4 g/100 ml albumin and 5 mg/ml meclofenamate (PSS). Lungs perfused with PSS containing 5.5 mM 2-deoxyglucose-0 mM glucose or 0 mM glucose alone exhibited greater pressor sensitivity to hypoxia than did lungs perfused with PSS containing 5.5 or 11 mM glucose. PSS with 0.1 mM iodoacetate - 5.5 mM glucose increased responses to low levels of hypoxia, but reduced those to more severe hypoxia. We conclude that inhibition of glycolysis increases pressor sensitivity of rat lungs to hypoxia. These findings provide indirect support for the idea that hypoxic vasoconstriction is initiated by depression of oxidative phosphorylation in some lung cell. (Supported by NIH Grant HL 14985 and a Grant from the Parker B. Francis Foundation.)

The "Mixing-Method" *in Vivo*: Is Arterial PO_2 a Function of Arterial Saturation in the Presence of Shunts?

Stephen C. Wood

ABSTRACT

The oxygen equilibrium curve (O_2EC) of blood is conventionally drawn with percentage oxyhemoglobin saturation as a function of oxygen partial pressure, i.e., % Sat=f(PO_2). This is the correct relationship of these variables in an open system. When the O_2EC is determined, *in vitro*, by the "mixing-method," the PO_2 of a known saturation is measured, i.e., PO_2=f(% Sat). The present hypothesis is that the principle of the "mixing-method" will apply *in vivo* when venous admixture occurs. Then, for a given O_2EC, the PO_2 of the mixed (arterial) blood is a function of saturation of the mixed blood. Thus, the independent and dependent variables applicable to an open system (pulmonary capillaries) are reversed in a closed system (central shunt). For a family of O_2ECs, the arterial PO_2 for a given saturation should be inversely related to Hb-O_2 affinity. If the O_2EC is shifted to the right, the arterial PO_2 for a given saturation will increase. This effect would be saturation dependent, being increasingly pronounced in the middle saturation range and disappearing where the curves converge. The limiting factor for this hypothetical advantage is the requirement for O_2 equilibration, by diffusion, in the gas exchange capillaries. A comparison of the Hb-O_2 affinities of blood among vertebrate groups, while not a direct test of this hypothesis, reveals a trend of right-shifted O_2ECs in amphibians and reptiles, the two groups with pronounced central shunts. Limited experimental evidence shows that a temperature-induced right shift of the O_2EC causes an increase in arterial PO_2 in an amphibian and a reptile. (Supported by NSF Grant PCM–77–24246 and Battelle Centres de Recherche, Geneva.)

Index